Treatise on Ocular Drug Delivery

Editor

Ashim K. Mitra

Division of Pharmaceutical Sciences
University of Missouri-Kansas City
USA

CONTENTS

FOREWORD

Therapeutic efficacy of pharmacotherapy in the eye necessitates delivering complex drug substances to sequestered active sites for the appropriate duration. Achieving this is fraught with challenges from issues of bioavailability to simple non-compliance, whether that's due to physical limitation such as in the elderly, lifestyle factors or simply not self-administering medication. Drug delivery can greatly improve the therapeutic outcome in these cases. Moreover, in certain diseases drug delivery may not only enhance performance of an active, but is an absolute requite for function.

Despite new and novel therapies for posterior segment diseases there is still a very large unmet medical need to treat serious ocular conditions. Vision threatening back of the eye diseases such as wet age-related macular degeneration, diabetic macular edema, uveitis and geographic atrophy are leading causes of blindness. Various therapeutic classes of drugs are showing promise at a receptor or ligand level for affecting these diseases. Promising new drug substances range from antibodies, antibody fragments and peptides to aptamers and siRNAs. In the case of some drugs, such as siRNAs, the lack of an effective delivery system may prevent fulfilling the promise of an entire therapeutic class.

Unfortunately, delivering these drugs to their intended target; the choroid, RPE and vitreoretinal space remains illusory. Without new and novel drug delivery strategies, effective pharmacologic intervention in these diseases may never come to fruition. Drug delivery to the eye is multifactorial and poses significant challenges. Bioavailability to the anterior segment of the eye remains low from topical administration despite decades of research. In fact, the challenges to ocular drug delivery are becoming exponentially greater with therapies directed towards posterior segment diseases and a much broader palette of drug substances to be delivered. The present eBook not only covers these issues in significant detail, but the leading experts in the field authored the chapters. The present eBook offers an integrated understanding of anatomy and physiology, disease state, drug absorption and disposition and drug delivery.

The first five chapters of the eBook lay the foundation for ocular drug delivery and the current state of the art. Chapter 1 nicely deals with the anatomic and physiologic constraints to drug delivery. Chapter 2 explores delivery beyond conventional topical and systemic approaches. Taking advantage of non-conventional routes of delivery minimizes some of the issues with conventional topical therapy including tear dilution, rapid precorneal drainage and may also buffer systemic absorption to some extent. Additionally, these novel routes offer new and novel opportunities for sustained and controlled delivery to the eye. This chapter differentiates conventional and novel routes and discusses their relative merits. Chapters 3 and 4 deal with anterior and posterior segment drug delivery, respectively. The various attempts to improve anterior segment drug delivery are described. Static and dynamic barriers to drug delivery are discussed. A decade ago little consideration was given to the dynamic barriers to penetration as well as the role of enzymes and transporters in posterior segment drug delivery. The field is just now realizing the impact of these factors and Chapter 4 describes these critical and newly defined variables.

Specific strategies for achieving effective drug delivery to the eye are detailed in Chapter 5 through 7 and Chapter 10. In Chapter 5, biodegradable polymers for drug delivery are reviewed. This class of polymers represents a significant component of many posterior segment drug delivery strategies. Unfortunately, a detailed understanding as it relates to the eye is often missing from the ocular formulator's arsenal. This is a crucial chapter for anyone interested in ocular drug delivery. Drug delivery in a broader context is dealt with in chapter 6 and includes erodible and non-erodible systems. Implants, microspheres, liposomes and semi-solids as well as more complex delivery systems are discussed. These strategies have been shown to be effective in circumventing many of the barriers to ocular absorption, but none are without potential side effects. Chapter 7 addresses enhancing the permeation of these barriers, rather than circumvention, through techniques such as ultrasound, microneedles and prodrug modification.

The next two chapters cover critical areas for the field. The eye is not readily amenable to serial sampling and as such it is difficult to reasonably power ocular pharmacokinetic studies. Microdialysis as a tool to address the limitations of classic ocular pharmacokinetic techniques is discussed in Chapter 8. This is a tool that will go a long way in facilitating the development of effective treatments for ocular diseases. However, getting new delivery systems approved and protected is as important as innovating new technologies. Unmet patient needs are not addressed until a drug delivery system is shown to be safe and effective in well-controlled clinical trials, approved through the relevant regulatory bodies and commercialized for use. Chapter 9 discusses US regulatory requirements and guidelines relevant to ophthalmics as well as recent patents in the field. The final chapter of the eBook, Chapter 10, discusses the exiting new area of nanotechnology in drug delivery. Nanotechnology advances such as liposomes, niosomes, nanoparticles and dendrimers among others are fully explored

The present eBook covers in significant detail the issues and resolutions with developing drug delivery systems for the eye. Moreover, key researchers in the field authored this eBook. This eBook serves as a great reference for anyone involved in treating ocular disease including: ophthalmologists and other clinicians, pharmaceutical formulation scientists, ocular pharmacokineticist and pharmacists amongst others. This reference should be in the armamentarium of any scientist serious about drug delivery to the ocular tissues.

Patrick M. Hughes

Formulations and Drug Delivery Sciences
Allergan, Inc.

PREFACE

Over the last three decades, considerable attention has been paid to the field of ocular drug delivery due to challenges encountered in delivery of ocular drugs. The global market for ocular therapeutics in 2008 was approximately $ 12.5 billion, which has been rising at a constant rate of 9% every year. This result was achieved from significant research efforts provided by ocular drug delivery scientists and researchers across the globe. Despite the complex anatomy and physiology of the eye, drug delivery to this globe has been widely explored with many novel drug delivery systems, devices and newly developed technologies such as nanotechnology, iontophoresis and phonophoresis. The primary objective of this eBook is to provide a comprehensive understanding of ocular barriers and highlight current progress in the field of ocular drug delivery.

In this eBook, recent advances and developments in ocular drug delivery systems have been specifically addressed. Ocular anatomy and physiology along with a distinctive comparison between conventional and novel routes for drug delivery have been described. A detailed review on the development of liposomes, nanoparticles, implants and nanomicelles which has revolutionized drug delivery to both anterior and posterior segment of the eye has also been discussed. Novel strategies such as ocular iontophoresis, phonophoresis and transporter targeted prodrug delivery which are being currently investigated for improving ocular drug delivery have also been provided. This eBook will definitely serve as an excellent reference to all future ocular researchers and scientists striving to improve drug delivery to the eye.

Ashim K. Mitra

Division of Pharmaceutical Sciences
University of Missouri-Kansas City
USA

List of Contributors

Sai HS. Boddu Department of Pharmacy Practice, College of Pharmacy and Pharmaceutical Sciences, The University of Toledo, Toledo, Ohio, USA

Aarika L. Menees School of Medicine, University of Missouri-Kansas City, Kansas City, Missouri 64108, USA

Animikh Ray Division of Pharmaceutical Sciences, University of Missouri-Kansas City, Kansas City, Missouri 64108, USA

Ashim K. Mitra Division of Pharmaceutical Sciences, University of Missouri-Kansas City, Kansas City, Missouri 64108, USA

Deep Kwatra Division of Pharmaceutical Sciences, University of Missouri-Kansas City, Kansas City, Missouri 64108, USA

Ramya Krishna Vadlapatla Division of Pharmaceutical Sciences, University of Missouri-Kansas City, Kansas City, Missouri 64108, USA

Varun Khurana Division of Pharmaceutical Sciences, University of Missouri-Kansas City, Kansas City, Missouri 64108, USA

Dhananjay Pal Division of Pharmaceutical Sciences, University of Missouri-Kansas City, Kansas City, Missouri 64108, USA

Jwala Renukuntla Division of Pharmaceutical Sciences, South College School of Pharmacy, Tennessee, USA

Sujay Shah Division of Pharmaceutical Sciences, University of Missouri-Kansas City, Kansas City, Missouri 64108, USA

Aswani Dutt Vadlapudi Division of Pharmaceutical Sciences, University of Missouri-Kansas City, Kansas City, Missouri 64108, USA

Mitesh Patel Division of Pharmaceutical Sciences, University of Missouri-Kansas City, Kansas City, Missouri 64108, USA

Ripal J. Gaudana Division of Pharmaceutical Sciences, University of Missouri-Kansas City, Kansas City, Missouri 64108, USA

Megha Barot Division of Pharmaceutical Sciences, University of Missouri-Kansas City, Kansas City, Missouri 64108, USA

Ashaben Patel Division of Pharmaceutical Sciences, University of Missouri-Kansas City, Kansas City, Missouri 64108, USA

Viral Tamboli Division of Pharmaceutical Sciences, University of Missouri-Kansas City, Kansas City, Missouri 64108, USA

Sulabh Patel Division of Pharmaceutical Sciences, University of Missouri-Kansas City, Kansas City, Missouri 64108, USA

Gyan P. Mishra Division of Pharmaceutical Sciences, University of Missouri-Kansas City, Kansas City, Missouri 64108, USA

Ashish Thakur Department of Pharmaceutical Sciences and Department of Ophthalmology, University of Colorado Anschutz Medical Campus, Aurora, Colorado 80045, USA

Uday B. Kompella Department of Pharmaceutical Sciences and Department of Ophthalmology, University of Colorado Anschutz Medical Campus, Aurora, Colorado 80045, USA

Pradeep K. Karla Division of Pharmaceutical Sciences, School of Pharmacy, Howard University, Washington D.C. 20059, USA

Ann-Marie Ako-Adouno Division of Pharmaceutical Sciences, School of Pharmacy, Howard University, Washington D.C. 20059, USA

Kay D. Rittenhouse Translational Medicine Ophthalmology, Specialty Care Business Unit, Pfizer Inc., New York 10027, USA

Harisha Atluri Xeno Port Inc. Santa Clara, California 95050, USA

Soumyajit Majumdar Department of Pharmaceutics, University of Mississippi, Mississippi 38677, USA

Tushar Hingorani Department of Pharmaceutics, University of Mississippi, Mississippi 38677, USA

Ketan Hippalgaonkar Department of Pharmaceutics, University of Mississippi, Mississippi 38677, USA

Walter G. Chambliss Department of Pharmaceutics, University of Mississippi, Mississippi 38677, USA

Xiaoyan Yang Division of Pharmaceutical Sciences, University of Missouri-Kansas City, Kansas City, Missouri 64108, USA

2

Send Orders of Reprints at reprints@benthamscience.net

CHAPTER 1

A Brief Overview of Ocular Anatomy and Physiology

Sai H.S. Boddu[1], Aarika L. Menees[3], Animikh Ray[2] and Ashim K. Mitra[2,*]

[1]Department of Pharmacy Practice, College of Pharmacy and Pharmaceutical Sciences, The University of Toledo, Ohio, USA – 43614; [2]Division of Pharmaceutical Sciences, School of Pharmacy, University of Missouri-Kansas City, Kansas City, Missouri-64108, USA and [3]School of Medicine, University of Missouri-Kansas City, Kansas City, Missouri-64110, USA

Abstract: Ocular globe is a very complex organ consisting of many tissues which protect optic nerve and photoreceptor cells. It sits in the skull cavity and is surrounded by fibrous muscle and lipoidal tissues. The eye is protected from external environment, infection and bright light by eyelids and eyelashes. Moreover, continuous tear production removes foreign objects from the eye. The anterior segment consists of a refractive system while the posterior segment consists of a visual light perceptive mechanism. Light rays entering the eye are focused onto the retina producing continuous images that are spontaneously transmitted to the brain. In this chapter, we discuss the anatomy and physiology of various ocular structures commencing from the anterior segment. Most of the aspects mentioned in this chapter describe the human eye unless otherwise specified.

Keywords: Eye, anatomy, physiology, cornea, retina, drug delivery, aqueous humor, vitreous humor, conjunctiva, lens, sclera, macula, choroid.

DEFINITION AND DEVELOPMENT OF THE EYE

The eye is defined as a photoreceptor which is shielded by a shading pigment on one side. This pigment helps in recognition of the light source direction [1]. Eyes can be broadly classified into two categories- simple eyes or compound eyes. Simple eyes are found in unicellular organisms and help to distinguish between bright and dark surroundings that are sufficient enough in carrying out circadian rhythms. The simplest form of eye, which is found in algae and flatworm, consists of just one photoreceptor and pigment cell [2-4]. Compound eyes consist of

*Address correspondence to Ashim K. Mitra: University of Missouri Curators' Professor of Pharmacy, Chairman, Division of Pharmaceutical Sciences, Vice-Provost for Interdisciplinary Research, University of Missouri - Kansas City, School of Pharmacy, 2464 Charlotte Street, Kansas City, MO 64108, USA; Tel: 816-235-1615; Fax: 816-235-5779; E-mail: mitraa@umkc.edu

thousands of photoreception units and can distinguish shapes and colors (human eye can distinguish ~10 million colors). Moreover, they have the capacity to detect fast movements and view very wide angles compared to simple eyes. Development of eye involves six stages. These include: a) growth of photoreceptor cells, b) depressed/folded area allowing limited directional sensitivity of light, c) formation of the pinhole, increasing directional sensitivity and imaging, d) formation of transparent humor enclosed in a chamber, e) development of a distinct lens and f) development of the iris and cornea [4-6].

Early stages are marked by the formation of "eyespots" which are simple patches of photoreceptor cells. These eyespots can only distinguish bright light from dim light. The eyespots gradually depress into a shallow cup granting the ability to slightly discriminate directional brightness. This cup deepens into a pit over time resulting in the formation of an effective pinhole camera. The photoreceptor cells gradually grow in number and increase the capability to distinguish dim shapes [7]. Thin transparent cells, which are originally formed to prevent damage to the eyespot, segregate into a transparent humor. This has the property of color filtering and improving ocular refractive index. An increase in the concentration of crystalline proteins inside these cells results in the formation of lens [8]. A transparent layer (cornea) and a nontransparent layer (iris) split forward from the lens in an independent fashion. Separation of these two layers by aqueous humor increases refractive power and eases circulatory problems. Six extraocular muscles which include medial rectus, lateral rectus, superior rectus, inferior rectus, superior oblique and inferior oblique control the vertical and horizontal movement of the eye. Various functions of the muscle are shown in Table **1** [9].

Table 1: Function of various orbit muscles

Muscle	Functions of the muscle	Innervations
Medial rectus	Adduction or movement of the eye inward	Cranial nerve **III** or Oculomotor
Lateral rectus	Abduction or movement of the eye outward	Cranial nerve **VI** or Abducens
Superior rectus	Elevation or upward movement of the eye Intorsion or rotates the top portion of the eye towards the nose, Adduction or inward movement of the eye	Cranial nerve **III** or Oculomotor
Inferior rectus	Depression or downward movement of the eye Extortion or movement of the eye away from the nose Adduction or inward movement of the eye	Cranial nerve **III** or Oculomotor

Superior oblique	Intorsion or rotates the top of the eye towards the nose Depression or downward movement of the eye Abduction or outward movement of the eye	Cranial nerve **IV** or Trochlear
Inferior oblique	Extorsion or movement of the eye away from nose elevation or upward movement of the eye abduction or outward movement of the eye	Cranial nerve **III** or Oculomotor

The diameter of eyeball in a newborn is approximately 1.8 cm which gradually increases to 2.54 cm in adulthood. The eye is a two piece system consisting of the cornea (smaller unit) and sclera (larger unit). The cornea and sclera are connected by a ring called the limbus. The eye attains its full size at the age of thirteen years. The volume of a fully grown eye is approximately 6.5 milliliters and weight 7.5 grams. The eye wall is composed of three major layers. The outermost layer is fibrous tunica consisting of cornea, sclera and corneoscleral limbus. The intermediate vascular layer is pigmented tunica consisting of choroid, ciliary body and iris. The innermost layer is nervous tunica consisting of the retina, photoreceptor cells, modulator cells, transmitter cells and supporting cells. Aqueous humor, lens and vitreous humor are responsible for refraction of light. The sclera is a white protective coat lining the entire eyeball except the cornea. It is made up of dense interlacing white fibrous tissue which protects the delicate structures of the eye and prevents any injury. Various parts of the eye are shown in Fig. **1**. The complete description of anatomy and physiology of the eye is beyond the scope of this eBook; hence we have curtailed our discussion to some of the major ocular tissues starting with the anterior segment (Fig. **2**).

CONJUNCTIVA

The conjunctiva is a mucous membrane composed of non-keratinizing squamous epithelium that covers the external surface of the eye and inner surface of the eyelids. The former is defined as bulbar conjunctiva and the latter as the palpebral conjunctiva. The bulbar conjunctiva moves freely and blends with Tenon's capsule and anteriorly it inserts into the limbus [10]. The conjunctiva located in the fornices is referred to as the fornical conjunctiva. The majority of the conjunctiva is made up of specialized stratified squamous cells. Goblet cells are interspersed within this epithelium and assist in production of mucin. This helps

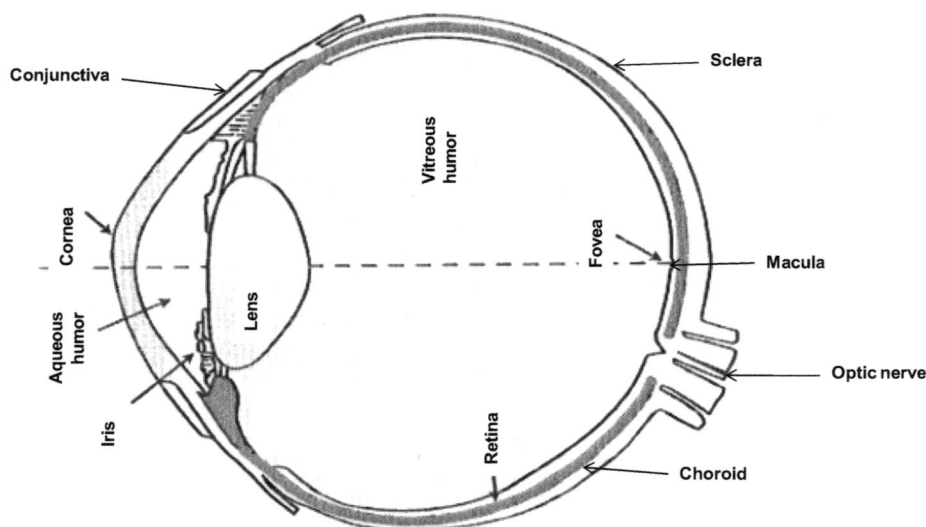

Figure 1: The structure of the eye. Modified with permission from reference [11].

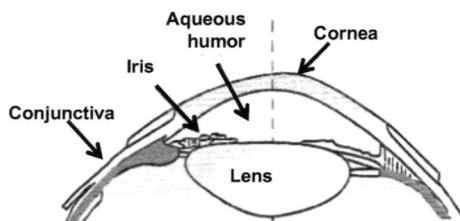

Figure 2: Anterior segment of the eye reproduced with permission from reference [11].

in nourishing the cornea and decreasing friction and drying of the opposing palpebral and bulbar conjunctiva. In addition to goblet cells, the conjunctiva also contains lymphatic vessels, plasma cells, macrophages and mast cells. There is a lymphoid layer that exists from the bulbar conjunctiva to the subtarsal folds of the lids which contain specialized aggregations of conjunctiva-associated lymphoid tissue (CALT) responsible for antigen processing. Furthermore, the conjunctiva is innervated by free nerve endings derived from the ophthalmic division of cranial nerve five. It contains no specialized sensory receptors. The bulbar conjunctiva is supplied by the anterior ciliary arteries, anterior conjunctival arteries and posterior conjunctival arteries. The marginal arcades of eyelids supply the palpebral conjunctiva [10].

CORNEA

The cornea is an avascular, transparent structure continuous with the sclera at the limbus. It is composed of five layers. From the anterior to the posterior surface of the cornea these layers are: surface epithelium, Bowman's layer, stroma, Descemet's membrane and endothelium (Fig. **3**) [11]. Given its avascularity, the anterior surface epithelial cells obtain oxygen and nutrients from tears whereas the posterior corneal endothelium depends on the aqueous humor [11-13]. cornea is the most sensitive portion of the eye and is innervated by free nerve endings [10, 14]. The surface epithelium is derived from the surface ectoderm and consists of non-keratanized, stratified squamous epithelium continuous with the bulbar conjunctiva [10, 14, 15]. Bowman's layer is located just beneath the basal lamina of the epithelial layer, consisting of collagen fibrils that are not restored if injured, resulting in scar formation [14, 15]. The stroma, or body of the cornea, is the largest portion of the cornea and is approximately 90% of the total thickness. It is anchored to the epithelium by type VII collagen and is otherwise primarily composed of types I, III, V and VI collagen lamellae, produced by keratocytes. Interspersed with the collagen and keratocytes is ground substance. This layer allows for the cornea's transparency due to the oblique orientation of the collagen lamellae in the anterior third and the parallel lamellae in the posterior two thirds. Corneal clouding occurs when excess fluid causes separation of the collagen fibrils from their normal orientation [10, 14, 15]. Descemet's membrane is a true basement membrane composed of type IV collagen. It is extremely thin and highly elastic with a tendency to curl up; furthermore, it is the basal lamina of the corneal endothelium and increases in thickness throughout life [10, 14]. The endothelium is composed of a single layer of polygonal, transparent nucleated cells whose primary function is to maintain corneal transparency through fluid balance within the stroma. The apical surfaces are in direct contact with the anterior chamber and its aqueous solution, while the basal surface is secured in Descemet's membrane. This structure and placement of the cells allow for active transport of ions and therefore the transfer of water from the corneal stroma into the anterior chamber. With age, the number of endothelial cells declines causing the residual cells to spread and enlarge to permit continuance of fluid balance [10, 14].

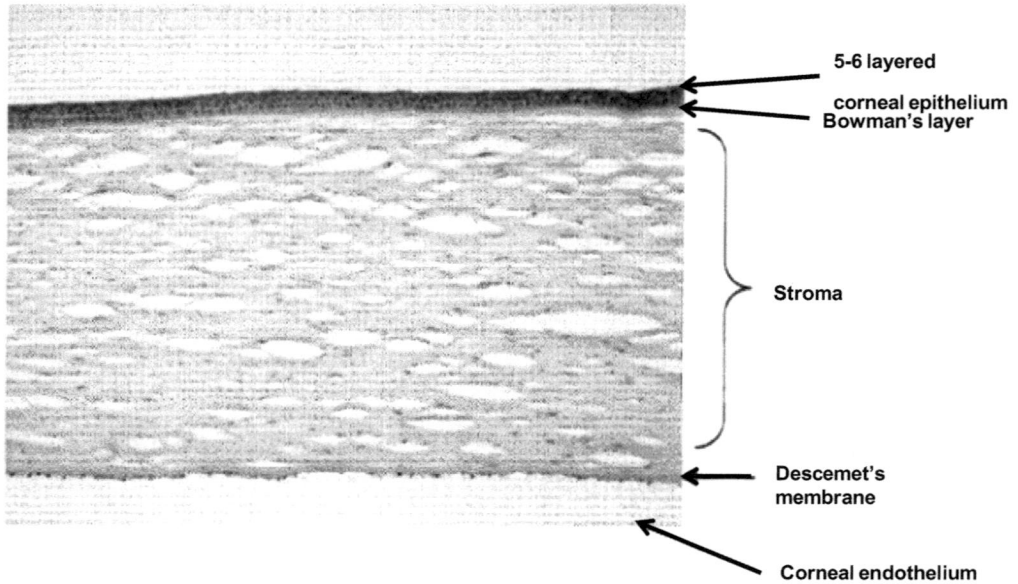

Figure 3: Layers of the cornea reproduced with permission from reference [12].

The cornea and crystalline lens are mainly responsible for focusing of incident light entering the eye. The cornea contains the highest concentration of nerve fibers (they enter on the margins and radiate towards the center) making it extremely sensitive to pain. These fibers are mainly associated with very low threshold pain receptors.

ANTERIOR CHAMBER & AQUEOUS HUMOR

The anterior chamber varies in depth and is bordered by cornea in the front and the pupil and iris diaphragm in the back. It is filled with aqueous humor produced by the ciliary epithelium in the posterior chamber. Aqueous humor is formed from blood plasma by mechanisms of diffusion, ultrafiltration and active transport [16]. The rate of aqueous humor formation is ~ 2-3 μL/min with the total volume of the anterior chamber averaging 250 μL. Before entering into the anterior chamber, the aqueous humor flows through the posterior chamber with a small resistance from the posterior iris and the anterior lens (Fig. **4**). The production of aqueous humor decreases with sleep, age, uveitis, retinal detachment and ciliochoroidal detachment.

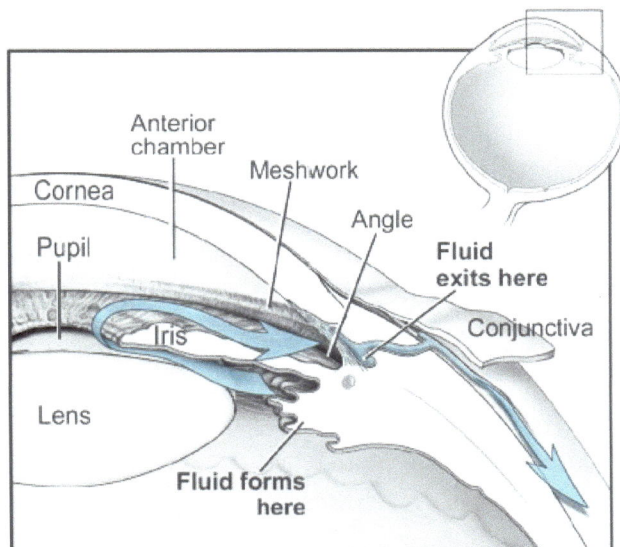

Figure 4: Flow of aqueous humor (Courtesy of National Eye Institute and National Institutes of Health).

IRIS

The iris is a circular structure with a circular aperture, the pupil, located at its center. It is located in the aqueous humor behind the cornea and anterior to the lens. It is part of the uveal tract attached to the ciliary body. All irides, independent of color, have the same stromal structure composed of melanocytes, non-pigmented cells, collagen fibrils and a matrix containing hyaluronic acid. The anterior border of the iris contains multiple crypts and crevices with variable sizes, shapes and depths through which aqueous humor flows. The unique color of individuals' irides is dependent upon amount of pigmentation in the anterior border layer and the deep stroma. People with blue irides have a lightly pigmented stroma, whereas those with brown irides are densely pigmented leading to increased absorption of light. Albinos lack any pigmentation in their stroma [9]. There are numerous blood vessels and nerves throughout stroma. Of note, in a normal human iris, anterior border layer is avascular with the remainder of stroma being primarily composed of vasculature which arises and radiates from the major arterial circle to the pupil. At the thickest portion of iris, the collarette, arteriovenous anastomoses form a minor vascular circle. Also found within stroma are myelinated and non-myelinated nerve fibers. The majority of the stroma is composed of blood vessels that arise and radiate from the major arterial circle to the pupil. In addition, a normal anterior border layer of the iris in humans is avascular. The posterior surface of the iris is densely pigmented and is known as the posterior pigmented layer. This layer shows an attachment with the non-pigmented epithelium of the ciliary body and thus with the neurosensory portion of the retina. While the basal surface of the pigmented layer borders the posterior chamber, the apical surface faces the stroma and adheres to the anterior pigmented layer [14]. The pupil is capable of changing size through activity of the iris sphincter and dilator muscles, both of these muscles are derived from the neuroectoderm. The sphincter muscle is composed of smooth muscle fibers circumferentially located in the deep stroma near the pupillary margin, anterior to the pigment epithelium on the posterior surface of the iris [14]. Innervation is primarily from parasympathetic nerve fibers that originate from cranial nerve III which leads to contraction of the muscle fibers and constriction of the pupil [10, 14, 17]. Pharmacologically, the sphincter muscles contract with muscarinic stimulation. The sphincter muscle does have sympathetic innervation, but an inhibitory action leads to relaxation of the muscle. The dilator muscles cause dilation with contraction and its muscle fibers radiate from iris' outer circumference toward the papillary margin on the posterior surface of iris [10, 14]. The smooth muscle fibers are innervated by both sympathetic and parasympathetic autonomic systems with sympathetic α1-adrenergic stimulation leading to contraction. The iris is mainly responsible for controlling the pupil diameter and size. Depending on the amount of light reaching the retina, iris muscles expand or contract aperture at the pupil (center of the iris).

LENS

The lens is composed of concentric layers of cells which form a biconvex structure that functions to focus images on the retina. It is located directly behind posterior chamber and pupil and is enclosed in a fibrous, elastic capsule suspended from the ciliary body by suspensory ligaments. The lens capsule is rich in type IV collagen and other matrix proteins as it is a basal lamina. Throughout life, the anterior lens capsule increases in thickness unlike the posterior capsule which remains constant. This is important because thinness of the posterior capsule creates an increased risk of rupture during extracapsular cataract extraction. The lens has an outer cortex and an inner nucleus. The nuclear component of the lens is a mass of fibers already formed at birth, whereas the cortex is formed by fibers postnatally. Cytoplasm of cell fibers is mostly homogeneous with few organelles permitting a high concentration of lens crystallins within the cytoplasm and thus creates a high refractive index for the lens. The lens is positioned for distant vision at rest as the suspensory ligaments' tension causes the elastic capsule containing the lens to flatten. With accommodation, the ciliary muscle contracts and decreases tension in the suspensory ligaments leading the elastic lens to resume a curved shape [14]. Accommodative power is steadily lost with age secondary to increased lens size and stiffness of the lens nucleus. The lens lacks innervation and blood supply leading to a much lower oxygen concentration than that found in other parts of the body [18]. Metabolic activity for majority of the lens is reliant on glycolytic metabolism of glucose from the aqueous humor to produce the reducing equivalents and ATP necessary for energy production [14, 18]. There are also lens epithelial and superficial fiber cells which contain mitochondria and permit cells located at the surface of lens to use oxidative pathways in addition to the glycolytic pathway for energy production [19, 20].

SCLERA

Sclera is the opaque or white portion (except horses and lizards which can have black sclera) of the eye which is fibrous in nature. It is also known as white of the eye. The development and differentiation of the sclera starts during 6th week of human embryonic stage from the neural crest and mesoderm regions [13, 21]. It is an opaque, fibrous tissue which forms the external protective coat (posterior five sixths of the connective tissue that coats the globe) [22]. Sclera is mainly composed of collagen (~28.8%), proteoglycans (~0.9%), elastin (~1-2%), proteins and cellular components (~3%) and water (~68%) [23]. Recent studies demonstrated the presence of types III, IV, V, VI, VIII, XII and XIII, XVIII collagen in addition to type I [22, 24]. Each subtype of collagen acts in a unique manner providing a robust framework which supports the visual apparatus of inner eye. Table **2** presents the type and function of various collagens present in the sclera.

Table 2: Type and function of collagen present in the sclera

Collagen	Function
Type I	Interacts with Type V collagen and helps in maintaining fibril diameter during fibrillogenesis [25]
Type III	Present in the major D-periodic interstitial fibrils along with Type I collagen [26]
Type V	Present at the fibril perimeter [26]
Type VI	Assembles into the filamentous structure between the fiber bundles [26]
Type VIII	Responsible for the formation of the hexagonal lattice in Descemet's membrane [27]
Type XII	Mediates interfibrillar interactions and development of ocular connective tissues [28]
Type XVIII	Collagen gene has been implicated in the development of high myopia and is known to be expressed in the human eye

Elastin fibers consist of microfibrillar and amorphous components which support the collagen framework in sclera. These fibers are synthesized by scleral fibroblasts and are mainly present in the inner layers of the stroma and lamina fusca (Fig. **5**) [29].

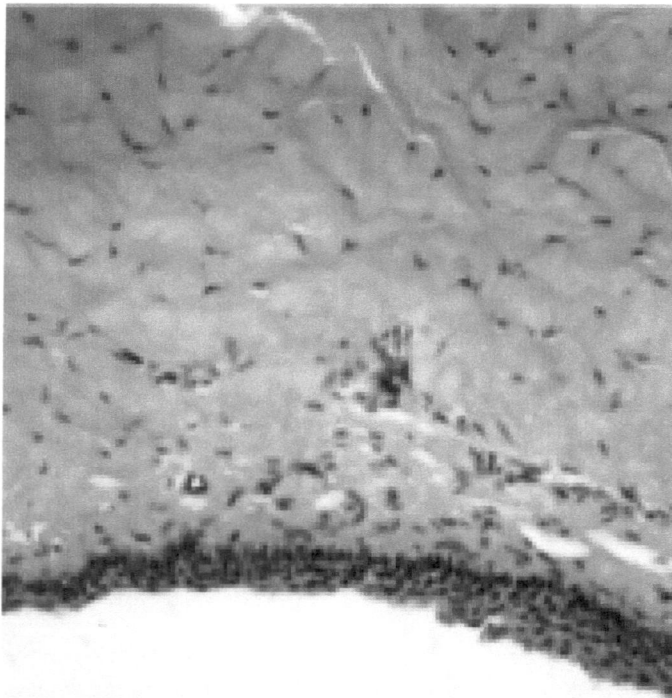

Figure 5: Histology of the sclera.

RETINA

The retina is a multi-layered sensory tissue that forms the innermost layer of the eye Fig. **6**.

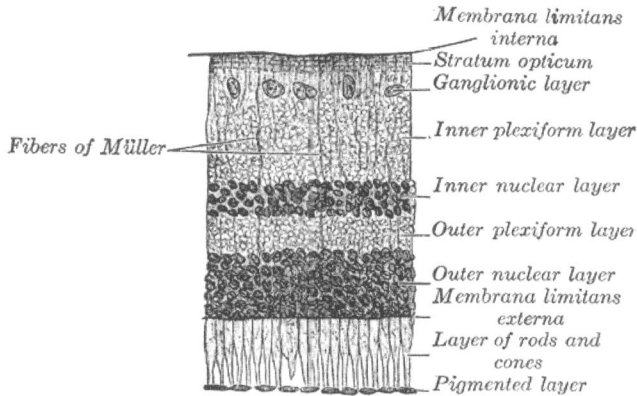

Figure 6: Structure of the retina. This diagram has been reproduced from Gray's Anatomy 20th US edition which has now lapsed into the public domain. (http://en.wikipedia.org/wiki/File: Gray881.png).

It contains millions of photoreceptors which can be divided into rods and cones. The photoreceptors are present in the macula, the portion of retina responsible for central vision. Retina is mainly divided into two layers: neural retina (inner layer) and retinal pigment epithelium (outer layer). These two layers are separated by the fluid filled subretinal space [30]. The neural retina is a highly organized and multi-layered membrane which consists of rods, cones, bipolar cells and ganglionic cells. Light rays entering the eye converge at the cornea and the crystalline lens makes them intersect at a point just behind the lens (in the vitreous humor). These rays again passes through nine layers and diverges back to the outermost retinal layer (pigmented epithelium) which is reflected back to the rods and cones. Rods are mainly responsible for peripheral and night vision. Cones and rods capture light rays and convert them into electrical impulses. These impulses travel along the optic nerve to the brain where they are turned into images. The bipolar cells synapse with the ganglionic cells whose axons course horizontally forming the optic nerve. Ganglionic cells conduct the signals from the retina to the brain. RPE is a non visual portion located between the neural portion of the retina and choroid. It consists of a layer of melanin-containing epithelial cells (except in albinos). Melanin helps in absorption of stray light rays entering the eyeball and hence prevents the reflection of scattering of light [31]. The RPE forms the outer blood–retinal barrier and has tight junctions that enable the epithelium to form a barrier by connecting the neighboring cells [32]. RPE cells are polarized and well differentiated on both the apical and basolateral portions. These cells regulate the trans-epithelial transport of various molecules similar to other epithelia and endothelia. This is facilitated by apical tight junctions (retards diffusion through the paracellular spaces) and asymmetric distribution of proteins (regulates vectorial transport) [33, 34]. Numerous microvilli are found on the apical or the neural retinal portion while small convoluted infoldings are present on the basolateral or choroid facing portion. This helps in the absorption of various nutrients and thereby maintains the viability of the neural retina. RPE expresses certain efflux proteins which prevent the entry of xenobiotics from the extravascular space of the retina.

FORMATION OF AN IMAGE ON THE RETINA

Light rays tend to diverge in all directions from the source and hence the set of rays from all points in space that reach the pupil should be focused. Refraction of light by the cornea and lens results in focusing the image on the photoreceptor cells of the retina. The cornea is responsible for major portion of refraction while the lens has considerably less refractive power. However, refraction by the lens can be adjusted according to convenience but refraction of cornea cannot be adjusted. This adjusting property of the lens is responsible for bringing objects situated at various distances from the eye onto the surface of the retina. This dynamic change in the refractive power of lens is known as accommodation. While distant objects are being viewed, the lens becomes comparatively thin and flattened with least refractive power. The lens becomes thicker and rounder when viewing near objects and acquires high refractive power. These changes are facilitated by ciliary muscles surrounding the lens. The circular opening in the iris, which is referred to as pupil, undergoes adjustment in its size. This immensely contributes to clarity of images which are formed on the retina. Images generated by the eye are affected by chromatic and spherical aberrations which blur the retinal image. These aberrations mostly occur in the light rays which are farthest from the center of lens. When the pupil is narrowed, these aberrations are minimized and thus the image quality is improved. This is similar to the closure of the iris diaphragm on a camera lens which enhances the sharpness of a photograph. Light rays falling on the photoreceptor cells of the retina stimulate a series of electrical signals that are transmitted to the brain *via* optic nerve. The photoreceptor cells consist of rods and cones which communicate with three distinct layers of cells *via* junctions known as synapses. In fact, the actual image formed on the retina is inverted and small; nevertheless, the brain interprets the image and it becomes upright.

OPTIC NERVE

The optic nerve, also known as Cranial nerve II, is responsible for transmission of visual information from retina to brain. It is composed of ~1.2 million myelinated axons of retinal ganglion cells of a single retina and has a varying diameter (1-10 μm).

It is located within the orbit and it extends from eyeball to optic foramen. Length of the optic nerve varies from 20-30 mm with a diameter of ~5 mm. Fibers of the optic nerve are made up of retinal ganglionic and Portort cells. These fibers are covered with three meningeal layers (dura, arachnoid and pia mater) produced by oligodendrocytes. Within the ocular bulb, the fibers converge to the optic papilla where they are accumulated into a rounded bundle known as the optic nerve. The nerve pierces the choroid and sclerotic coats and enters the orbital fat present in the back of the eye towards the optic foramen. Later, it enters the middle fossa of the cranium and joins its fellow nerve from the other side forming the optic chiasma. The optic nerve can be classified under four subdivisions for convenience:

1. Intraocular portion: It is less than 1mm in length and consists of the optic nerve head, optic discand the optic papilla

2. Intraorbital portion: It emerges from the sclera ~3 mm below and extends into the medial side of the posterior pole of the bulbus. It is ~25 mm long and passes in the backward and medial direction up to

the optic foramen. This tissue is surrounded by the posterior part of the fascia bulbi (tenon's capsule) and orbital fat.

3.   Intracanalicular portion: It is ~5 mm in length and is located within the optic canal. The tissue receives blood supply from the pial plexus.

4.   Intracranial portion: It is ~10 mm in length and runs backward, upward and medially and merges into the optic chiasm present in the subarachnoid space [35].

Fiber tracks are incapable of regeneration; hence optic nerve damage results in irreversible blindness. Functionally, the optic nerve begins in the retinal ganglion cells. The axons which arise at these cells move towards exit of the optic nerve from the eye, while axons arising from the nasal side go towards the head of optic nerve. The axons which arise from around fovea (in the macular region) form a spindle-shaped papillomacular bundle which enters the temporal sector of optic nerve head. The fovea is usually situated underneath middle of the nerve head. The papillomacular bundle makes its entry into the optic disc inferior to its equator. Axons from the remaining retinal region take a curved route around the papillomacular bundle to make entry into the optic nerve head at the superior and inferior poles. The layer of retinal nerve fiber is thickest in these curved bundles as they near the upper and lower sector of optic disc.

VITREOUS HUMOR

Approximately 80% of volume of the eye is made up of a clear gel-like substance known as vitreous humor. This fluid fills up the space between the lens and the retina. Vitreous humor consists of water (99%), hyaluronic acid, hyalocytes, inorganic salts, sugar, ascorbic acid and a network of collagen fibrils [36]. The network of non-branching collagen fibers with hyaluronic acid imparts viscosity to the vitreous humor which is two to four times higher than pure water and has a refractive index of 1.336. Hyalocytes help in the removal of unwanted cellular debris. Unlike the aqueous humor which is continuously replenished, vitreous humor is stagnant [37]. It is produced by certain retinal cells and has a similar composition to the cornea. The vitreous humor is in continuous contact with the retina; nevertheless, it adheres to the retina only at three places: the macula, optic nerve disc and fovea.

MACULA

Macula is a Latin word which means "spot". It is an oval-shaped, yellow spot which is highly pigmented and is present in the center of the retina. It has a diameter of around 5 mm with two or more layers of ganglionic cells. The fovea is located at the center of the macula and it has the largest concentration of cone cells which are responsible for most visual acuity. The macular/foveal area is mainly responsible for color discrimination. Moreover, the yellow color of the macula helps in absorption of excess light entering the eye and thus acts as a natural form of protection.

CONCLUSION

Eye is a very complex organ associated with a wide array of physiological processes. In this chapter, we have briefly described the anatomy and physiology of various structures. However, for a more detailed study, the readers are encouraged to refer the articles and books cited throughout this chapter. An understanding of ocular anatomy and physiology plays an important role in the development and delivery of drugs. Entry of a drug into the eye is prevented by various natural protective mechanisms thus leading to insufficient therapeutic concentrations. The cornea and BRB act as a major barrier for the treatment of anterior and posterior segment diseases respectively. A thorough anatomical study at the cellular level involving the functional identification of various transporters that can increase ocular bioavailability *via* prodrug derivatization has been discussed in the subsequent chapters.

ACKNOWLEDGEMENTS

The authors are thankful to the National Eye Institute, National Institutes of Healthand Gray's Anatomy of the Human Body (1918), 20th edition for providing some figures. The authors are thankful to the National Institutes of Health grants (R01 EY 09171-16 and R01 EY 10659-12 and the research start-up funds from The University of Toledo.

CONFLICT OF INTEREST

The author(s) confirm that this chapter content has no conflict of interest.

REFERENCES

[1]   Gehring WJ, Ikeo K. Pax 6: mastering eye morphogenesis and eye evolution. Trends Genet 1999; 15(9) :371-7.
[2]   Arendt D, Wittbrodt J. Reconstructing the eyes of Urbilateria. Philos Trans R Soc Lond B Biol Sci 2001; 356(1414): 1545-63.
[3]   Plachetzki DC, Serb JM, Oakley TH. New insights into the evolutionary history of photoreceptor cells. Trends Ecol Evol 2005; 20(9): 465-7.
[4]   Fernald RD. The evolution of eyes. Brain Behav Evol 1997; 50(4): 253-9.
[5]   Fernald RD. Casting a genetic light on the evolution of eyes. Science 2006; 313(5795): 1914-8.
[6]   Fernald RD. Eyes: variety, development and evolution. Brain Behav Evol 2004; 64(3): 141-7.
[7]   Land MF, Fernald RD. The evolution of eyes. Annu Rev Neurosci 1992; 15 :1-29.
[8]   Doolittle RF. Lens proteins. More molecular opportunism. Nature 1988; 336(6194) :18.
[9]   Reeves AG. Disorders of the nervous system: a primer. Chicago, Ill.: Year Book Medical Publishers; 1981. xi, 240 p. p.
[10]   Martini F, Timmons MJ, Tallitsch RB. Human anatomy. 6th ed. San Francisco: Pearson Benjamin Cummings; 2003. 487-501 p.
[11]   Dey S, Anand BS, Patel J, Mitra AK. Transporters/receptors in the anterior chamber: pathways to explore ocular drug delivery strategies. Expet Opin Biol Ther 2003;3(1):23-44.
[12]   Dey S, Mitra AK. Transporters and receptors in ocular drug delivery: opportunities and challenges. Expert Opin Drug Deliv 2005; 2(2): 201-4.
[13]   Trotter RR. Cornea and sclera. Arch Ophthalmol 1968; 79(3): 338-48.
[14]   Gray H, Carter HV. Anatomy, descriptive and surgical. St. Louis: Mosby Year Book; 1991. xxxii, 750 p. p.
[15]   Kolb H. Gross Anatomy of the Eye. In: Kolb H, Fernandez E, Nelson R, editors. Webvision: The Organization of the Retina and Visual System. Salt Lake City (UT)1995.
[16]   Civan MM, Macknight AD. The ins and outs of aqueous humour secretion. Exp Eye Res 2004; 78(3): 625-31.
[17]   Imesch PD, Wallow IH, Albert DM. The color of the human eye: a review of morphologic correlates and of some conditions that affect iridial pigmentation. Surv Ophthalmol 1997; 41(Suppl 2): S117-23.
[18]   Kaufman PL, Alm A, Adler FH. Adler's physiology of the eye: clinical application. 10th ed. St. Louis: Mosby; 2003. xvii, 876 p. p.
[19]   Kirsch RE. The lens. Arch Ophthalmol 1975; 93(4): 284-314.
[20]   Henkind P, Hansen RI, Szalay J. Physiology of the human eye and visual system. In: Records RE, editor. Hagerstown, Md.: Harper & Row; 1979. p. 98-155.
[21]   Johnston MC, Noden DM, Hazelton RD, Coulombre JL, Coulombre AJ. Origins of avian ocular and periocular tissues. Exp Eye Res 1979; 29(1): 27-43.
[22]   Rada JA, Shelton S, Norton TT. The sclera and myopia. Exp Eye Res 2006; 82(2): 185-200.

[23]   Sandberg-Lall M, Hagg PO, Wahlstrom I, Pihlajaniemi T. Type XIII collagen is widely expressed in the adult and developing human eye and accentuated in the ciliary muscle, the optic nerve and the neural retina. Exp Eye Res 2000; 70(4): 401-10.

[24]   Watson PG, Young RD. Scleral structure, organisation and disease. A review. Exp Eye Res 2004; 78(3): 609-23.

[25]   Norton TT, Rada JA. Reduced extracellular matrix in mammalian sclera with induced myopia. Vision research 1995; 35(9): 1271-81.

[26]   Marshall GE, Konstas AG, Lee WR. Collagens in the aged human macular sclera. Curr Eye Res 1993; 12(2): 143-53.

[27]   Sawada H, Konomi H, Hirosawa K. Characterization of the collagen in the hexagonal lattice of Descemet's membrane: its relation to type VIII collagen. J Cell Biol 1990; 110(1): 219-27.

[28]   Shaw LM, Olsen BR. FACIT collagens: diverse molecular bridges in extracellular matrices. Trends Biochem Sci 1991; 16(5): 191-4.

[29]   Marshall GE. Human scleral elastic system: an immunoelectron microscopic study. Br J Ophthalmol 1995; 79(1): 57-64.

[30]   Thomas OE. Retina. In: Ryan SJ, editor. St. Louis: Mosby; 1989.

[31]   Tortora GJ, Derrickson B. Principles of anatomy and physiology. 12th ed: Hoboken John Wiley & Sons; 2009. 1 v. (various pagings) p.

[32]   Rizzolo LJ. Development and role of tight junctions in the retinal pigment epithelium. Int Rev Cytol 2007; 258 :195-234.

[33]   Rizzolo LJ. Polarity and the development of the outer blood-retinal barrier. Histol Histopathol 1997; 12(4): 1057-67.

[34]   Williams CD, Rizzolo LJ. Remodeling of junctional complexes during the development of the outer blood-retinal barrier. Anat Rec 1997; 249(3): 380-8.

[35]   Snell RS, Lemp MA. Clinical anatomy of the eye. Cambridge, MA: Blackwell Scientific Publications; 1989. 379-412 p.

[36]   Sebag J. The vitreous: structure, functionand pathobiology. New York: Springer-Verlag; 1989. xi, 173 p. p.

[37]   Tolentino FI. The vitreous. Arch Ophthalmol 1974; 92(4): 350-8.

Send Orders of Reprints at reprints@benthamscience.net

CHAPTER 2

Routes of Ocular Drug Delivery - Conventional *vs.* Novel Routes

Deep Kwatra, Ramya Krishna Vadlapatla, Varun Khurana, Dhananjay Pal and Ashim K. Mitra*

Division of Pharmaceutical Sciences, School of Pharmacy, University of Missouri-Kansas City, 2464 Charlotte Street, Kansas City, MO 64108-2718, USA

Abstract: Drug delivery to the eye has conventionally involved two basic methods of drug administration *i.e.* the topical route and the systemic route. Both of these orthodox methods of drug delivery face a number of barriers limiting their effectiveness in attaining therapeutic levels at the target site. The tight junctions, tear dilution and rapid clearance by the blood supply in both the anterior and posterior segments of the eye, act as the major barriers. To overcome these barriers, novel routes for drug delivery have been tried out by ophthalmologists that can bypass these barriers. The novel routes possess multiple advantages on the conventional routes such as increased drug concentration at the target site. Some of the routes are less invasive than the conventional routes and also cause fewer side effects. Some of these routes when used for delivering specialized formulations can also allow for better controlled/sustained/targeted drug delivery. In this chapter the comparisons between these conventional and novel routes of drug delivery have been made describing the advantages and disadvantages of each route.

Keywords: Ocular drug delivery, anterior segment, posterior segment, routes, corneal pathway, non-corneal route, systemic route, blood-aqueous barrier, blood-retinal barrier, intravitreal, periocular.

INTRODUCTION

Improving ocular bioavailability of a therapeutic agent has always been a major challenge for scientists involved in field of ophthalmic drug delivery. The presence of blood-aqueous barrier in the anterior chamber and blood-retinal barrier in the posterior chamber of the eye, collectively known as the blood-ocular

---

***Address correspondence to Ashim K. Mitra:** University of Missouri Curators' Professor of Pharmacy, Chairman, Division of Pharmaceutical Sciences, Vice-Provost for Interdisciplinary Research, University of Missouri - Kansas City, School of Pharmacy, 2464 Charlotte Street, Kansas City, MO 64108, USA; Tel: 816-235-1615; Fax: 816-235-5779; E-mail: mitraa@umkc.edu

barriers, limit the accessibility of therapeutic agents in ocular compartments *via* systemic circulation. Some of the vision-threatening disorders including age related macular degeneration, diabetic retinopathy and CMV retinitis require sufficient transport of drug molecules into the posterior segment for successful therapy. Delivery of therapeutic agents to the anterior segment by topical administration is challenged by factors including precorneal constraints such as tear turnover, solution drainage and limited precorneal residence time. Moreover, anatomical barriers prevent active molecules from reaching the deep ocular tissues following topical administration [1]. The search for better, non invasive and therapeutically efficient routes have resulted in many new routes for ocular drug delivery. Recent advances in conventional drug delivery strategies including topical administration through the application of novel drug delivery system or devices appear to be very promising. In this chapter we have described various conventional and non conventional routes of ocular drug administration along with concerns associated with such methods.

The routes for oculars drug delivery can be classified as:

a) Conventional Route

a.1) Topical Route

a.2) Systemic Route

b) Novel Routes

b.1) Subconjunctival Route

b.2) Sub-Tenon Route

b.3) Retrobulbar Route

b.4) Peribulbar Route

b.5) Intracameral Route

CONVENTIONAL ROUTES OF OCULAR DRUG DELIVERY

Topical Route

This conventional route of drug delivery is widely applicable for non-invasive treatment of the anterior segment. It is commonly recommended for treating both surface as well as intraocular pathologies. Many advantages of this route are obvious: noninvasive, self administered, relatively high ratio of ocular to systemic drug levels and cost effective. Various types of dosage forms like solutions, suspensions, ointments, soluble gels and rate controlled release systems are administered by this route. This preferred route of ocular drug delivery is not free from limitations. Bioavailability in the aqueous humor is only 5% for lipophilic molecules and less than 0.5% for hydrophilic molecules [2]. Due to this lower bioavailability from eye drops (less than 1-7%), frequent administrations are needed [3]. Inefficiency stems mainly from physiological and anatomical constraints. The fate of a drug following topical administration is depicted in Fig. **1**.

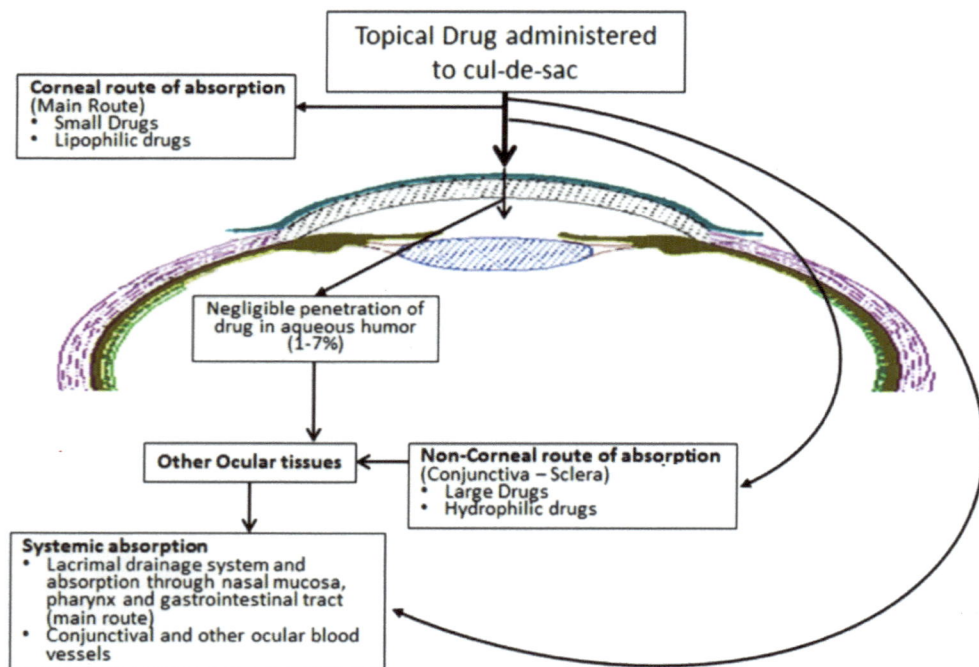

Figure 1: Schematic diagram showing the fate of a drug following topical administration.

Anatomical Barriers

Following topical administration, absorption can be either through the corneal or non-corneal route. The cornea is composed of five layers: epithelium, bowman's membrane, stroma, descement's membrane and endothelium (Fig. **2**). Among these anatomical structures, the corneal epithelium is considered a major barrier to most topically administered drugs. It is composed of 5-6 layers of columnar cells with tight junctions, which impart a paracellular resistance of 12-16 kΩ.cm. Lipophilic drugs can easily be transported through the lipid structures of the epithelium (transcellular route) whereas hydrophilic drugs need to permeate through intercellular spaces (paracellular route) [4]. Thus the epithelium is considered to be a major barrier to hydrophilic drugs. The anterior layer of stroma is modified into Bowman's membrane which is an acellular layer separating the epithelium from stroma. It is composed of randomly arranged collagen fibrils. The stroma is composed of multiple layers of hexagonally arranged collagen fibers and constitutes 90% of the total corneal thickness. This layer is highly hydrophilic with water filled porous channels, which allow the the rapid movement of hydrophilic drugs. This layer can also acts as a reservoir for hydrophilic drugs. The corneal endothelium consists of a monolayer of polygonal cells with large intercellular junctions. It is considered to be a leaky lipophilic layer [5]. This cell layer is in direct contact with aqueous humor and regulates the movement of molecules from inside into the stroma. Thus for a drug to reach into the eye, it should have optimum lipophilicity to permeate through the corneal epithelium as well as sufficient hydrophilicity to permeate across stroma.

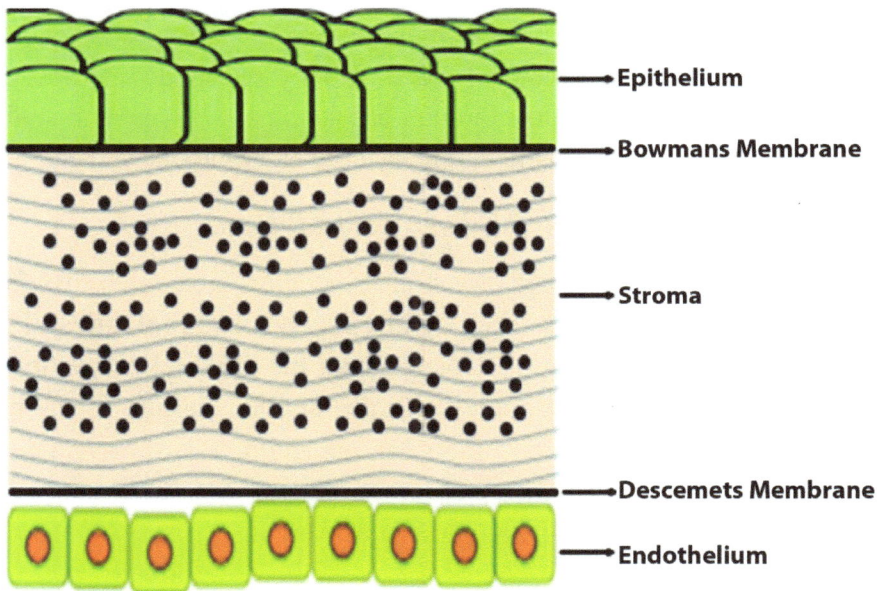

Figure 2: Structure of cornea.

Non-corneal route involves drug permeation across the conjunctiva and sclera into the vitreous humor. This route is considered to be important especially for large and hydrophilic molecules such as inulin and timolol [6]. Permeability of conjunctiva to hydrophilic molecules appears to be higher than cornea. Moreover, the conjunctival epithelium does not express tight junctions as corneal epithelium. This route is considered a minor pathway for drug absorption as the limbal area is rich in blood vessels which can potentially eliminate significant fraction of absorbed dose remove from the target site into the systemic circulation [7]. A small fraction of the dose that enters the sclera can penetrate through spaces within its randomly arranged collagen fibrils or through the perivascular openings [8]. The fraction that is absorbed through this pathway then enters the uveal tract and finally reaches the vitreous.

Physiological Barriers

Topically applied dosage forms exhibit poor bioavailability because of precorneal factors such as solution drainage, tear dilution, tear turnoverand increased lacrimation [9]. Rapid drainage from the precorneal area reduces ocular contact time, which lowers bioavailability. The tear volume under normal conditions is 7-9 μL with a turnover rate of 16% per minute [10]. Following topical application, the solution is diluted due to increased lacrimation and tear secretion. This process significantly lowers drug amounts in the precorneal space, thereby reducing drug absorption. A large portion of the dose is also lost through nasolacrimal drainage and spillage. All these factors can act synergistically lowering the drug entry into the cornea.

Factors Affecting Bioavailability Through Topical Route

Apart from the above mentioned constraints, ocular bioavailability following topical administration is also governed by physicochemical properties of the drug molecule. The rate of absorption is dependent on the physical properties of drug molecule and structure of the tissue. Topically applied dosage forms penetrate across the cornea either by transcellular or paracellular pathway. The rate of transport depends on physicochemical properties of the drug *i.e.*, solubility, lipophilicity, degree of ionization and molecular weight.

Solubility: Solubility is stated as the maximum amount of solute that can be dissolved in a solvent at standard temperature, pressure and pH. It depends on the pKa of the drug and the pH of the solution which further determines the ratio of ionized to unionized molecules. It is only the unionized molecules that can permeate across the biological membrane. Mitra *et al.*, have shown that the permeability of free unionized pilocarpine is approximately two fold greater than that of its ionized form [11]. The ratio of unionized to ionized molecules in a solution is given by Henderson-Hasselbach equation, *i.e.*, Eqs. 1 and 2.

$$\text{For weak acids, } pH = pka + \log\frac{[ionized\ drug]}{[unionized\ drug]} \tag{1}$$

$$\text{For weak bases, } pH = pka + \log\frac{[unionized\ drug]}{[ionized\ drug]} \tag{2}$$

In case of ionized molecules, the charge also effects the transcorneal permeation. Above its isoelectric point (pI 3.2) the corneal epithelium is negatively charged. Hence cationic species can penetrate easier than the anionic species.

Lipophilicity: A sigmoidal relationship exists between lipophilicity and corneal permeability [12]. For a drug to permeate through the corneal epithelium, it must be highly lipophilic. This is measured in terms of partition coefficient which is the ratio of unionized solute concentration in octanol and water as shown in Eqs.3 and 4.

$$Partition\ coefficient = \frac{[Solute]_{octanol}}{[Solute]_{Water}^{Unionized}} \tag{3}$$

$$Log\ P = log\left(\frac{[Solute]_{octanol}}{[Solute]_{Water}^{Unionized}}\right) \tag{4}$$

Log octanol buffer coefficient in the range of 2-4 is considered to be optimum for corneal permeation [13]. But the inner layer of cornea (stroma) being hydrophilic requires a degree of hydrophilicity for optimal permeation. Therefore a drug must be in the unionized form with optimum aqueous solubility and lipophilicity for corneal permeation.

Molecular weight and size: Hydrophilic drugs can also permeate the cornea through the paracellular route. Molecular weight and particularly size (molecular radius) are important in determining the permeability characteristics. Tight junctions on the apical cell layers of corneal epithelium have a paracellular pore diameter of 2 nm [14]. Hence this layer allows permeation of molecules having less than 500 Dalton molecular weight. Moreover, the pore density of corneal epithelium is $4.3*10^6/cm^2$, further limiting paracellular diffusion. Studies on isolated stroma have indicated that permeability of drug molecules across stroma is not dependent on partition coefficient but it is a function of molecular size and radius [5]. Nevertheless, stroma is often considered as a rate limiting factor for highly lipophilic compounds. The endothelium because of its wide intercellular junctions is not considered a rate limiting factor for drug transport relative to epithelium and stroma. However permeability across conjunctival epithelium does not depend on lipophilicity [5]. Conjunctiva offers a larger paracellular pore diameter compared to cornea. The conjunctival epithelia had 2 times larger pores and 16 times higher pore density than the cornea. Such total paracellular space is large enough to allow permeation of small peptides and oligonucleotides with molecular weights upto 5000-10000 Daltons [15]. Hence permeability of conjunctiva to large hydrophilic molecules is much higher relative to cornea. Permeation through sclera occurs through the aqueous pores or channels occupying the space between randomly arranged collagen fibrils [16]. Studies have shown that permeation across sclera is dependent mainly on the molecular size of the solute [5]. For example, the permeation of sucrose (molecular weight-342 Daltons) is 16 times faster than inulin (molecular weight-5000 Daltons) across sclera [17]. Scleral permeability is approximately half of conjunctiva but much higher than cornea.

Formulations for Enhancing Topical Delivery

An increase in ocular residence time accelerates ocular bioavailability. Hence attempts have been made to prolong drug retention time in the cul-de-sac. Some of them include increasing ocular contact time by viscosity enhancers, mucoadhesive polymers, penetration enhancers and complexing agents such as cyclodextrins.

Viscosity enhancers: Hydrophilic polymers such as methylcellulose, polyvinyl alcohol (PVA), hydroxypropylmethylcellulose (HPMC) have been added to increase viscosity of ophthalmic formulations. An optimum viscosity of 12-15 cps is suitable for ophthalmic solutions [18]. Highly viscous solutions may cause ocular irritation and rapid blinking. An extremely viscous solution can also cause blurred vision as well as blockade of puncti and canaliculi [19]. George *et al.* have shown that an increase in the viscosity for drugs having a log P value of 1-4, did not improve ocular bioavailability. It may be possible since drugs are highly lipophilic and readily permeate the corneal membrane. For molecules with low log P values, a rise in viscosity leads to higher ocular bioavailability. Among various polymers, PVA is highly preferred in ophthalmic formulations as it reduces the surface tension of water and interfacial tension at the oil-water interface besides promoting the tear film stability [18]. PVA-tropicamide solution appears to be 3.7 times more effective than tropicamide solution alone and 2 times more effective than other polymers examined [28].

Mucoadhesive polymers: Bioadhesion is referred to a process in which a drug carrier adheres to biological tissue. Mucoadhesion is a process by which drug conjugate is attached to cell surface mucus. Mucoadhesives are generally represented by macromolecular hydrocolloids with several hydrophilic functional groups capable of forming hydrogen bonds. These polymers are high molecular weight compounds that cannot easily cross biological membrane. Mucoadhesives can be natural, synthetic or semi synthetic. Robinson *et al.* have shown that cationic and anionic polymers bind more effectively to corneal epithelium than neutral polymers [20]. These mucoadhesive polymers adhere to the mucin coat covering the conjunctival and corneal surfaces. These physical and chemical forces *i.e.*, ionic, hydrophobic and hydrogen bonding allow enhanced retention and prolong contact time [21]. In addition the clearance is also reduced since the mucus turnover rate is much slower than the tear turnover rate. This increased residence time results in high drug concentration at the site leading to enhanced absorption. Some of the mucoadhesive agents commonly added in ophthalmic drug delivery are hyaluronic acid, chitosan, carboxymethylcellulose and polyacrylic acid derivatives such as carbopols and polycarbophils. Hyaluronic acid is a natural polymer present in both vitreous and aqueous humor. It is the widely preferred mucoadhesive because of its high water binding capacity and non irritant properties [22]. Chitosan is also suitable for ophthalmic formulations as it is biodegradable, biocompatible and non toxic. It has been hypothesized that mucoadhesive polymers in a viscous solution can further enhance ocular residence time, thus boosting ocular bioavailability [23].

Penetration enhancers: Penetration enhancers transiently raise the permeability of cornea resulting in higher drug penetration. There are several classes of penetration enhancers such as calcium chelators, surfactants and preservatives. These compounds act either by altering the permeability of the cell membrane or by disrupting tight junctions [24]. Calcium is required for maintaining the integrity of the tight junctions. Calcium chelators like EDTA disrupt tight junctions thus promoting paracellular transport. Surfactants include non ionic surfactants and bile salts. These compounds act mainly by altering cell membrane permeability, although a few can act on tight junctions [25, 26]. These surfactants are incorporated into the lipid bilayer resulting in lipid phase transition in cell membrane. If the concentration of surfactant is raised above the critical micellar concentration, micelles are formed. These micelles remove phospholipids from the membrane by solubilization.

Preservatives like benzalkonium chloride (BAC) are known to increase the permeability of certain ophthalmic drugs [9, 27]. It may be due to widening the intercellular spaces in tight junctions of corneal epithelial cells [28, 29]. Similarly compounds like azones are known to increase the transcorneal permeation of hydrophilic drugs. These penetration enhancers aid in lowering the drop size of the instilled formulation. Such reduction in drop size lowers drainage and ensures enhanced bioavailability [30]. However these enhancers should be used with extreme caution because these surfactants can damage the integrity of the epithelial tissue. EDTA can reach the iris-ciliary body and alter the permeability of the vasculature in the uvea [31]. Bile salts and surfactants may cause ocular irritation. Similarly, BAC can accumulate leading to toxicity.

Cyclodextrins: Cyclodextrins are truncated or bucket shaped molecules with a hydrophilic outer surface and central hydrophobic cavity (Fig. **3**). These molecules can form inclusion complexes with many guest molecules by incorporating them into inner cavity. Complexation with cyclodextrins is an effective way to increase the solubility of a water insoluble drug without altering its structure and biological activity. Cyclodextrins act as true carriers by incorporating hydrophobic molecules into cavity and delivering at the corneal epithelium. Since no covalent bond is formed, the complex is reversible and dissociates at the surface of the membrane. Cyclodextrins being hydrophilic cannot cross the biological membrane and are drained away by the nasolacrimal fluid. The resultant systemic exposure is undetectable and toxicity of these cyclodextrins is considered negligible.

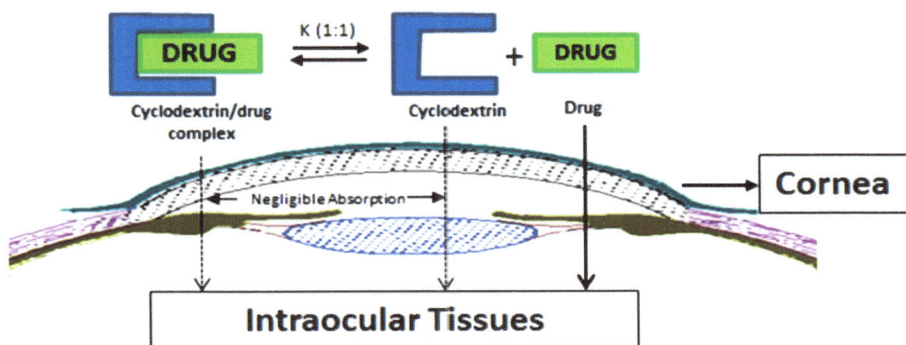

Figure 3: Complexation with cyclodextrins.

In comparison with other penetration enhancers, cyclodextrins do not disrupt the integrity of the corneal membrane. Cyclodextrins are thus good adjuvants in ophthalmics as these molecules can increase the solubility of the drug, stabilize in aqueous solution and reduce ocular irritation [32]. Cyclodextrins have been reported to increase the solubility of many compounds such as steroids and carbonic anhydrase inhibitors [33, 34]. However, at high concentrations cyclodextrins show toxicological responses. At a concentration exceeding 25%, cyclodextrins can form complexes with components of biological membranes such as cholesterol and phospholipids [35]. In patients with dry eye, topical administration of cyclodextrins can further cause crusting of the eyelids. Furthermore, evaporation of water can result in hypertonic cyclodextrin solution, which can be irritating to the eye. This phenomenon is rarely observed in patients with normal tear production.

Examples of Topically Administered Dosage Forms

Ocular drugs are typically administered as liquid dosage forms. Based on the consistency, content and concentration of the formulation the drug retention time in the ocular cul-de-sac can be significantly altered resulting in significantly altered bioavailability. The most commonly used dosage forms for topical drug delivery are:

Solutions: Solutions are most widely preferred ophthalmic dosage forms. These products can be self administered by patients. Once the drug is in a dissolved state it can be readily absorbed. However, short residence time lowers the amount of drug that can partition into the corneal epithelium. The rate controlling parameters for the ocular bioavailability in case of solutions are physicochemical properties of drug and its concentration in tissue. Retention of the drug in eyes is also altered by viscosity, osmolality, hydrogen ion concentration and the amount of drug instilled [36].

Suspensions: A sparingly water soluble drug in finely divided state is suspended in a liquid to form a suspension. Following topical administration a small fraction of the suspended particles are retained while a large amount is drained into the nasolacrimal ducts [37]. The particle size is the main determinant of the fraction retained. An increase in the particle size generally prolongs the retention time. Studies have shown that 25μm polystyrene beads are retained for about 12 hours whereas 3μm particles are drained immediately. However larger particles can also cause irritation. So an optimum particle size should be maintained. Particles ideally may have slow dissolution in tear fluid which can prolong and provide once a day administration.

Ointments: Ointments are widely applied for sustaining drug release. With ophthalmic ointments, precorneal clearance of the drug is reduced to 0.5% per minute relative to tear turnover of 16% per minute [38]. This formulation reduces frequency of drug administration in comparison to eye drops. However, these formulations are still less preferred due to their potential ocular irritation and vision interference [39]. Ointments are prepared by dispersion of an active in the base which can be a simple one (petroleum jelly, paraffin, mineral oil) or a compound base (emulsion of either oil in water (o/w) or water in oil (w/o)). Drug release from the ointment is governed by its solubility within the base. For example, pilocarpine (water soluble drug) is rapidly released as compared to fluorometholone (oil soluble drug) from an oleaginous ointment [40]. As the nasolacrimal drainage is minimized with the use of ointments, systemic toxicity is extremely low.

Systemic Route

Since a very low drug fraction from plasma enters the eye, systemic route for ocular drug delivery requires large doses. Hence, it is a less favored route for the treatment of ocular infections due to potential systemic side effects.

Barriers in Systemic Delivery to the Eye

Systemic delivery of drugs to ocular components is limited by the presence of Blood Ocular Barrier (BOB) which restricts the entry of xenobiotics and other toxins into the eye. BOB is composed of Blood Aqueous Barrier (BAB) and Blood Retinal Barrier (BRB) in the anterior and posterior segments respectively.

Blood aqueous barrier: The structures involved in the formation of BAB are the ciliary body and the iris. The blood vessels of the ciliary body are larger in diameter and show fenestrations. Hence molecules such as plasma proteins can escape into the ciliary stroma through these vessels. The ciliary epithelium consists of non-pigmented and pigmented cell layers. Studies indicate that pigmented epithelium has only few sealing strands and hence is leaky [41-44]. Macromolecules that pass through the intercellular clefts of the pigmented epithelium are finally blocked by the tight junctions of non-pigmented epithelium. The blood vessels of iris lack fenestrations and are joined by tight junctions through their epithelia [45]. The anterior epithelium of iris stroma shows large openings making it a discontinuous layer [41]. The posterior epithelium of iris being a continuation of non-pigmented layer of ciliary epithelium has the same anatomical features. Thus, the BAB is composed of two parts: non-pigmented layer of ciliary body and posterior iris as well as endothelial epithelium of iridial blood vessels.

Blood retinal barrier: BRB regulates the homeostatic microenvironment in the retina and is composed of two components, the outer and inner BRB. The outer BRB is formed by tight junctions in between retinal pigment epithelial cells (RPE). RPE has a number of receptors on basolateral membrane facilitating nutrient transport from the fenestrated choriocapillaries. In addition, it also regulates the removal of waste products formed during retinal metabolism in an apico-basal direction to the choroid. Inner BRB has tight junctions between capillary endothelial cells of retina. These capillary cells are surrounded by pericytes which regulate the vascular tone and support capillary wall [46]. Number of pericytes to vascular endothelial cells is greater in retina which further limits permeability [47]. Astrocytes and Muller cells are also associated with inner BRB. Muller cells regulate homeostasis and signaling of various molecules, whereas astrocytes stimulate the expression of tight junction proteins such as zonula occludens [48, 49]. Thus systemic delivery of drugs into the eye is associated with poor bioavailability due to the presence of these barriers which restricts BAB transport.

Intravitreal Injection

Intravitreal injections (IVI) provide treatment of many retinal diseases. In IVI, therapeutic agents are introduced directly into the vitreous fluid through pars plana. Poor outcomes associated with systemic drug delivery, blood ocular barrier and inaccessibility of vitreous through topical drops led to the development of IVI. It was initially selected to experimentally create endophthalmitis in rabbits in early 1940's. Agents can be introduced into the vitreous either as a solution or a depot formulation or dispersion of microparticles. After reaching equilibrium, drug concentration decreases following first order kinetics either across the retinal surface or across the anterior hyaloid surface through the aqueous humor [50]. The retention of drugs within the vitreous is affected by the molecular weight. Inner limiting membrane protecting photoreceptor cells is impermeable to relatively high molecular weight substances (>40kDa for linear molecules and >70kDa for globar molecules). Hence, macromolecules have longer retention time of several weeks as compared to less than 3 days for low molecular weight compounds (<500 Da) [51].

Even though this route is preferred for the entry of drug into posterior segment, it has major limitations. Most therapies for posterior segment require repetitive IVI which might lead to retinal detachment, cataract, hyperemia and endophthalmitis [52]. Sustained release drug delivery systems can avoid frequent administration of therapeutic agents and thus can offer patient compliance. Macugen® (pegaptanib sodium) - an agent that targets Vascular Endothelial growth factor – is administered once every six weeks as an IVI in the treatment of neovascular (wet) age-related macular degeneration (AMD). Similarly, Iluvien® - an injectable implant of fluocinolone acetonide intended for the treatment of Diabetic Macular Edema, is under Phase III clinical trial. This non-erodible, injectable implant is intended to release the drug for the period of three years.

NOVEL ROUTES OF OCULAR DRUG DELIVERY

Delivery of small molecules including various therapeutic agents and large molecules like proteins to the eye still remains a major challenge. During the past few years, an intense research in the field of novel drug delivery systems coupled with better understanding of intricate physiology of eye has produced promising results solving some of the delivery issues. Drug delivery to the posterior segment through the subconjunctival and periocular route are gaining popularity [53]. Other novel routes are also being examined for successful posterior delivery. The novel routes have been depicted in Fig. **4**.

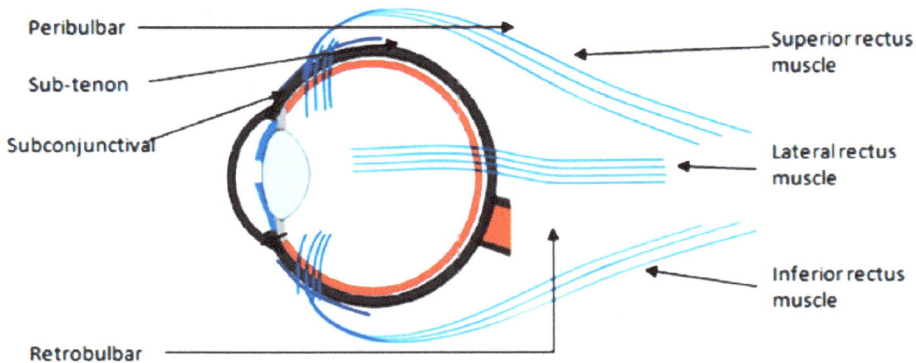

Figure 4: Novel routes of ocular drug delivery.

Subconjunctival Route

This route deposits the active agent beneath the conjunctiva, a mucous membrane that lines the inner surface of eyelid. The subconjunctival injection allows circumvention of the barriers imposed by cornea and conjunctiva, resulting in higher levels in vitreous. The conjunctival epithelium serves as a rate-limiting barrier to the permeability of hydrophilic drugs. Therefore, it is more prudent to administer such hydrophilic drugs avoiding the diffusion across conjunctival epithelium. Also administration of micro/nanoparticles by this route sustains release of the active ingredient for a prolonged period of time and thus aid in minimizing the dosing frequency [54]. This route is less invasive when compared to intravitreal route [55]. In a case report published by Erdurmus and Totan, the subconjunctival injection of bevacizumab (recombinant monoclonal antibody against VEGF) was very effective in reducing the degree of corneal neovascularization [56]. Similarly Kompella *et al.*, have reported that subconjunctivally administered nano- and microparticles of budesonide (a corticosteroid for treatment of inflammatory disorders) reduced the VEGF expression in retinal pigmented epithelial cells. Application of this biodegradable polymer based drug delivery system *via* this route sustains drug delivery compared to the solution [57]. Misra *et al.*, has recently utilized this route to deliver insulin hydrogels for the prevention and treatment of retinal neurovascular degeneration in diabetic retinopathy [58]. In order to maintain prolonged functional activity and effective transscleral permeation, PEGylated aptamer pegaptanib in PLGA microspheres have also been administered through subconjunctival injection [59, 60].

Sub-Tenon Route

Sub-tenon space represents a cavity bound by tenon's capsule and sclera. Sub-tenon route has emerged as a better alternative to retrobulbar and peribulbar route for administration of anesthesia due to less complications and avoidance of sharp needles [61]. Posterior sub-tenon injections of steroids have been utilized in the treatment of uveitis and cystoid macular edma complicating uveitis [62]. Sub-tenon injections of triamcinolone acetonide (TA) were effective against pain and scleral inflammation in nonnecrotizing scleritis [63]. Toda *et al.*, reported that low risk of endophthalmitis has been associated with sub-tenon injection of TA compared to IVI. An increase in the blood glucose levels and blood pressure was reported, but its association with TA injections still remains unclear [64-66]. According to Li *et al.*, sub-tenon anesthesia is the safest and most effective way to achieve local anesthesia. This approach uses a blunt cannula thus avoiding any danger associated with sharp needles. Further, pre-operative deep sedation is not required in this procedure [67].

Retrobulbar Route

Retrobulbar route is generally employed for administrating anesthesia and other drugs including antibiotics and corticosteroids behind the globe. The retrobulbar injection enters the eye through eyelid and orbital fascia that installs the drug in retrobulbar space. There is a possibility of damaging the optic nerve during the procedure that can be avoided by limiting the penetration of needle to not more than 1.5 cm behind the globe [52, 68]. The retrobulbar infusion of triamcinolone was found to be safe and effective for the treatment of uveitis in patients, with minor complications as compared to sub-tenon delivery [69]. It is considered as the most efficient route for delivery of anesthetic agents with minor or no change in intraocular pressure. Administration of anesthetic through retrobulbar route may lead to elevated levels of intraocular pressure in orbital diseases and may also cause inadvertent laceration of orbital vessels resulting in retrobulbar hemorrhage [70-72].

Peribulbar Route

This route is a preferred route for the delivery of anesthesia in cataract surgery due to its reduced injury rate to the intraorbital structure compared to the retrobulbar route of administration [73]. A study conducted by Rizzo *et al.* on several patients, suggests that the peribulbar anesthesia administered by medial percutaneous single injection is safe and effective alternative to classical techniques for ocular regional anesthesia [74]. Several reports suggest that the chance of retrobulbar hemorrhage recurrence with peribulbar blocks is very low. Although, incidence of elevated levels of intraocular pressure, proptosis, bleeding into extraocular muscles or within the muscle cone after peribulbar injection have been reported [70, 75, 76].

Intracameral Route

Intracameral route is intended to inject the drug in anterior chamber of the eye and has its own limitations in terms of accessibility of therapeutic agent to the posterior segment. It is generally employed in cataract surgery [52]. A clinical study conducted by Chang *et al.* demonstrated its effectiveness of intracamerally administered dexamethasone in reducing the post-operative inflammation in glaucomatous and non-glaucomatous eye in humans [77]. Moreover, intracameral bevacizumab injections have also been shown to reduce the aqueous VEGF level in patient with neovascular glaucoma [78]. Intracameral injection of amphotericin B is very effective in patients suffering from fungal keratitis [79]. Post-operative endophthalmitis is a serious consequence that may arise from cataract surgery. Intracameral administration of agents like cefuroxime has shown promising results in the prevention of post-operative endophthalmitis relative to subconjunctival administration. It is cost-effective over most commonly applied topical antibiotics [80, 81]. The most effective and direct method for the treatment of fungal endophthalmitis is the administration of voriconazole (broad spectrum antifungal agent) through intracameral route [82]. Moxifloxacin is administered intracamerally in order to prevent the occurrence of endophthalmitis after cataract surgery [83, 84].

CONCLUDING REMARKS

Invention of new drug molecules and novel drug delivery systems for the treatment of ocular diseases are accelerating in a fast pace. But achieving required levels at the targeted ocular tissues is still a challenge. A lot of progress has been made through development of formulations to improve the bioavailability of the drugs delivered *via* the conventional routes of ocular drug delivery. Simultaneously a lot of work has also been done in identifying novel routes of drug delivery that are less invasive, achieve better targetability, better retention and bioavailability at the targeted ocular tissue. It's through the combination of the use of these novel routes and novel drug delivery systems that the holy grail of optimum ocular bioavailability can be achieved.

ACKNOWLEDGEMENTS

We would like to acknowledge NIH grants R01EY09171-16 and R01EY010659-14 for financial support.

CONFLICT OF INTEREST

The author(s) confirm that this chapter content has no conflict of interest.

REFERENCES

[1]   Duvvuri S, Gandhi MD, Mitra AK. Effect of P-glycoprotein on the ocular disposition of a model substrate, quinidine. Curr Eye Res 2003; 27(6): 345-53.

[2]   Zhang W, Prausnitz MR, Edwards A. Model of transient drug diffusion across cornea. J Control Release 2004; 99(2): 241-58.

[3]   Ghate DA, Holley G, Dollinger H, *et al.* Evaluation of endothelial mucin layer thickness after phacoemulsification with next generation ophthalmic irrigating solution. Cornea 2008; 27(9): 1050-6.

[4]   Grass GM, Robinson JR. Mechanisms of corneal drug penetration. II: Ultrastructural analysis of potential pathways for drug movement. J Pharm Sci 1988; 77(1) :15-23.

[5]   Prausnitz MR, Noonan JS. Permeability of cornea, sclera, and conjunctiva: a literature analysis for drug delivery to the eye. J Pharm Sci 1998; 87(12) :1479-88.

[6]   Ahmed I, Patton TF. Importance of the noncorneal absorption route in topical ophthalmic drug delivery. Invest Ophthalmol Vis Sci 1985; 26(4): 584-7.

[7]   Barar J, Javadzadeh AR, Omidi Y. Ocular novel drug delivery: impacts of membranes and barriers. Expert Opin Drug Deliv 2008; 5(5): 567-81.

[8]   Ahmed I, Gokhale RD, Shah MV, Patton TF. Physicochemical determinants of drug diffusion across the conjunctiva, sclera, and cornea. J Pharm Sci 1987; 76(8): 583-6.

[9]   Lee VH, Robinson JR. Topical ocular drug delivery: recent developments and future challenges. J Ocul Pharmacol 1986; 2(1): 67-108.

[10]   Hughes P. Overview of ocular drug delivery and iatrogenic ocular cytopathologies. In: Mitra AK, editor. Ophthalmic Drug Delivery Systems. New York: Marcel Dekker, Inc. ; 1993. p. pp. 1–27.

[11]   Mitra AK, Mikkelson TJ. Mechanism of transcorneal permeation of pilocarpine. J Pharm Sci 1988; 77(9): 771-5.

[12]   Wang W, Sasaki H, Chien DS, Lee VH. Lipophilicity influence on conjunctival drug penetration in the pigmented rabbit: a comparison with corneal penetration. Curr Eye Res 1991; 10(6): 571-9.

[13]   Schoenwald RD, Ward RL. Relationship between steroid permeability across excised rabbit cornea and octanol-water partition coefficients. J Pharm Sci 1978; 67(6): 786-8.

[14]   Aronow WS. Indications for surgical treatment of stable angina pectoris. Arch Intern Med 1979; 139(6): 690-2.

[15]   Hamalainen KM, Kananen K, Auriola S, Kontturi K, Urtti A. Characterization of paracellular and aqueous penetration routes in cornea, conjunctiva, and sclera. Invest Ophthalmol Vis Sci 1997; 38(3): 627-34.

[16]   Doane MG, Jensen AD, Dohlman CH. Penetration routes of topically applied eye medications. Am J Ophthalmol 1978; 85(3): 383-6.

[17]   Huang AJ, Tseng SC, Kenyon KR. Paracellular permeability of corneal and conjunctival epithelia. Invest Ophthalmol Vis Sci 1989; 30(4): 684-9.

[18]   Patton TF, Robinson JR. Ocular evaluation of polyvinyl alcohol vehicle in rabbits. J Pharm Sci 1975; 64(8): 1312-6.

[19]   Ghate D, Edelhauser HF. Ocular drug delivery. Expert Opin Drug Deliv 2006; 3(2): 275-87.

[20]   Park K, Robinson JR. Bioadhesive polymers as platforms for oral-controlled drug delivery: method to study bioadhesion. Int J Pharm 1984; 19(2): 107-27.

[21]   Kurz D, Ciulla TA. Novel approaches for retinal drug delivery. Ophthalmol Clin North Am 2002; 15(3): 405-10.

[22]   Saettone MF, Chetoni P, Tilde Torracca M, Burgalassi S, Giannaccini B. Evaluation of muco-adhesive properties and *in vivo* activity of ophthalmic vehicles based on hyaluronic acid. Int J Pharm 1989; 51(3): 203-12.

[23]   Davies NM, Farr SJ, Hadgraft J, Kellaway IW. Evaluation of mucoadhesive polymers in ocular drug delivery. I. Viscous solutions. Pharm Res 1991; 8(8): 1039-43.

[24]   Liaw J and Robinson J R. Ocular penetration enhancers. In: Mitra AK, editor. Ophthalmic Drug Delivery Systems. New York: Marcel Dekker, Inc.; 1993. p. pp. 369–82.

[25]   Hosoya K, Lee VH. Cidofovir transport in the pigmented rabbit conjunctiva. Curr Eye Res 1997; 16(7): 693-7.

[26]   Anderberg EK, Artursson P. Epithelial transport of drugs in cell culture. VIII: Effects of sodium dodecyl sulfate on cell membrane and tight junction permeability in human intestinal epithelial (Caco-2) cells. J Pharm Sci 1993; 82(4): 392-8.

[27]   Burstein NL. Preservative alteration of corneal permeability in humans and rabbits. Invest Ophthalmol Vis Sci 1984; 25(12): 1453-7.

[28]   Tonjum AM. Permeability of rabbit corneal epithelium to horseradish peroxidase after the influence of benzalkonium chloride. Acta Ophthalmol (Copenh) 1975; 53(3): 335-47.

[29]   Tonjum AM, Green K. Quantitative study of fluorescein iontophoresis through the cornea. Am J Ophthalmol 1971; 71(6): 1328-32.

[30]   Van Santvliet L, Ludwig A. The influence of penetration enhancers on the volume instilled of eye drops. Eur J Pharm Biopharm 1998; 45(2): 189-98.

[31]   Grass GM, Robinson JR. Relationship of chemical structure to corneal penetration and influence of low-viscosity solution on ocular bioavailability. J Pharm Sci 1984; 73(8): 1021-7.

[32]   Kaur IP, Chhabra S, Aggarwal D. Role of cyclodextrins in ophthalmics. Curr Drug Deliv 2004; 1(4): 351-60.

[33]   Loftsson T, Stefansson E. Cyclodextrins in eye drop formulations: enhanced topical delivery of corticosteroids to the eye. Acta Ophthalmol Scand 2002; 80(2): 144-50.

[34]   Loftsson T, Frithriksdottir H, Stefansson E, *et al.* Topically effective ocular hypotensive acetazolamide and ethoxyzolamide formulations in rabbits. J Pharm Pharmacol 1994; 46(6): 503-4.

[35]   Irie T, Uekama K. Pharmaceutical applications of cyclodextrins. III. Toxicological issues and safety evaluation. J Pharm Sci 1997; 86(2): 147-62.

[36]   Lee VHL. Precorneal Corneal and Postcorneal factors. In: Mitra AK, editor. Ophthalmic Drug Delivery systems. New York: Marcel Dekker, Inc.; 1993. p. pp. 59–82.

[37]   Sieg JW, Robinson JR. Vehicle effects on ocular drug bioavailability i: evaluation of fluorometholone. J Pharm Sci 1975; 64(6): 931-6.

[38]   Massey JY, Hanna C, Goodart R, Wallace T. Effect of drug vehicle on human ocular retention of topically applied tetracycline. Am J Ophthalmol 1976; 81(2): 151-6.

[39]   Newton DW, Becker CH, Torosian G. Physical and chemical characteristics of water-soluble, semisolid, anhydrous bases for possible ophthalmic use. J Pharm Sci 1973; 62(9): 1538-42.

[40]   Sieg JW, Robinson JR. Vehicle effects on ocular drug bioavailability III: Shear-facilitated pilocarpine release from ointments. J Pharm Sci 1979; 68(6): 724-8.

[41]   Raviola G. The structural basis of the blood-ocular barriers. Exp Eye Res 1977; 25 (Suppl.): 27-63.

[42]   Raviola G. Effects of paracentesis on the blood-aqueous barrier: an electron microscope study on Macaca mulatta using horseradish peroxidase as a tracer. Invest Ophthalmol 1974; 13(11): 828-58.

[43]   Smith RS. Ultrastructural studies of the blood-aqueous barrier. I. Transport of an electron-dense tracer in the iris and ciliary body of the mouse. Am J Ophthalmol 1971; 71(5): 1066-77.

[44]   Shiose Y, Oguri M. Electron microscopic studies on the blood-retinal barrier and the blood-aqueous barrier. Nihon Ganka Gakkai Zasshi 1969; 73(9): 1606-22.

[45]   Vegge T. An electron microscopic study of the permeability of iris capillaries to horseradish peroxidase in the vervet monkey (Cercopithecus aethiops). Z Zellforsch Mikrosk Anat 1971; 121(1): 74-81.

[46]   Sims DE. Recent advances in pericyte biology--implications for health and disease. Can J Cardiol 1991; 7(10): 431-43.

[47]   Balabanov R, Dore-Duffy P. Role of the CNS microvascular pericyte in the blood-brain barrier. J Neurosci Res 1998; 53(6): 637-44.

[48]   Bringmann A, Skatchkov SN, Pannicke T, et al. Muller glial cells in anuran retina. Microsc Res Tech 2000;50(5):384-93.

[49]   Gardner TW, Lieth E, Khin SA, et al. Astrocytes increase barrier properties and ZO-1 expression in retinal vascular endothelial cells. Invest Ophthalmol Vis Sci 1997; 38(11): 2423-7.

[50]   Maurice D. Review: practical issues in intravitreal drug delivery. J Ocul Pharmacol Ther 2001; 17(4): 393-401.

[51]   Marmor MF, Negi A, Maurice DM. Kinetics of macromolecules injected into the subretinal space. Exp Eye Res 1985; 40(5): 687-96.

[52]   Raghava S, Hammond M, Kompella UB. Periocular routes for retinal drug delivery. Expert Opin Drug Deliv 2004; 1(1): 99-114.

[53]   Short BG. Safety evaluation of ocular drug delivery formulations: techniques and practical considerations. Toxicol Pathol 2008; 36(1): 49-62.

[54]   Ghate D, Edelhauser HF. Barriers to glaucoma drug delivery. J Glaucoma 2008; 17(2): 147-56.

[55]   Hosoya K, Lee VH, Kim KJ. Roles of the conjunctiva in ocular drug delivery: a review of conjunctival transport mechanisms and their regulation. Eur J Pharm Biopharm 2005; 60(2): 227-40.

[56]   Erdurmus M, Totan Y. Subconjunctival bevacizumab for corneal neovascularization. Graefes Arch Clin Exp Ophthalmol 2007; 245(10): 1577-9.

[57]   Kompella UB, Bandi N, Ayalasomayajula SP. Subconjunctival nano- and microparticles sustain retinal delivery of budesonide, a corticosteroid capable of inhibiting VEGF expression. Invest Ophthalmol Vis Sci 2003; 44(3): 1192-201.

[58]   Misra GP, Singh RS, Aleman TS, et al. Subconjunctivally implantable hydrogels with degradable and thermoresponsive properties for sustained release of insulin to the retina. Biomaterials 2009; 30(33): 6541-7.

[59]   Anderson OA, Bainbridge JW, Shima DT. Delivery of anti-angiogenic molecular therapies for retinal disease. Drug Discov Today 2010; 15(7-8): 272-82.

[60]   Carrasquillo KG, Ricker JA, Rigas IK, *et al.* Controlled delivery of the anti-VEGF aptamer EYE001 with poly(lactic-co-glycolic)acid microspheres. Invest Ophthalmol Vis Sci 2003; 44(1): 290-9.

[61]   Faure C, Faure L, Billotte C. Globe perforation following no-needle sub-Tenon anesthesia. J Cataract Refract Surg 2009; 35(8): 1471-2.

[62]   Lafranco Dafflon M, Tran VT, Guex-Crosier Y, Herbort CP. Posterior sub-Tenon's steroid injections for the treatment of posterior ocular inflammation: indications, efficacy and side effects. Graefes Arch Clin Exp Ophthalmol 1999; 237(4): 289-95.

[63]   Johnson KS, Chu DS. Evaluation of sub-Tenon triamcinolone acetonide injections in the treatment of scleritis. Am J Ophthalmol 2010; 149(1): 77-81.

[64]   Toda J, Fukushima H, Kato S. Systemic complications of posterior subtenon injection of triamcinolone acetonide in type 2 diabetes patients. Diabetes Res Clin Pract 2009; 84(2): e38-40.

[65]   Moshfeghi DM, Kaiser PK, Scott IU, *et al.* Acute endophthalmitis following intravitreal triamcinolone acetonide injection. Am J Ophthalmol 2003; 136(5): 791-6.

[66]   Benz MS, Murray TG, Dubovy SR, Katz RS, Eifrig CW. Endophthalmitis caused by Mycobacterium chelonae abscessus after intravitreal injection of triamcinolone. Arch Ophthalmol 2003; 121(2): 271-3.

[67]   Li HK, Abouleish A, Grady J, Groeschel W, Gill KS. Sub-Tenon's injection for local anesthesia in posterior segment surgery. Ophthalmology 2000; 107(1): 41-6; discussion 46-7.

[68]   Wadhwa S, Paliwal R, Paliwal SR, Vyas SP. Nanocarriers in ocular drug delivery: an update review. Curr Pharm Des 2009; 15(23): 2724-50.

[69]   Okada AA, Wakabayashi T, Morimura Y, *et al.* Trans-Tenon's retrobulbar triamcinolone infusion for the treatment of uveitis. Br J Ophthalmol 2003; 87(8): 968-71.

[70]   Nassr MA, Morris CL, Netland PA, Karcioglu ZA. Intraocular pressure change in orbital disease. Surv Ophthalmol 2009; 54(5): 519-44.

[71]   Netland PA, Siegner SW, Harris A. Color Doppler ultrasound measurements after topical and retrobulbar epinephrine in primate eyes. Invest Ophthalmol Vis Sci 1997; 38(12): 2655-61.

[72]   Yung CW, Moorthy RS, Lindley D, Ringle M, Nunery WR. Efficacy of lateral canthotomy and cantholysis in orbital hemorrhage. Ophthal Plast Reconstr Surg 1994; 10(2): 137-41.

[73]   Janoria KG, Gunda S, Boddu SH, Mitra AK. Novel approaches to retinal drug delivery. Expert Opin Drug Deliv 2007; 4(4): 371-88.

[74]   Rizzo L, Marini M, Rosati C, *et al.* Peribulbar anesthesia: a percutaneous single injection technique with a small volume of anesthetic. Anesth Analg 2005; 100(1): 94-6.

[75]   Gock G, Francis IC, Mulligan S. Traumatic intramuscular orbital haemorrhage. Clin Experiment Ophthalmol 2000; 28(5): 391-2.

[76]   Ahmad S, Ahmad A, Benzon HT. Clinical experience with the peribulbar block for ophthalmologic surgery. Reg Anesth 1993; 18(3): 184-8.

[77]   Chang DT, Herceg MC, Bilonick RA, *et al.* Intracameral dexamethasone reduces inflammation on the first postoperative day after cataract surgery in eyes with and without glaucoma. Clin Ophthalmol 2009; 3: 345-55.

[78]   Grover S, Gupta S, Sharma R, Brar VS, Chalam KV. Intracameral bevacizumab effectively reduces aqueous vascular endothelial growth factor concentrations in neovascular glaucoma. Br J Ophthalmol 2009; 93(2): 273-4.

[79]   Yoon KC, Jeong IY, Im SK, Chae HJ, Yang SY. Therapeutic effect of intracameral amphotericin B injection in the treatment of fungal keratitis. Cornea 2007; 26(7): 814-8.

[80]   Sharifi E, Porco TC, Naseri A. Cost-effectiveness analysis of intracameral cefuroxime use for prophylaxis of endophthalmitis after cataract surgery. Ophthalmology 2009; 116(10): 1887-96.

[81]   Yu-Wai-Man P, Morgan SJ, Hildreth AJ, Steel DH, Allen D. Efficacy of intracameral and subconjunctival cefuroxime in preventing endophthalmitis after cataract surgery. J Cataract Refract Surg 2008; 34(3): 447-51.

[82]   Shen YC, Wang CY, Tsai HY, Lee HN. Intracameral voriconazole injection in the treatment of fungal endophthalmitis resulting from keratitis. Am J Ophthalmol 2010; 149(6): 916-21.

[83]   Lane SS, Osher RH, Masket S, Belani S. Evaluation of the safety of prophylactic intracameral moxifloxacin in cataract surgery. J Cataract Refract Surg 2008; 34(9): 1451-9.

[84]   Espiritu CR, Caparas VL, Bolinao JG. Safety of prophylactic intracameral moxifloxacin 0.5% ophthalmic solution in cataract surgery patients. J Cataract Refract Surg 2007; 33(1): 63-8.

Send Orders of Reprints at reprints@benthamscience.net

CHAPTER 3

Drug Delivery to Anterior Segment of the Eye

Jwala Renukuntla[1], Sujay J. Shah [2], Mitesh Patel[2], Aswani Dutt Vadlapudi[2] and Ashim K. Mitra[2,*]

[1]*Division of Pharmaceutical Sciences, South College School of Pharmacy, 400 Goody's Lane Knoxville, TN 37922, USA and* [2]*Division of Pharmaceutical Sciences, School of Pharmacy, University of Missouri-Kansas City, Kansas City, Missouri-64108, USA*

Abstract: Transport of therapeutic agents into the anterior segment of the eye is highly restricted by various anatomical and physiological barriers. Topical administration is the most convenient method of drug delivery for the treatment of anterior segment eye diseases. The global market for eye care products is approximately $12.5 billion and is growing at a rate of 9% every year. Eye drops account for 90% of all conventional ophthalmic formulations. However, it suffers from several disadvantages such as nasolacrimal drainage, loss in conjunctival blood circulation, tear dilution, normal tear drainage and reflux blinking. There is a need for alternate drug delivery systems which can address poor ocular absorption associated with conventional drug delivery systems. In this chapter, we have made an attempt to briefly describe various drug delivery systems employed in the treatment of anterior segment eye diseases such as nanoemulsions, collagen corneal shields, hydrogels, vesicular systems (liposomes and niosomes), iontophoresis, phonophoresis, punctal plugs and contact lenses.

Keywords: Eye, anterior segment, novel systems, drug delivery, nanoemulsions, collagen corneal shields, hydrogels, vesicular systems, iontophoresis, phonophoresis, punctal plugs, contact lenses.

INTRODUCTION

Drug delivery to the eye is one of the most challenging tasks owing to its complex anatomy and physiology. Topical drug administration is the most preferred method for the treatment of ocular infections due to the accessibility of anterior segment of the eye [1, 2]. It is composed of cornea, conjunctiva, iris, ciliary body

*Address correspondence to Ashim K. Mitra: University of Missouri Curators' Professor of Pharmacy, Chairman, Division of Pharmaceutical Sciences, Vice-Provost for Interdisciplinary Research, University of Missouri - Kansas City, School of Pharmacy, 2464 Charlotte Street, Kansas City, MO 64108, USA; Tel: 816-235-1615; Fax: 816-235-5779; E-mail: mitraa@umkc.edu

and lens. Human cornea and several precorneal constraints limit ocular drug bioavailability following topical administration [3, 4]. Following topical administration, less than 5% of the instilled dose is absorbed into the eye [5].

A first order process measuring a significant change in a biological, physical or chemical activity, may be described by a traditional Eq. 1.

$$C = C_0 * e^{-kt} \text{ or } C = C_0 * e^{(-t/T)} \tag{1}$$

T= time constant or referred as the inverse of the rate constant, (k).

t= time period for a particular interval

Time constant for a specific activity during this process is the ratio of measurable change in activity to the average rate of change of that activity. It is represented by $T = \Delta f/(\partial f/\partial t)_{avg}$

Where, Δf defines change in activity over a definite time

$(\partial f/\partial t)_{avg}$ represents average rate of that change

The time constant for tear turnover is: $T = V/Q = 7.0/1.2 = 5.8$ minutes

V defines volume of the tear pool (~7.0 μl)

Q = tear turnover rate (1.2 μl/min).

Substituting the value of T in Eq. 1 we can compare the difference in initial concentration between a 5.8 minute delay (C=36.7%) and 17.5 minute delay(C<5%) [5]. Such low residence time is responsible for low drug concentrations in the cornea. Other constraints such as blinking, irritation, increased lacrimal flow rate may further diminish drug levels to less than 5% of applied dose within a few minutes of instillation [4-6].

CONVENTIONAL DRUG DOSAGE FORMS

Though topical administration is the most preferred route, it suffers from several disadvantages such as nasolacrimal drainage, loss of medication into conjunctival blood circulation, tear dilution, normal tear drainageand reflux blinking (Fig. **1**). Structural barriers such as the cornea and the conjunctiva limit drug absorption in the anterior segment of the eye [7]. Corneal epithelium is approximately 35-50 μm thick and offers a high shunt resistance of 12-16 kohm-cm^2. The resistance offered by the cornea to the intraocular drug absorption is the sum of resistances offered by all three layers; $R_{cornea} = R_{epithelium} + R_{stroma} + R_{endothelium}$. The human cornea consists of three layers: the outer lipophilic epithelium, middle hydrophilic stroma and inner endothelium. Hence, cornea poses a formidable barrier to transcorneal permeation of both hydrophilic and hydrophobic compounds [8]. Moreover, hydrophilic drugs are absorbed through the conjunctival circulation and drained into the systemic circulation *via* the scleral-conjunctival route [9]. Schoenwald *et al.* studied the effect of octanol-water partition coefficients on the permeability of eleven steroids across rabbit cornea. Investigators observed that the optimum permeability is generated at a value of the log octanol-water partition coefficient of 2.9 [10]. This observation clearly indicates that compounds with moderate lipophilicity can readily permeate through the corneal epithelium.

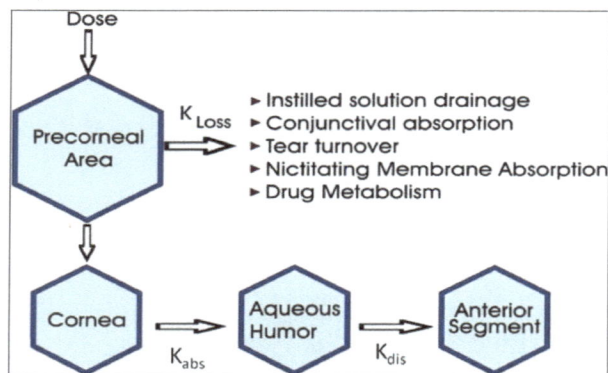

Figure 1: Fate of a topically administered drug.

Various topical dosage forms such as ocular drops, aqueous suspensions, emulsions and ointments have been utilized to enhance ocular drug absorption. Eye drops account for ~90% of ophthalmic products currently available in the market due to its high patient compliance. A single dose of timolol/pilocarpine eye drops has been found effective at controlling intraocular pressure for 12 hr [11]. The effect of levocabastine eye drops on allergic conjunctivitis has been previously investigated in clinical trials. In 94% of patients, symptoms were relieved in 15 min following instillation of levocabastine eye drops [12]. Liou *et al*. have demonstrated intraoperative miosis prevention and postoperative corneal edema reduction following topical administration of 0.1% indomethacin eye drops [13].

Inspite of its high application, the ocular bioavailability of therapeutic agents following topical administration of ocular drops has been a major concern. Ocular drug absorption following topical administration is governed by a number of factors. The retention of the dosage form in the pre-corneal region greatly influences the volume and amount available for drug absorption. The human eye can accommodate about 30 µL of solution [14], however, nearly all marketed ocular dispensers deliver a volume of 30-50 µL to the eye. A study conducted by File *et al*. [15] demonstrated that both 20 and 50 µL drops of 0.5% pilocarpine hydrochloride produce similar miotic response in human volunteers. This investigation clearly suggests that marketed dispensers probably deliver higher drug solution than required for eliciting pharmacological response. Moreover, rapid tear turnover rate has been one of the major reasons for inadequate ocular drug bioavailability following topical administration [16]. Under normal physiological conditions, the tear turnover rate in human is approximately 16% per min. The normal tear volume (7 µL) is quickly restored in about 2-3 min. As a result, nearly 80% of the administered dose is quickly drained within the first 15-30 sec. This process reduces the contact time of the drug with the corneal epithelium thereby decreasing its absorption [16].

In order to avoid these limitations, penetration enhancers (surfactants, bile acids, bile salts, calcium chelators), viscosity enhancers (hydroxypropyl methylcellulose, carboxy methylcellulose (CMC), polyvinyl alcohol)and drug solubilizers (cyclodextrins) are usually incorporated in eye drops to improve ocular drug absorption [1, 3]. Surfactants are amphiphilic in nature and can readily diffuse inside the lipid bilayer of the cell membrane. On reaching saturation, mixed micelles are formed which results in the removal of phospholipids and membrane solubilization. This effect increases the transcellular transport of therapeutic agents. Bile salts enhance drug permeability by altering the rheological properties of membrane lipid. These agents increase absorption by producing a transient change in lipid structure and integrity of the cell membrane. Chelators such as EDTA enhance paracellular drug transport by binding to calcium ions, thereby loosening tight epithelial junctions [17]. Other penetration enhancers such as saponin, digitonin and fatty acids enhance transcellular drug transport by transiently opening the phospholipid bilayer [18, 19].

Several penetration/absorption enhancers such as benzalkonium chloride (BAC), ethylene diamine tetraacetic acid (EDTA), non-ionic surfactants, surface-active heteroglycosides, lysophosphatidyl lipids and bile salts have been have been investigated for their potential in improving ocular drug absorption [18]. Surfactants with a hydrophilic-lipophilic balance in the range of 16-17 have exhibited high efficacy in increasing corneal drug permeability. Tween 20 and Brij 35 at a concentration of 1% increased the corneal permeation of fluorescein by five-fold without generating any toxic effects [20]. Bile salts such as sodium taurodeoxycholate (2 and 10mM) have also significantly enhanced the corneal permeability of 6-carboxyfluorescein, glutathione, FITC-dextran (mol. wt 4000Da) and insulin [21]. Clinically significant concentrations of cyclosporine have been generated in allografted rabbit's cornea following topical instillation in the presence of azone [22]. Azone has also displayed a high potential for increasing the transcorneal permeation of levobunolol by 20 fold [23]. Saponin, EDTA, benzalkonium chloride and paraben significantly increased the corneal absorption of macromolecules such as thyrotropin-releasing hormone and luteinizing hormone-releasing hormone relative to conjunctival absorption [24]. Similarly, benzalkonium chloride, EDTA, taurocholic acid and saponin demonstrated high potential in improving the corneal absorption of FITC-dextrans (molecular weights 4400 and 9400Da) [25]. Eye drops containing 0.02% BAC solution generated seven fold higher corneal inulin levels [26, 27]. However, BAC has been reported to accumulate in the corneal epithelium leading to severe toxicity [28, 29].

Various polymers such as CMC, low molecular weight hydroxypropyl cellulose (HPC), medium molecular weight HPC, methyl cellulose (MC), hydroxyethyl cellulose (HEC), polyvinyl pyrrolidone (PVP), polyvinyl alcohol (PVA)and hyaluronic acid (HA) have demonstrated high efficacy in enhancing corneal drug absorption. Sasaki *et al.* investigated the effect of CMC on the ocular absorption of tilisolol in rabbits. In the presence of CMC, high hevels of Tilisolol was generated in tear fluids and the aqueous humor [30]. Cyclodextrins such as hydroxypropyl-β-cyclodextrin (HP-β-CD) has displayed high efficacy in increasing the ocular absorption of baicalein [31]. In the presence of HP-β-CD, baicalein concentration in the aqueous humor was enhanced 2.1 fold relative to baicalein suspension. In the cornea, the peak concentration of baicalein was achieved within 5 min and was nearly 4.5 times higher relative to baicalein suspension.

In addition to eye drops, ophthalmic ointments have been extensively studied as a drug vehicle owing to their improved drug retention, resistance to nasolacrimal drainage and inhibition of drug dilution by tears [32]. Acyclovir ointment (3%) has achieved a C_{max} of 3.38 and 45.73 μg/mL in the aqueous humor and the cornea at 60 and 30 min, respectively [33]. Miconazole ointment (1%) has demonstrated high efficacy in the treatment of fungal ulcers and associated lesions caused by Candida, Aspergillus and Fusarium organisms in experimental keratomycosis [34]. Despite their high efficacy, inaccurate dose delivery, blurred vision, the requirement for preservativesand manufacturing difficulties are challenges associated with the use of ointments. Several ointments such as Erythromycin (Ilotycin®), gentamicin (Gentak®) and tobramycin (Tobrex®) are available for night time administrations.

The use of mucoadhesive polymers has also been proposed as a viable approach for improving ocular bioavailability of poorly permeable drugs. These polymers increase ocular drug absorption by prolonging drug contact time with corneal epithelium. At physiological pH, mucoadhesive polymers have been demonstrated to interact with mucin, a negatively charged glycoprotein with a high molecular weight. The hypothesis of electrostatic interactions between mucin and cationic mucoadhesives is supported by the evidence of selective and preferential uptake of cationic liposomes by the cornea. On the other hand, mucoadhesion of anionic polymers to the corneal epithelium primarily occurs due to extensive hydrogen bonding [35]. Previously, it has been demonstrated that cationic and anionic polymers exhibit excellent mucoadhesive properties compared to non-cellulose esters or PVA.

Saettone *et al.* [36] evaluated the efficacy of polyanionic natural and semi-synthetic polymers such as polygalacturonic acid, hyaluronic acid, carboxymethylamylose, carboxymethylchitin, chondroitin sulfate, heparin sulfate and mesoglycan in enhancing the ocular absorption of pilocarpine and cyclopentolate. Investigators demonstrated a strong correlation between the *in vivo* and *in vitro* mucoadhesive interactions of these polymers with mucin with hyaluronic acid exhibiting optimal interaction. Several other mucoadhesive polysaccharides such as polygalactouronic acid [36], xyloglucan [37], xanthan gum [38], gellan gum [39], pullulan, guar gumand scleroglucan have also been examined for their suitability in enhancing ocular drug absorption [40]. However, challenges such as difficulties in sterilization by ultra filtration and possible blurred vision discourage the extensive application of mucoadhesive polymers for improving corneal drug absorption.

Recently, CMC and sodium alginate gel containing 1% w/v atenolol displayed high potential in prolonging the IOP reducing effect of atenolol (8 h) relative to atenolol solution [41]. Pilocarpine hydrogels were formulated with poly (ethylene glycol) (PEG)-based copolymers with multiple thiol (SH) groups. These pilocarpine hydrogels markedly sustained pupillary constriction for 24 hrs relative to pilocarpine solution (3 hrs) [42]. Pluronic F-127 based *in situ* gelling systems demonstrated temperature dependent sol-gel phase transition and increased retention time of forskolin in a rabbit model. The IOP reducing effect of forskolin was achieved after 12 h following topical administration of the formulation [43]. Gel formulation containing Pluronic F127 and chitosan significantly enhanced the transcorneal transport and ocular retention time of timolol maleate [44]. Liu *et al.* studied the effect of a formulation containing alginate (gelling agent) and HPMC (viscosity enhancer) on the release and pre-corneal retention of gatifloxacin [45]. Investigators observed that alginate along with HPMC demonstrated high potential in retaining gatifloxacin compared to alginate or HPMC solution respectively. Recently, a novel ophthalmic solution containing a combination of Gelrite and alginate has been proposed as an *in situ* gelling vehicle for increasing the ocular retention of matrine [46].

Drug delivery to ocular tissues from systemic circulation has been proposed as an alternative approach to topical administration. However, following systemic administration, ocular absorption is highly restricted by the blood aqueous barrier (BAB) composed of non-pigmented epithelial layer of ciliary body and endothelial blood vessels of the iris [47, 48]. Hence, designing an efficient drug delivery system might be beneficial in increasing ocular drug bioavailability and reducing systemic side effects and dosing frequency [49]. An ideal drug delivery system for the treatment of anterior segment indications should a) facilitate higher drug absorption b) provide zero order drug release c) be easy to manufacture and d) meet the regulatory demands [50, 51]. Improved delivery can also be ascribed to the development of various drug delivery systems like contact lenses, nanoemulsions, corneal collagen shields, hydrogels and vesicular systems (liposomes and niosomes).

Contact Lenses

Recently, there has been a growing interest in the development of drug loaded contact lenses to provide sustained release. An advantage of this method of administration is that it requires smaller doses and resulting in very low systemic drug exposure. Also, this method is simple and improves compliance [52]. The complexity to design lenses with vision correction as well as therapeutic delivery has been an insuperable obstacle for many years. However, new approaches and technologies have opened a pathway to introduce therapeutic contact lenses into mainstream practice [53].

Currently, researchers are focusing on developing contact lenses with the capacity to absorb and deliver high amounts of drugs in a controlled manner. The work is mainly based on the following concepts:

1. Use of nanometric particles or vesicles to entrap drug and disperse monomers that constitute contact lenses. Therefore, with polymerization, the drug loaded particles remain entrapped in the lens structure. Drug release is regulated by colloidal particles and lenses maintain their optical transparency if the dimensions of colloidal particles are suitable and such particles are in moderate concentrations [54]. However, low stability of colloidal structures during sterilization and premature release of drugs due to storage in lens soaking solution are two major drawbacks of this approach.

2.   The second approach is to functionalize the hydrogel to allow for non-covalent bonds with drug molecules. This technique aims to design structure so as to allow drug molecules to directly interact with the polymer chains. The main drawback is that the neutralization of ionic groups involves large changes in volumes which can be undesirable for lens optical properties.

3.   Molecular imprinting is another important technique. The procedure involves synthesis of contact lenses in the presence of drug molecules which act as a molding causing monomers to arrange themselves according to their affinity. When the process is completed the spatial arrangement becomes permanent due to monomer polymerization. Due to this process, the lens structure develops specific receptors with adequate size which can capture drug molecules with highest affinity [53].

In 2007, Danion *et al.* studied the antibacterial activity of levofloxacin loaded liposomes which were surface immobilized on contact lenses. The entire cargo was released in a period of 6 days [55]. Santos *et al.* in the year 2009 developed acrylic hydrogels containing high proportions of cyclodextrins to maintain the mechanical properties and biocompatibilities of hydrogels as well as to increase drug loading and capacity rates. Poly(hydroxyethylmethacrylate) hydrogels were copolymerized with glycidyl methacrylate (GMA) at different proportions and then grafted onto beta-cyclodextrins to create a network. Loading efficiency of diclofenac was improved by 1300% and its drug affinity increased by 15 fold with these hydrogels. The lenses prepared from these hydrogels are able to prevent drug leakage and conserve fluid of soft contact lenses causing sustained delivery over two weeks [56]. Vasurfilcon A or lotrafilcon A (containing silicone) were used to prepare contact lenses which were incubated in a solution containing 0.4ppm epidermal growth factor (EGF) for 7 hours. Uptake and release of EGF was demonstrated by lenses made of vasurfilcon A but not lotrafilcon A. Schultz *et al.* showed lens material composed of silicone may not be a suitable candidate for delivering EGF to ocular tissues [57]. Most recently, Garhwal *et al.* used pullulan and polycaprolactone (PCL) to synthesize core-shell nanospheres to entrap ciprofloxacin. These nanospheres were then incorporated into HEMA based contact lenses and were tested for bacterial growth inhibition. The results showed that less than 2μg/mL of nanospheres were needed to inhibit bacterial growth [58].

Nanoemulsions/Microemulsions

Nanoemulsions are isotropic colloidal dispersions similar to conventional emulsions. These thermodynamically unstable systems are composed of oil and water. Generally a mixture of surfactants and co-surfactants are added to attain thermodynamic stability. Such dispersions are transparent and the sizes of the dispersed particles range from 50 to 1000 nm [59]. Advantages such as ease in manufacturing, sterilization and dissolution of both hydrophilic and lipophilic drugs make nanoemulsions a viable alternative system for topical drug delivery [60]. Moreover, the presence of penetration enhancers (surfactants) facilitate corneal absorption [61]. Nanoemulsions offer sustained drug release and achieve higher drug levels in aqueous humor which often mimics their absorption enhancement activity. It also helps in reducing the dosing frequency [60]. Drugs like indomethacin and timolol exhibit longer retention times in ocular tissues and improved bioavailability when formulated into nanoemulsions. A three-fold rise is observed in indomethacin concentration in the cornea, aqueous humor and iris-ciliary body at 0.5 and 1 h post-instillation in rabbit eye [62]. Pilocarpine based nanoemulsions/microemulsions reduced the frequency of instillation from four to two times compared to conventional eye drops. A prolonged suppression in intraocular pressure in normotensive rabbits was observed following a single dose application of pilocarpine emulsion 1.7% (equivalent to 2% pilocarpine hydrochloride) which reached a maximal value of 6.0 +/- 0.2 mmHg at 29 hours [63]. Fialho *et al.* [64] developed a stable microemulsion based formulation which generated higher penetration of dexamethasone in the anterior segment and also prolonged drug release relative to conventional preparations. The area under the curve obtained for the microemulsion system was two-fold higher than a conventional preparation ($p < 0.05$) (Fig. **2**). Moreover, low surface tension of nanoemulsions provides more spreading over the cornea which in turn improves the contact between the corneal epithelium and instilled drug molecules and provides higher therapeutic levels in the anterior segment [64].

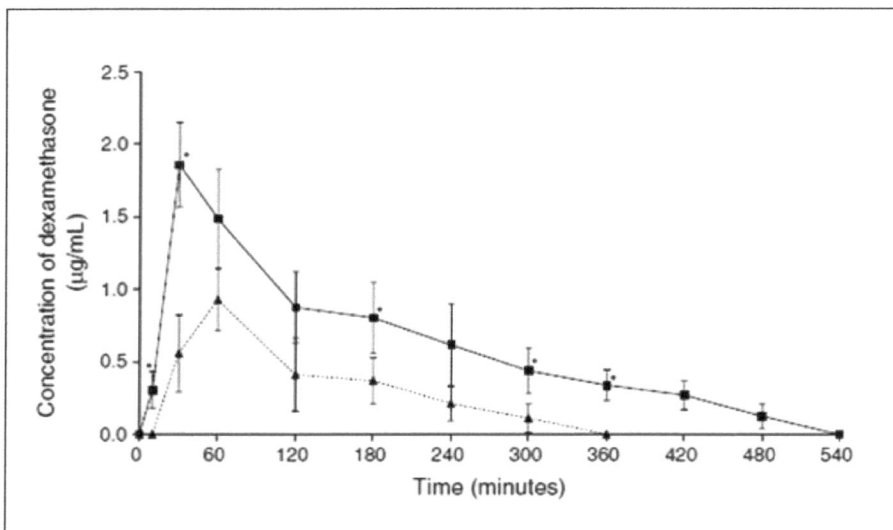

Figure 2: Concentration of dexamethasone in the aqueous humour after administration of the developed microemulsion and the conventional preparation. *Significantly different from the value of conventional formulation using unpaired t-test, $P < 0.05$. (■) microemulsion; (▲) conventional. Reproduced with permission from [64].

Corneal Collagen Shields

Corneal collagen shields were primarily developed as temporary protective corneal bandage lenses to promote wound healing following surgery in traumatic and non-traumatic conditions. In mammals, 25% of the total body protein consists of collagen and it is the major protein of connective tissue, cartilage and bone. A similarity in the secondary and tertiary structures of human, porcine and bovine collagens enable formulators to use collagen from animal origin [65]. Though corneal collagen shields produce some discomfort as well as interfere with vision, a comparable bioavailability from collagen shields and eye drops make it an attractive device for ocular delivery (Fig. **3**) [66]. Several reports describe the application of antibiotics, antifungal, anti-inflammatory, antiviral and immunosuppressive agents in the form of corneal shields for drug delivery to the eye. Corneal shields consists of cross-links between collagen subunits in a process controlled by exposure to ultraviolet light as the degree of cross linking is related to the dissolution time of the collagen shield on the cornea. The effect of collagen cross-linking on bioavailability of ofloxacin which serves as a drug depot has been investigated at dissolution times of 24 and 72 h and found to achieve higher drug concentrations in the aqueous humor and the cornea [67]. Presoaked collagen shields in solutions of gatifloxacin and moxifloxacin achieved higher concentrations of topically delivered drugs into the anterior segment without altering the structure of rabbit cornea. Initial concentrations of antibiotics were 5.43 +/- 0.16 mg/mL and 3.14 +/- 0.22 mg/mL, respectively. After 6 hours, concentrations receded but remained relatively affective after 6 h (1.39 +/- 1.13 μg/mL for gatifloxacin and 0.816 +/- 0.6 μg/mL for moxifloxacin) [68]. Three different collagen shields manufactured from porcine and bovine collagens are currently available with dissolution times of 12, 24 and 72 h. These materials are fabricated as a corneal bandage lens for protecting ocular surfaces during surgical, traumatic and non-traumatic corneal conditions. Thus it is clearly evident that corneal collagen shields can be utilized as a drug delivery device particularly in the promotion of corneal epithelial and stromal healing [66].

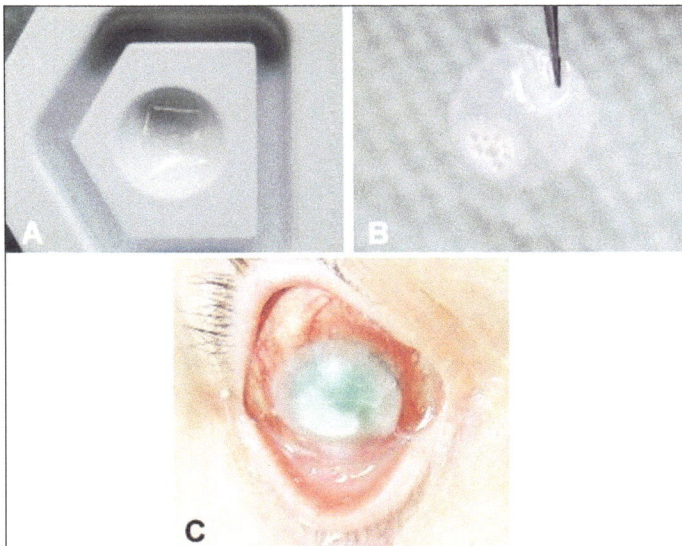

Figure 3: A) Corneal collagen shield in sterile packaging prior to re-hydration. B) Re-hydrated corneal collagen shield (72-hour) following 5-minute soak in prednisolone acetate (1%). C) Corneal collagen shield (72-hour) presoaked in ciprofloxacin (0.3%) in a patient with bacterial keratitis. Reproduced with permission from [66].

Hydrogels

Hydrogels can be defined as polymeric networks that absorb large amounts of water and form a gel like structure as a result of physical or chemical cross-linking of individual polymer chains. Gelation usually occurs at ambient temperatures and the use of organic solvents is very rare. Both natural and synthetic polymers are indicated in the preparation of hydrogels [69]. Hydrogels made from natural polymers offer advantages like biodegradability and biocompatibility. However, such materials do not offer sufficient mechanical strength and may harbor pathogens which may trigger auto-immune response. Synthetic hydrogels do not possess such intrinsic bioactive properties but can be tailored to a desired degradability and functionality. There are two distinct groups of hydrogels, namely preformed and *in situ* forming gels. Preformed hydrogels are simple viscous solutions which do not undergo any alterations in their structure or properties after administration whereas, *in situ* forming gels undergo gelation upon administration due to changes in physicochemical properties depending on the ocular environment [70]. The swelling property of hydrogels in water or aqueous solvents causes higher solution viscosity, inducing a liquid-gel transition to prolong drug contact time with the cornea.

These viscous systems fall under two categories: Newtonian and Non-Newtonian depending on their behavior with change in shear rate. Newtonian systems are independent of the shear rate and thus have a constant viscosity during the blinking of the eye which is the shear stress factor. On the other hand, some Non-Newtonian systems lower the viscosity due to shear stress created by blinking and other ocular movements. Pseudoplasticity is of particular interest in ocular delivery since it aids in blinking by reducing the viscosity and thus permits the application of highly viscous systems like gels and ointments, which would not be possible with Newtonian systems [70].

Pilocarpine has long been used for the treatment of glaucoma. However, it is often associated with low ocular bioavailability. Hence, researchers have successfully prepared rapidly forming hydrogels with poly (ethylene glycol) based copolymers comprising multiple thiol groups to efficiently deliver pilocarpine into the eye. The resulting formulation showed high drug loading capacity (~74%). A biphasic release pattern was observed over duration of 8 days with release half lives of 2 and 94 h. When this formulation was compared to an aqueous solution of pilocarpine in rabbits, the pilocarpine hydrogel formulation exhibited sustained pupillary constriction for 24 h compared to 3 h for the aqueous solution [42].

These results suggest that hydrogels significantly improve ocular bioavailability and the IOP lowering activity of pilocarpine.

Vesicular Systems

Vesicular systems are also known as liquid-retentive delivery systems containing a drug in a vesicle. Several promising agents failed in clinical trials due to limited permeation into cells. A vesicular system can address this issue. It can also provide sustained and prolonged drug release thus eliminating the need for repeated dosing. Vesicular systems are generally prepared with lipids and have the ability to deliver both hydrophilic and lipophilic drugs. Such a system can prevent drug metabolism by the tear fluids or corneal enzymes [71]. Liposomes, niosomes and pharmacosomes are three types of vesicular drug delivery systems studied as ocular colloidal carriers [1, 72].

Liposomes: A liposome can be defined as a microscopic vesicle composed of one or more phospholipid bilayer membranes with a diameter ranging from 0.01 - 10μm (Fig. **4**). Based on the size, liposomes can be classified into small unilamellar vesicles (SUV) (10-100 nm), large unilamellar vesicles (LUV) (100-300 nm) and multilamellar vesicles (MUV) (contains more than one bilayer). Liposomes consist of an aqueous inner core enclosed by a membrane, composed of phospholipids.

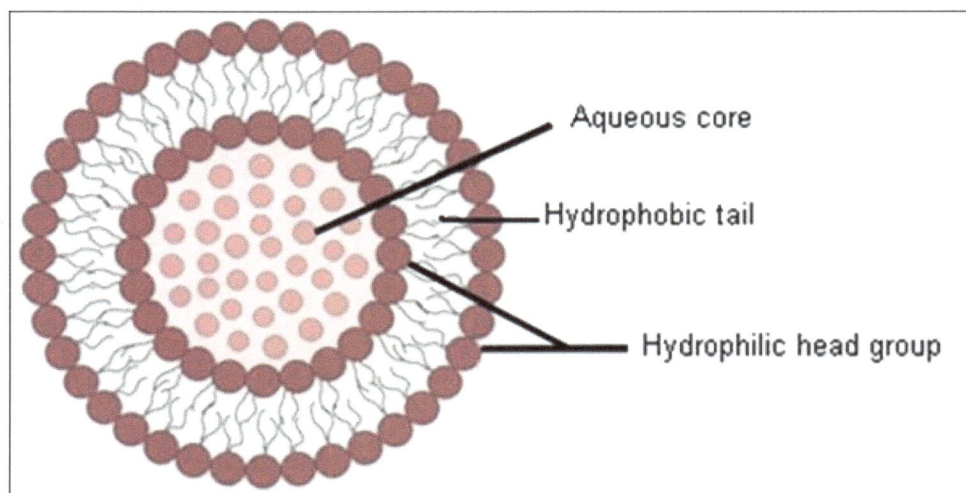

Figure 4: Structure of liposome.

Hydrophilic drugs can be encapsulated in the inner aqueous core while the hydrophobic drugs tend to bind to the lipid bilayer [73]. Liposomes have been successfully utilized in the delivery of a wide range of therapeutics including nucleotides, proteins and plasmids [74]. These vesicles are made of naturally derived phospholipids such as egg phosphatidylethanolamine or dioleoylphosphatidylethanolamine (DOPE) which make them suitable for ophthalmic drug delivery [75]. Liposomes have been successfully utilized for delivery to the anterior segment of the eye. Therapeutic efficiency of liposomes depends on various factors, including size, charge, encapsulation efficiency, retention and stability in the conjunctival sac, other ocular tissues and affinity towards the corneal surface [76]. The surface charge of liposomes plays a key role in determining their affinity towards the cornea. According to Felt *et al.* [77] the negatively charged corneal surface has higher affinity towards positively charged liposomes. This study also suggested that drug elimination due to lacrimal flow is significantly reduced because the cationic liposomes increased the viscosity as well as provided stronger interactions with the negatively charged mucus. Liposomes loaded with pilocarpine hydrochloride were prepared by Monem *et al.* This study concluded that neutral MLVs exhibit a more prolonged effect relative to negatively charged MLVs and free drug [78]. Acyclovir (ACV) liposomes were formulated and evaluated for their *in vitro* permeation and *in vivo* absorption across the cornea in rabbits. Positively charged liposomes formed a coating on the corneal surface. Morphology showed that the vesicles bound tightly to the corneal tissue prolonging residence time and improving ACV absorption [79]. Ocular pharmacokinetics of ganciclovir (GCV) encapsulated in liposomes was studied in albino rats and the results were compared with GCV solution. Transcorneal permeability of GCV liposomes was 3.9 fold higher than GCV solution. AUC of GCV in the aqueous humor was found to be 1.7 fold higher with GCV liposomes. GCV tissue distribution following liposomal delivery suggested 2-10 times higher concentration in the sclera, cornea, iris, lens and vitreous humor relative to drug solution. These results suggest that liposomes may efficiently deliver GCV to the eye [80]. Ciprofloxacin loaded liposomes suspended in hydrogels were formulated using two phospholipids, soya bean phosphatidyl choline and cholesterol. Encapsulation efficiency of the drug was measured to be 82.01± 0.52%. Transcorneal permeation of ciprofloxacin from 0.3% aqueous solution,

0.3% liposomal suspension and 0.3% liposomal hydrogels were studied over 6 h. Cumulative drug permeated across cornea appears to be 201 ± 8.7 µg with aqueous solution thereby providing only 6.7 % absorption; while the cumulative amount permeated from liposomal suspension was 614 ± 14.2 µg and percentage permeation was 20.4 %. However, liposomal hydrogel formulation caused ciprofloxacin permeation to be 918 ± 25.11 µg and the percentage permeation was 30.6 %. From these results it is clear that liposomal suspensions can produce a three-fold increase in permeation compared to aqueous solutions [81]. This observation may be attributed to the electrostatic interactions between positively charged liposomes and the negatively charged corneal membrane. Liposomes are well adsorbed onto the corneal surface and can transfer their membrane associated drug directly into the corneal epithelial cell membranes, thereby enhancing drug transport across the cornea [82]. Similarly, liposomes containing ofloxacin and gatifloxacin were evaluated [83, 84]. In the case of ofloxacin liposomal hydrogel, permeation was increased sevenfold *versus* aqueous solution. Hence liposomal hydrogels can overcome most of the precorneal barriers ensuring steady and prolonged transcorneal permeation [83]. Although liposomes are potential ophthalmic drug delivery systems, their use has not been well accepted due to their potential drawbacks such as difficulties in sterilization, limited drug loading capacity and very short shelf lives. More work still needs to be done for ocular purposes before liposomes can be clinically introduced.

Niosomes: Niosomes are bilayered non-ionic surfactant vesicles. Similar to liposomes, these vesicles have the ability to entrap hydrophilic as well as hydrophobic molecules either in an aqueous layer or in a lipoidal vesicular membrane [73, 85]. Niosomes have several advantages over other drug delivery systems. They are composed of biodegradable and non-immunogenic materials, have a lower cost of production and do not require expensive handling techniques. Niosomes are also known to be more chemically stable than liposomes and they can provide better physical stability and controlled drug delivery at the site of action [86]. Physical properties of these carrier systems can be altered to generate various drug distribution patterns and release profiles. Timolol maleate containing niosomal formulations which were coated with chitosan or carbopol exhibited significant IOP lowering effects in rabbits relative to timolol solution [87]. In

2005, Guinedi *et al.* prepared niosomes using Span 40 or Span 60 and cholesterol and were successful in entrapping the IOP lowering drug, acetazolamide. Results showed that higher entrapment was achieved with Span 60 and cholesterol in a 7:6 molar ratio (Fig. **5**). Acetazolamide niosomes showed a significant decrease in IOP compared to solution of free drug [71]. Niosomes have been reported to be successful ocular vehicle for cyclopentolate by Sattone *et al.* These niosomes were prepared by sonication of equimolar mixture of polysorbate-20 and cholesterol. *In vivo* studies showed niosomes to increase the ocular bioavailability of cyclopentolate when compared to a reference buffer. The researchers concluded that this increased absorption of cyclopentolate may be due to the modified permeability characteristics of conjunctival and scleral tissues [88]. A local antibiotic, gentamicin sulphate, was entrapped in niosomes to provide controlled delivery. Tween 60 and 80 or Brij 35 and cholesterol were used to prepared gentamicin sulphate loaded niosomes. Results showed entrapment efficiencies to be as high as 92% and a release of about 66% in 8 hours [89].

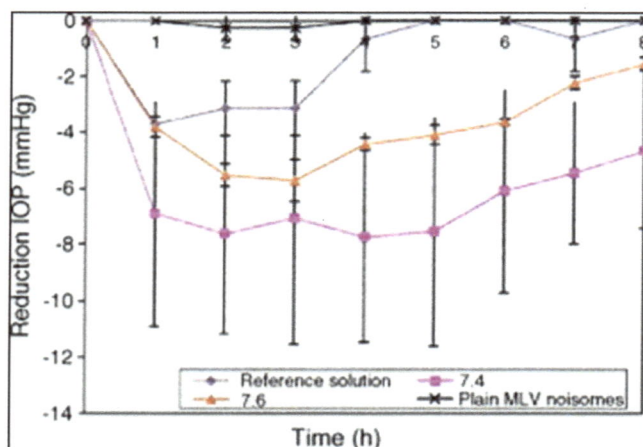

Figure 5: Reduction in IOP after topical administration of acetazolamide multilamellar niosomes composed of Span 60 and cholesterol in 7:4 and 7:6 molar ratios compared to acetazolamide solution 1% and plain MLV niosomes. Reproduced with permission from [71].

OTHER STRATEGIES TO ENHANCE ANTERIOR SEGMENT DELIVERY

In spite of the development of various drug delivery systems for topical delivery, it still remains a potential challenge for drug delivery to the anterior segment. In addition to these strategies, iontophoresis, phonophoresis and punctual plugs have also been investigated for enhancing drug delivery through the cornea. These systems are described below.

Iontophoresis

Iontophoresis is a viable non-invasive strategy designed to facilitate drug entry into the target site. This technique which is based on electrorepulsion and electroosmosis, makes use of a mild electrical current to enhance tissue penetration of ionized drug molecules [90, 91]. Ocular iontophoresis is a fast, safe and painless (non-invasive) approach for delivering impermeable substances. Iontophoresis may be accomplished by two approaches: 1) transcorneal iontophoresis, which aids in generating high drug concentration in the anterior segment and 2) transscleral iontophoresis, which aids in achieving high and sustained drug concentrations in the vitreous and retina [92]. Von Sallmann, a pioneer in the clinical use of ocular iontophoresis demonstrated modest success in achieving relatively high levels of penicillin in the aqueous humor through transcorneal iontophoresis compared to a subconjunctival route of administration [93, 94]. Iontophoretic delivery of antibiotics like gentamicin, tobramycin and ciprofloxacin resulted in appreciable lowering of a pseudomonas colony growth relative to eye drops [95-97]. Transcorneal iontophoresis leads to a 100 fold increase in permeability of gentamicin in cornea and aqueous humor of the rabbit eye compared to control eyes in which topical application was performed under the same conditions [98]. Hence, transcorneal iontophoresis of antibiotics can be considered as an effective way of treating bacterial keratitis and other anterior segment infections. Further studies are needed to establish the safety and efficacy of ocular iontophoresis as it is known to cause corneal and endothelial damage [99]. Though drug delivery by iontophoretic technique can overcome potential side effects associated with ocular implants and intraocular injections, the time course of the drug action is comparatively less than controlled release systems [47].

Phonophoresis

Phonophoresis involves the use of ultrasonic sound for enhancing drug permeability. This technique was first used by Griffin and Touchstone for studying the movement of cortisol in swine skeletal muscles [100]. The researchers observed that the application of ultrasonic sound of 1 watt/cm^2 can effectively transport cortisol through the skeletal muscles. The implication of this technique in drug delivery to the cornea was enunciated by Zderic *et al.* in 2002 [101]. This group studied the effect of the application of 1second bursts of 20 kHz ultrasound, at I (SAPA) of 14 W/cm^2 (I (SATA) of 2 W/cm^2, to improve corneal permeation of anti-glaucoma drugs with varying lipophilicities (atenolol, carteolol, timolol and betaxolol). Following application of ultrasonic sound for 60 min, permeability across the rabbit cornea increased by 6 fold for atenolol, 2.8 fold for carteolol, 1.9 fold for timolol and 4.4 fold for betaxolol. This study also found that exposure of ultrasound to the cornea resulted in epithelial disorganization and produced small structural changes in the stroma. The exact mechanism involved is yet unclear. However, it is considered that minor structural change of the cornea may be involved in enhanced drug permeation. This technique is currently undergoing further investigation.

Punctal Plugs

Punctal plugs are minute and biocompatible devices are inserted into tear ducts to obstruct drainage and overcome short precorneal residence time of an eye drop. These devices reduce tear drainage by occluding the nasolacrimal duct. An extension of occlusion ranges from 7-180 days depending on the material used for the punctal plug [102, 103]. Devices made from silicone, Teflon, hydroxyethyl methacrylate (HEM), polycaprolactone (PCL) or polydioxanone may be utilized for 180 days while those prepared from animal collagen can only last for 7-10 days [104]. Plugs inserted into the upper punctum of the eye extrude spontaneously from the puncta relative to the one inserted in the lower punctum. Recently, Medennium Inc has developed a punctal plug (SmartPlug™) made from a thermosensitive, hydrophobic acrylic polymer which transforms into a soft cohesive gel at body temperature from its solid rod state at room temperature. This novel plug allows better retention and avoids extrusion. Punctal plugs may be valuable delivery systems for delivering drugs indicated for the chronic treatment of diseases such as glaucoma and dry eye [105]. Also, dose reduction and controlled drug delivery can be achieved by the use of punctal plugs thus improving the efficacy and patient compliance. Punctal plugs can be molded from various polymers in many different shapes and sizes. Diffusion from the polymeric core to the tear fluid is a major contributing factor for drug release. Drugs trapped in the solution, suspension, microemulsion, nanoparticle, microparticle or liposome or any other carrier can easily be loaded. Efficacy of an anti-glaucoma drug formulated as eye-drops in conjunction with occlusion by punctual plug has been evaluated in patients with primary open angle glaucoma. Silicone punctal plugs were employed in this study to occlude the inferior punctum of one eye and block the nasolacrimal duct. Even though a significant decrease of 2 mmHg of IOP was observed in the plugged eyes, this study concluded that such an IOP decrease was not clinically significant [106, 107]. Recent data suggests that silicone plugs can provide symptomatic relief in severe dry eye condition [108].

Anti-glaucoma drugs such as latanoprost and bimatoprost were loaded into punctal plugs by QLT Inc. (Vancouver, Canada) and Vistakon Pharmaceuticals, LLC, respectively. Latanoprost punctal plugs with doses of 44 µg, 81 µg and 95 µg were studied in a Phase II study by QLT Inc. Preliminary results with 44 µg punctal plugs showed a mean IOP reduction by 3.5 mmHg at the end of 4 weeks. There is a plan for a similar clinical trial for punctal plug containing olopatadine, an antihistamine and anti-inflammatory drug, indicated for the treatment of allergic conjunctivitis. Phase II results of bimatoprost punctal plug (Vistakon Pharmaceuticals, LLC) have revealed no dose-response for IOP reduction. Side effects including itchiness, irritation, increased lacrimation and ocular discomfort were commonly observed. Though some side effects were observed, it is encouraging to see new drug delivery systems like punctal plugs moving into clinical trials which provide enhanced and sustained topical drug delivery [109].

CONCLUSION

Over the last two decades there has been a significant growth in the development of novel drug delivery systems which would efficiently incorporate drugs and sustain their release following topical ocular administration. Despite many efforts by the scientists, eye drops account for 90% of all ophthalmic formulations. It can be attributed to stringent regulatory demands for new ophthalmic chemical entities/delivery systems. In the near future we may anticipate an amalgamation of existing drug delivery systems and newer strategies for the development of improved therapies for ocular diseases.

ACKNOWLEDGEMENTS

This work has been supported by Missouri Life Sciences Research Fund, NIH grants R01EY010659-14 and R01EY009171-16.

CONFLICT OF INTEREST

The authors declare no conflict of interest.

REFERENCES

[1]   Kaur IP, Kanwar M. Ocular preparations: the formulation approach. Drug Dev Ind Pharm 2002; 28(5): 473-93.
[2]   Bourlais CL, Acar L, Zia H, Sado PA, Needham T, Leverge R. Ophthalmic drug delivery systems--recent advances. Prog Retin Eye Res 1998; 17(1): 33-58.
[3]   Gaudana R, Jwala J, Boddu SH, Mitra AK. Recent perspectives in ocular drug delivery. Pharm Res 2009; 26(5): 1197-216.
[4]   Boddu SH, Gunda S, Earla R, Mitra AK. Ocular microdialysis: a continuous sampling technique to study pharmacokinetics and pharmacodynamics in the eye. Bioanalysis 2010; 2(3): 487-507.
[5]   Joshi A. Microparticulates for ophthalmic drug delivery. J Ocul Pharmacol 1994; 10(1): 29-45.
[6]   Urtti A, Salminen L. Minimizing systemic absorption of topically administered ophthalmic drugs. Surv Ophthalmol 1993; 37(6): 435-56.
[7]   Dey S, Mitra AK. Transporters and receptors in ocular drug delivery: opportunities and challenges. Expert Opin Drug Deliv 2005; 2(2): 201-4.
[8]   Prausnitz MR, Noonan JS. Permeability of cornea, sclera, and conjunctiva: a literature analysis for drug delivery to the eye. J Pharm Sci 1998; 87(12): 1479-88.
[9]   Romanelli L, Valeri P, Morrone LA, Pimpinella G, Graziani G, Tita B. Ocular absorption and distribution of bendazac after topical administration to rabbits with different vehicles. Life Sci 1994; 54(13): 877-85.
[10]   Schoenwald RD, Ward RL. Relationship between steroid permeability across excised rabbit cornea and octanol-water partition coefficients. J Pharm Sci 1978; 67(6): 786-8.
[11]   Lofors KT, Hovding G, Viksmoen L, Aasved H, Bergaust B, Bulie T. Twelve-hour IOP control obtained by a single dose of timolol/pilocarpine combination eye drops. Acta Ophthalmol (Copenh) 1990; 68(3): 323-6.
[12]   Janssens MM, Vanden Bussche G. Levocabastine: an effective topical treatment of allergic rhinoconjunctivitis. Clin Exp Allergy 1991; 21 (Suppl 2): 29-36.
[13]   Liou SW, Yen RJ. The effect of 0.1% Indomethacin eyedrops on cataract surgery. J Ocul Pharmacol 1991; 7(1): 77-81.

[14]   Mishima S, Gasset A, Klyce SD, Jr., Baum JL. Determination of tear volume and tear flow. Invest Ophthalmol 1966; 5(3): 264-76.

[15]   File RR, Patton TF. Topically applied pilocarpine. Human pupillary response as a function of drop size. Arch Ophthalmol 1980; 98(1): 112-5.

[16]   Ahmed I, Patton TF. Importance of the noncorneal absorption route in topical ophthalmic drug delivery. Invest Ophthalmol Vis Sci 1985; 26(4): 584-7.

[17]   Grass GM, Wood RW, Robinson JR. Effects of calcium chelating agents on corneal permeability. Invest Ophthalmol Vis Sci 1985; 26(1): 110-3.

[18]   Kaur IP, Smitha R. Penetration enhancers and ocular bioadhesives: two new avenues for ophthalmic drug delivery. Drug Dev Ind Pharm 2002; 28(4): 353-69.

[19]   Pillion DJ, Amsden JA, Kensil CR, Recchia J. Structure-function relationship among Quillaja saponins serving as excipients for nasal and ocular delivery of insulin. J Pharm Sci 1996; 85(5): 518-24.

[20]   Marsh RJ, Maurice DM. The influence of non-ionic detergents and other surfactants on human corneal permeability. Exp Eye Res 1971; 11(1): 43-8.

[21]   Morimoto K, Nakai T, Morisaka K. Evaluation of permeability enhancement of hydrophilic compounds and macromolecular compounds by bile salts through rabbit corneas *in vitro*. J Pharm Pharmacol 1987; 39(2): 124-6.

[22]   Newton C, Gebhardt BM, Kaufman HE. Topically applied cyclosporine in azone prolongs corneal allograft survival. Invest Ophthalmol Vis Sci 1988; 29(2): 208-15.

[23]   Tang-Liu DD, Burke PJ. The effect of azone on ocular levobunolol absorption: calculating the area under the curve and its standard error using tissue sampling compartments. Pharm Res 1988; 5(4): 238-41.

[24]   Sasaki H, Yamamura K, Mukai T, *et al.* Modification of ocular permeability of peptide drugs by absorption promoters. Biol Pharm Bull 2000; 23(12): 1524-7.

[25]   Sasaki H, Yamamura K, Tei C, Nishida K, Nakamura J. Ocular permeability of FITC-dextran with absorption promoter for ocular delivery of peptide drug. J Drug Target 1995; 3(2): 129-35.

[26]   Green K, Tonjum A. Influence of various agents on corneal permeability. Am J Ophthalmol 1971; 72(5): 897-905.

[27]   Keller N, Moore D, Carper D, Longwell A. Increased corneal permeability induced by the dual effects of transient tear film acidification and exposure to benzalkonium chloride. Exp Eye Res 1980; 30(2): 203-10.

[28]   Gasset AR, Ishii Y, Kaufman HE, Miller T. Cytotoxicity of ophthalmic preservatives. Am J Ophthalmol 1974; 78(1): 98-105.

[29]   Pfister RR, Burstein N. The effects of ophthalmic drugs, vehicles, and preservatives on corneal epithelium: a scanning electron microscope study. Invest Ophthalmol 1976; 15(4): 246-59.

[30]   Sasaki H, Yamamura K, Mukai T, *et al.* Pharmacokinetic prediction of the ocular absorption of an instilled drug with ophthalmic viscous vehicle. Biol Pharm Bull 2000; 23(11): 1352-6.

[31]   Zhang L, Zhang J, Wang L, Xia H. Ocular pharmacokinetics and availability of topically applied baicalein in rabbits. Curr Eye Res 2009; 34(4): 257-63.

[32]   Shell JW. Pharmacokinetics of topically applied ophthalmic drugs. Surv Ophthalmol 1982; 26(4): 207-18.

[33]   Kitagawa K, Fukuda M, Sasaki K. Intraocular penetration of topically administered acyclovir. Lens Eye Toxic Res 1989; 6(1-2): 365-73.

[34]   Gupta SK. Efficacy of miconazole in experimental keratomycosis. Aust N Z J Ophthalmol 1986; 14(4): 373-6.

[35]   Ludwig A. The use of mucoadhesive polymers in ocular drug delivery. Adv Drug Deliv Rev 2005; 57(11): 1595-639.

[36]   Saettone MF, Monti D, Torracca MT, Chetoni P. Mucoadhesive ophthalmic vehicles: evaluation of polymeric low-viscosity formulations. J Ocul Pharmacol 1994; 10(1): 83-92.

[37]   Burgalassi S, Chetoni P, Panichi L, Boldrini E, Saettone MF. Xyloglucan as a novel vehicle for timolol: pharmacokinetics and pressure lowering activity in rabbits. J Ocul Pharmacol Ther 2000; 16(6): 497-509.

[38]   Ceulemans J, Vinckier I, Ludwig A. The use of xanthan gum in an ophthalmic liquid dosage form: rheological characterization of the interaction with mucin. J Pharm Sci 2002; 91(4): 1117-27.

[39]   Sultana Y, Aqil M, Ali A. Ion-activated, Gelrite-based *in situ* ophthalmic gels of pefloxacin mesylate: comparison with conventional eye drops. Drug Deliv 2006; 13(3): 215-9.

[40]   Esposito P, Colombo I, Lovrecich M. Investigation of surface properties of some polymers by a thermodynamic and mechanical approach: possibility of predicting mucoadhesion and biocompatibility. Biomaterials 1994; 15(3): 177-82.

[41]   Hassan MA. A long acting ophthalmic gel formulations of atenolol. Drug Dev Ind Pharm 2007; 33(11): 1192-8.

[42]   Anumolu SS, Singh Y, Gao D, Stein S, Sinko PJ. Design and evaluation of novel fast forming pilocarpine-loaded ocular hydrogels for sustained pharmacological response. J Control Release 2009; 137(2): 152-9.

[43]   Gupta S, Samanta MK. Design and evaluation of thermoreversible in situ gelling system of forskolin for the treatment of glaucoma. Pharm Dev Technol 2010; 15(4): 386-93.

[44]   Gupta H, Jain S, Mathur R, Mishra P, Mishra AK, Velpandian T. Sustained ocular drug delivery from a temperature and pH triggered novel in situ gel system. Drug Deliv 2007; 14(8): 507-15.

[45]   Liu Z, Li J, Nie S, Liu H, Ding P, Pan W. Study of an alginate/HPMC-based in situ gelling ophthalmic delivery system for gatifloxacin. Int J Pharm 2006; 315(1-2): 12-7.

[46]   Liu Y, Liu J, Zhang X, Zhang R, Huang Y, Wu C. In situ gelling gelrite/alginate formulations as vehicles for ophthalmic drug delivery. AAPS PharmSciTech 2010; 11(2): 610-20.

[47]   Del Amo EM, Urtti A. Current and future ophthalmic drug delivery systems. A shift to the posterior segment. Drug Discov Today 2008; 13(3-4): 135-43.

[48]   Ghate D, Edelhauser HF. Ocular drug delivery. Expert Opin Drug Deliv 2006; 3(2): 275-87.

[49]   Behar-Cohen F. Drug delivery systems to target the anterior segment of the eye: fundamental bases and clinical applications. J Fr Ophtalmol 2002; 25(5): 537-44.

[50]   Boddu SH, Jwala J, Vaishya R, *et al.* Novel nanoparticulate gel formulations of steroids for the treatment of macular edema. J Ocul Pharmacol Ther; 26(1): 37-48.

[51]   Lee VH, Robinson JR. Topical ocular drug delivery: recent developments and future challenges. J Ocul Pharmacol 1986; 2(1): 67-108.

[52]   Alvarez-Lorenzo C, Hiratani H, Concheiro A. Contact Lenses for Drug Delivery: Achieving Sustained Release with Novel Systems. American Journal of Drug Delivery 2006; 4(3): 131-51.

[53] Alvarez-Lorenzo C, Concheiro-Nine A. Drug-loaded soft contact lenses. Arch Soc Esp Oftalmol 2008; 83(2): 73-4.

[54] Gulsen D, Chauhan A. Ophthalmic Drug Delivery through Contact Lenses. Invest Ophthalmol Vis Sci 2004; 45(7): 2342-7.

[55] Danion A, Arsenault I, Vermette P. Antibacterial activity of contact lenses bearing surface-immobilized layers of intact liposomes loaded with levofloxacin. J Pharm Sci 2007; 96(9): 2350-63.

[56] dos Santos JF, Alvarez-Lorenzo C, Silva M, *et al.* Soft contact lenses functionalized with pendant cyclodextrins for controlled drug delivery. Biomaterials 2009; 30(7): 1348-55.

[57] Schultz CL, Morck DW. Contact lenses as a drug delivery device for epidermal growth factor in the treatment of ocular wounds. Clin Exp Optom 2010; 93(2): 61-5.

[58] Garhwal R, Shady SF, Ellis EJ, *et al.* Sustained ocular delivery of ciprofloxacin using nanospheres and conventional contact lens materials. Invest Ophthalmol Vis Sci 2012; 53(3): 1341-52.

[59] Sarker DK. Engineering of nanoemulsions for drug delivery. Curr Drug Deliv 2005; 2(4): 297-310.

[60] Vandamme TF. Microemulsions as ocular drug delivery systems: recent developments and future challenges. Prog Retin Eye Res 2002; 21(1): 15-34.

[61] Lawrence MJ, Rees GD. Microemulsion-based media as novel drug delivery systems. Adv Drug Deliv Rev 2000; 45(1): 89-121.

[62] Calvo P, Alonso MJ, Vila-Jato JL, Robinson JR. Improved ocular bioavailability of indomethacin by novel ocular drug carriers. J Pharm Pharmacol 1996; 48(11): 1147-52.

[63] Naveh N, Muchtar S, Benita S. Pilocarpine incorporated into a submicron emulsion vehicle causes an unexpectedly prolonged ocular hypotensive effect in rabbits. J Ocul Pharmacol 1994; 10(3): 509-20.

[64] Fialho SL, da Silva-Cunha A. New vehicle based on a microemulsion for topical ocular administration of dexamethasone. Clin Experiment Ophthalmol 2004; 32(6): 626-32.

[65] Chvapil M, Kronenthal L, Van Winkle W, Jr. Medical and surgical applications of collagen. Int Rev Connect Tissue Res 1973; 6: 1-61.

[66] Willoughby CE, Batterbury M, Kaye SB. Collagen corneal shields. Surv Ophthalmol 2002; 47(2): 174-82.

[67] Kuwano M, Horibe Y, Kawashima Y. Effect of collagen cross-linking in collagen corneal shields on ocular drug delivery. J Ocul Pharmacol Ther 1997; 13(1): 31-40.

[68] Kleinmann G, Larson S, Neuhann IM, *et al.* Intraocular concentrations of gatifloxacin and moxifloxacin in the anterior chamber *via* diffusion through the cornea using collagen shields. Cornea 2006; 25(2): 209-13.

[69] Lin CC, Metters AT. Hydrogels in controlled release formulations: network design and mathematical modeling. Adv Drug Deliv Rev 2006; 58(12-13): 1379-408.

[70] Nanjawade BK, Manvi FV, Manjappa AS. *In situ* forming hydrogels for sustained ophthalmic drug delivery. J Control Release 2007; 122(2): 119-34.

[71] Guinedi AS, Mortada ND, Mansour S, Hathout RM. Preparation and evaluation of reverse-phase evaporation and multilamellar niosomes as ophthalmic carriers of acetazolamide. Int J Pharm 2005; 306(1-2): 71-82.

[72] Mahmoud SS, Gehman JD, Azzopardi K, Robins-Browne RM, Separovic F. Liposomal phospholipid preparations of chloramphenicol for ophthalmic applications. J Pharm Sci 2008; 97(7): 2691-701.

[73]   Kaur IP, Garg A, Singla AK, Aggarwal D. Vesicular systems in ocular drug delivery: an overview. Int J Pharm 2004; 269(1): 1-14.

[74]   Kurz D, Ciulla TA. Novel approaches for retinal drug delivery. Ophthalmol Clin North Am 2002; 15(3): 405-10.

[75]   Dharma SK, Fishman PH, Peyman GA. A preliminary study of corneal penetration of 125I-labelled idoxuridine liposome. Acta Ophthalmol (Copenh) 1986; 64(3): 298-301.

[76]   Elorza B, Elorza MA, Sainz MC, Chantres JR. Comparison of particle size and encapsulation parameters of three liposomal preparations. J Microencapsul 1993; 10(2): 237-48.

[77]   Felt O, Furrer P, Mayer JM, Plazonnet B, Buri P, Gurny R. Topical use of chitosan in ophthalmology: tolerance assessment and evaluation of precorneal retention. Int J Pharm 1999; 180(2): 185-93.

[78]   Monem AS, Ali FM, Ismail MW. Prolonged effect of liposomes encapsulating pilocarpine HCl in normal and glaucomatous rabbits. Int J Pharm 2000; 198(1): 29-38.

[79]   Law SL, Huang KJ, Chiang CH. Acyclovir-containing liposomes for potential ocular delivery. Corneal penetration and absorption. J Control Release 2000; 63(1-2): 135-40.

[80]   Shen Y, Tu J. Preparation and ocular pharmacokinetics of ganciclovir liposomes. AAPS J 2007; 9(3): E371-7.

[81]   Hosny KM. Ciprofloxacin as ocular liposomal hydrogel. AAPS PharmSciTech 2010; 11(1): 241-6.

[82]   Lee VH, Urrea PT, Smith RE, Schanzlin DJ. Ocular drug bioavailability from topically applied liposomes. Surv Ophthalmol 1985; 29(5): 335-48.

[83]   Hosny KM. Preparation and evaluation of thermosensitive liposomal hydrogel for enhanced transcorneal permeation of ofloxacin. AAPS PharmSciTech 2009; 10(4): 1336-42.

[84]   Hosny KM. Optimization of gatifloxacin liposomal hydrogel for enhanced transcorneal permeation. J Liposome Res 2009.

[85]   Wadhwa S, Paliwal R, Paliwal SR, Vyas SP. Nanocarriers in ocular drug delivery: an update review. Curr Pharm Des 2009; 15(23): 2724-50.

[86]   Abdelkader H, Ismail S, Kamal A, Alany RG. Design and evaluation of controlled-release niosomes and discomes for naltrexone hydrochloride ocular delivery. J Pharm Sci 2011; 100(5): 1833-46.

[87]   Aggarwal D, Kaur IP. Improved pharmacodynamics of timolol maleate from a mucoadhesive niosomal ophthalmic drug delivery system. Int J Pharm 2005; 290(1-2): 155-9.

[88]   Saettone MFGP, M. Carafa, E. Santucci, and F. Alhaique. Non-ionic surfactant vesicles as ophthalmic carriers for cyclopentolate a preliminary evaluation. STP Pharm. Sci. 1996; 6: 94–8.

[89]   Abdelbary G, El-Gendy N. Niosome-encapsulated gentamicin for ophthalmic controlled delivery. AAPS PharmSciTech 2008; 9(3): 740-7.

[90]   Guy RH, Kalia YN, Delgado-Charro MB, Merino V, Lopez A, Marro D. Iontophoresis: electrorepulsion and electroosmosis. J Control Release 2000; 64(1-3): 129-32.

[91]   Singh P, Maibach HI. Iontophoresis in drug delivery: basic principles and applications. Crit Rev Ther Drug Carrier Syst 1994; 11(2-3): 161-213.

[92]   Grossman RE, Chu DF, Lee DA. Regional ocular gentamicin levels after transcorneal and transscleral iontophoresis. Invest Ophthalmol Vis Sci 1990; 31(5): 909-16.

[93]   Dunnington JH, Von Sallmann L. Observations on Penicillin Therapy in Ophthalmology. Trans Am Ophthalmol Soc 1944; 42: 132-54.

[94]   Wright RE, Stuart-Harris CH. Penetration of Penicillin into the Eye. Br J Ophthalmol 1945; 29(8): 428-36.

[95]   Frucht-Pery J, Raiskup F, Mechoulam H, Shapiro M, Eljarrat-Binstock E, Domb A. Iontophoretic treatment of experimental pseudomonas keratitis in rabbit eyes using gentamicin-loaded hydrogels. Cornea 2006; 25(10): 1182-6.

[96]   Hobden JA, O'Callaghan RJ, Hill JM, Reidy JJ, Rootman DS, Thompson HW. Tobramycin iontophoresis into corneas infected with drug-resistant Pseudomonas aeruginosa. Curr Eye Res 1989; 8(11): 1163-9.

[97]   Hobden JA, Reidy JJ, O'Callaghan RJ, Insler MS, Hill JM. Ciprofloxacin iontophoresis for aminoglycoside-resistant pseudomonal keratitis. Invest Ophthalmol Vis Sci 1990; 31(10): 1940-4.

[98]   Hughes L, Maurice DM. A fresh look at iontophoresis. Arch Ophthalmol 1984; 102(12): 1825-9.

[99]   Rootman DS, Jantzen JA, Gonzalez JR, Fischer MJ, Beuerman R, Hill JM. Pharmacokinetics and safety of transcorneal iontophoresis of tobramycin in the rabbit. Invest Ophthalmol Vis Sci 1988; 29(9): 1397-401.

[100]   Griffin JE, Touchstone JC, Liu AC. Ultrasonic Movement of Cortisol into Pig Tissue. Ii. Movement into Paravertebral Nerve. Am J Phys Med 1965; 44: 20-5.

[101]   Zderic V, Vaezy S, Martin RW, Clark JI. Ocular drug delivery using 20-kHz ultrasound. Ultrasound Med Biol 2002; 28(6): 823-9.

[102]   Calonge M. The treatment of dry eye. Surv Ophthalmol 2001; 45 (Suppl 2): S227-39.

[103]   Balaram M, Schaumberg DA, Dana MR. Efficacy and tolerability outcomes after punctal occlusion with silicone plugs in dry eye syndrome. Am J Ophthalmol 2001; 131(1): 30-6.

[104]   Kompella UB, Kadam RS, Lee VH. Recent advances in ophthalmic drug delivery. Ther Deliv 2010; 1(3): 435-56.

[105]   Latkany R. Dry eyes: etiology and management. Curr Opin Ophthalmol 2008; 19(4): 287-91.

[106]   Bartlett JD, Boan K, Corliss D, Gaddie IB. Efficacy of silicone punctal plugs as adjuncts to topical pharmacotherapy of glaucoma--a pilot study. Punctal Plugs in Glaucoma Study Group. J Am Optom Assoc 1996; 67(11): 664-8.

[107]   Ariturk N, Oge I, Erkan D, Sullu Y, Sahin M. The effects of nasolacrimal canal blockage on topical medications for glaucoma. Acta Ophthalmol Scand 1996; 74(4): 411-3.

[108]   Ervin AM, Wojciechowski R, Schein O. Punctal occlusion for dry eye syndrome. Cochrane Database Syst Rev 2010; (9): CD006775.

[109]   Kuno N, Fujii S. Recent Advances in Ocular Drug Delivery Systems. Polymers 2011; 3(1): 193-221.

Send Orders of Reprints at reprints@benthamscience.net

CHAPTER 4

Barriers for Posterior Segment Ocular Drug Delivery

Ripal J. Gaudana[‡], Megha Barot[‡], Ashaben Patel[‡], Varun Khurana and Ashim K. Mitra[*]

Division of Pharmaceutical Sciences, School of Pharmacy, University of Missouri-Kansas City, Kansas City, Missouri-64108, USA

Abstract: Drug delivery for the treatment of posterior segment diseases has become a major challenge in the field of ophthalmology due to its restrictive barrier functionalities. Blood-ocular barriers act as a physical barrier between the local blood vessels, ocular tissues and fluids which restrict the passage of various solutes and fluids. Ocular barriers may be classified as static and dynamic barriers. Static barrier include sclera, Bruch's membrane-choroid (BC), retinal pigment epithelium (RPE) and conjunctiva while dynamic barriers include drug clearance mechanism through blood and lymphatic vessels. Apart from above mentioned barriers, it is also imperative to understand the role of enzymes and transporters in drug disposition. Overall, it is essential to understand anatomy, physiology and disposition mechanisms of eye and interaction between drug molecules/formulation with various ocular tissues in order to design a successful drug delivery system.

Keywords: Eye, static barrier, dynamic barrier, sclera, Bruch's membrane-choroid, Conjunctiva, Blood retinal barrier, transporters, metabolism, ocular drug delivery.

INTRODUCTION

Drug delivery, particularly to the posterior ocular segment remains an extremely challenging task due to its restrictive barrier functionalities. Blood-ocular barriers act as a physical barrier between the local blood vessels, ocular tissues and fluids. These barriers also control the passage of various solutes and fluids. Moreover they also effectively impede the transport of various ocular therapeutic agents [1]. Research on the posterior segment diseases, such as age-related macular

---
*Address correspondence to Ashim K. Mitra: University of Missouri Curators' Professor of Pharmacy, Chairman, Division of Pharmaceutical Sciences, Vice-Provost for Interdisciplinary Research, University of Missouri - Kansas City, School of Pharmacy, 2464 Charlotte Street, Kansas City, MO 64108, USA; Tel: 816-235-1615; Fax: 816-235-5779; E-mail: mitraa@umkc.edu
[†]First 3 authors have contributed equally for the preparation of eBook chapter.

degeneration (AMD), diabetic macular edema (DME), retinitis pigmentosa, endophthalmitis and proliferative vitreoretinopathy is of high clinical significance.

Drug delivery to the retina remains a challenging task due to various limitations and inefficiency associated with topical and systemic administrations. Various forms of local formulation strategies for intravitreal and transscleral drug delivery to the retina have recently emerged [2, 3]. While intravitreal delivery is the primary mode of therapy to the retina, it also carries various risks that include cataract, endophthalmitis, retinal puncture and detachment [3-7]. Transscleral delivery is an alternative form of local therapy to the retina which includes, sub-conjunctival, sub-tenon's, retrobulbar, peribulbar and intrascleral administrations. Transscleral offers localized drug delivery with a less invasive procedure compared to intravitreal administration [2].

Posterior segment drug delivery requires actives to permeate through various ocular tissue layers (sclera, Bruch's membrane-choroid and retinal pigment epithelium) before reaching the neural retina. As a result, a very steep drug concentration gradient is established and very low drug amounts are detected in the retina. This steep gradient is due to barriers that hinder molecules from successfully reaching the retina. Two types of barriers hinder posterior drug delivery *i.e.*, static and dynamic.

Static barriers comprise of those ocular tissues that pose a physical barrier to drug diffusion such as sclera, Bruch's membrane-choroid (BC), retinal pigment epithelium (RPE) and conjunctiva. Dynamic barriers include drug clearance mechanism through blood and lymphatic vessels, by bulk fluid flow due to intraocular drainage as well as active transport mechanism of RPE transporter proteins [2].

STATIC BARRIERS

Sclera

The sclera is elastic and microporous tissue and consists of proteoglycans and closely packed collagen fibers [2, 8]. Collagen fibrils embedded in a glycosaminoglycan (GAG) matrix are the major component of the sclera, with type I being the major collagen type [9, 10]. The structure of the sclera, pore diameter and intracellular space may help to determine the behavior of drug movement [2]. Due to the regional difference in collagen architecture, posterior sclera is almost twice as thick as the anterior sclera [11] and has only 60% of the stiffness of the anterior sclera [12]. Posterior sclera is composed of loose weave of collagen fibers having a greater degree of extensibility in comparison to the more uniform weave orientation of anterior sclera which explains its higher permeability for solutes [13]. Lateral orientation of the scleral fibers may also affect drug transport, as diffusion within the sclera in the lateral direction appears to be a slower process that produces localized drug distribution on a millimeter scale over hours to days [14]. Moreover due to hypocellular nature of the sclera, it has very low level of proteolytic enzymes or protein-binding sites that can degrade or sequester drugs. Slower hydrolysis of various prostaglandin ester prodrugs further indicate low protease activity in sclera compared to the cornea [10, 15].

Ex vivo permeability of sclera has been extensively reported in the literature suggesting relatively high scleral permeability compare to the cornea (Table **1**) [15-19]. This fact has resulted in delivery of several drug molecules *via* transscleral route especially for posterior segment ocular diseases. Several factors influence scleral permeability of molecules. It has a strong dependence on molecular weight (Table **2**), with smaller molecules exhibiting higher permeabilities then larger molecules [19-22]. However, Ambati *et al.* have demonstrated scleral permeability for higher molecular weight dextrans, IgG and bovine serum albumin [21, 23]. This anomaly may be explained by an orientation effect of asymmetrical particles in a matrix. Degree of asymmetry of molecules rise with ascending molecular weight [20]. Thus facilitated diffusion in the matrix will be more pronounced like an extended polymer such as dextrans [13, 23]. However, molecular radius was found to be much better predictor of scleral permeability than molecular weight. Globular protein albumin (3.62 nm) has higher scleral permeability than the linear dextran (4.5 nm) of the same molecular weight across rabbit sclera [10, 21]. Results from log-linear regression analysis shows that molecular radius is a better predictor of scleral permeability (r^2=0.87, P=0.001) than molecular weight (r^2=0.31, P=0.16). Experimental data (Table **2**) demonstrated that scleral permeability decreases roughly exponentially with molecular radius [21, 24].

Table 1: Comparison of scleral *versus* corneal drug permeability

Drug	Permeability Coefficient (10^{-6}cm/sec)		Scleral permeability (fold increase)	Species	Reference
	Cornea	Sclera			
Prostaglandins	1.65 (±0.48)	15.6 (±2.5)	upto 15 times	Human	[15]
Insulin and selected beta-blockers	1.87 (±0.21)	8.45 (±2.28)	upto 5 times	Rabbit	[19]
Hydrocortisone	4.5 (±0.7)	21.8 (±4.3)	5 times	Rabbit	[18]
Polyethylene glycol	1.03	8.80	9 times	Rabbit	[17]
Sulfonamide-based carbonic anhydrase inhibitors			upto 10 times	Human and rabbit	[16]

Table 2: Effect of solute's molecular weight and molecular radii on scleral permeability

Compound	Molecular Weight (D)	Radius (nm)	Permeability Coefficient (10^{-6}cm/sec)	Species	Reference
Sucrose	342	0.48	21.6 ± 6.0	Human	[22]
			42.2 ± 13.7	Rabbit	[19]
			39.7 ± 13.2	Rabbit	[20]
Dextran-10	10000	0.23	6.4 ± 1.7	Human	[22]
			4.5 ± 2.2	Rabbit	[20]
Dextran-40	40000	0.73	4.9 ± 2.4	Human	[22]
			2.8 ± 1.6	Rabbit	[21]
			2.2 ± 0.6	Rabbit	[20]
Dextran-70	70000	0.81	1.9 ± 0.4	Human	[22]
			1.4 ± 0.8	Rabbit	[21]
			2.6 ± 1.3	Rabbit	[20]
Sodium fluorescein	376	0.50	84.5 ± 16.1	Rabbit	[21]
FITC-D, 4	4400	1.30	25.2 ± 5.1	Rabbit	[21]
FITC-D, 20	19600	3.20	6.79 ± 4.18	Rabbit	[21]
FITC-D, 40	38900	4.50	2.79 ± 1.58	Rabbit	[21]
FITC-BSA	67000	3.62	5.49 ± 2.12	Rabbit	[21]
Rhodamine D,70	70000	6.40	1.35 ± 0.77	Rabbit	[21]
FITC-D, 70	71200	6.40	1.39 ± 0.88	Rabbit	[21]
FITC-IgG	150000	5.23	4.61 ± 2.17	Rabbit	[21]
FITC-D,150	150000	8.25	1.34 ± 0.88	Rabbit	[21]

Boubriak *et al.* have reported that a diffusion coefficient increases in the sclera as hydration increases [20]. Large surface area (16-17 cm^2) of the sclera and a high degree of hydration renders it conducive to water-soluble substances [9]. Increase in solute's lipid solubility is reported to lower the scleral permeability across rabbit and human sclera [25, 26]. Other authors also reported higher scleral permeability for hydrophilic molecules [27, 28]. Anionic molecules possess higher permeability then cationic molecules in bovine, porcine and rabbit sclera (Table **3**) [29-31].

Scleral permeability is also altered by physical changes such as surgical thinning, cryotherapy, transscleral diode laser and variations in transscleral pressure [22]. Surgical thinning of the sclera predictably increases permeability whereas cryotherapy and diode laser treatment may not alter the permeability or ultrastructure of sclera [22]. Effect of simulated transscleral pressure on scleral permeability has been demonstrated across human and rabbit sclera which suggest decreasing in scleral permeability at higher intraocular pressure despite the tendency for a lowering in scleral thickness with higher pressure [8, 32, 33].

Bruch's Membrane-Choroid (BC)

Choroid is a vascular tunic part of the eye that supplies blood to the outer two-thirds of the retina. Similar to sclera, the choroid is also made up of collagen and can be considered as a matrix. Higher melanin content of choroid differentiates it from sclera [29, 34]. In terms of solute permeability, choroid–Bruch's layer generally offers greater resistance than does the sclera due to the presence of melanin and lipodial plasma membranes of endothelial cells. Due to rapid blood flow, choroid–Bruch's layer could be even more formidable barrier *in vivo*, which can potentially remove solutes before reaching the neural retina [29, 35].

Bruch's membrane and choroid permabilities have always been studied in tandem due to the difficulty of separating the two tissue layers [2, 29]. Choroid-Bruch's layer permeability has been studied across the bovine and porcine tissue which has shown dependency on solute's lipophilicity and molecular radii [29, 36, 37]. A trend line of decreasing choroid–Bruch's layer permeability with increasing solute lipophilicity or molecular radii appear to be steeper than sclera. Overall results suggest that mechanistically transport across the choroid-Bruch's layer occurs in a fashion similar to transport across the sclera, differing only in magnitude, with the former being a more significant barrier for lipophilic solutes [2, 29, 37]. In addition to lipophilicity and molecular radii, molecular charge is another factor that should be taken into consideration. It has been shown that similar to sclera, choroid–Bruch's layer is also more permeable to negatively charged solutes over positively charged solutes (Table **3**) [29, 38].

Table 3: Effect of physicochemical properties of solutes on ocular tissue permeability

Ocular Tissue	Molecular Radius	Lipophilicity	Charge
Sclera	Permeability exponential decreases with increasing molecular radii [21, 24]	Permeability decrease with increasing lipophilicity [9, 25, 26]	Permeability increase with negatively charged solute [29-31]
Bruch's membrane-choroid (BC)	Permeability decreases with increasing molecular radii [36]	Permeability decrease with increasing lipophilicity [29, 37]	Permeability increase with negatively charged solute [29, 38]
Retinal pigment epithelium (RPE)	Permeability exponential decreases with increasing molecular radii [36]	Permeability increase with increasing lipophilicity [36]	

Resistance to solute transport across the choroid has been observed due to age-related changes in human Bruch's membrane [29, 39]. However, no significant change in permeability or ultrastructure of sclera has been observed due to ageing [22]. It has been reported that Bruch's membrane thickens (from 2 to 4.7 µm between first to tenth decade of life) and the choroidal layer thins out (11 µm per 10 years) with aging in the human eye [40]. Moreover, age-related linear diminution in hydraulic conductivity has been reported. Taurine and other amino acid transport across the choroid–Bruch's layer in humans has been studied [39, 41, 42]. These results indicated that the aged Bruch's membrane offers a major resistance to solute transport [39, 41]. Permeability of human Bruch's membrane to serum proteins was also reported to diminish about 10-fold from the first to ninth decade of life [43].

Taken together these reports indicate that the choroid–Bruch's layer is a significant barrier to transscleral delivery of drugs. If the choroid is the intended target for treatment such as choroidal neovascularization, higher level of free drug in the choroid can be achieved by designing hydrophilic and anionic drugs and/or prodrugs relatives to lipophilic and cationic ones [29]. If retina is the intended target in addition to choroid–Bruch's layer then there may be a further reduction in drug transport because of the presence of RPE which will be further discussed in the following section.

Retinal Pigment Epithelium (RPE)

The retina is a multilayered membrane of neuroectodermal origin and can be broadly divided into the neural retina and the RPE. Neural retina is involved in signal transduction, leading to vision. RPE, on the other hand, is a single cell layer lies at the interface between the neural retina and the choroid. It plays a vital role in supporting and maintaining the viability of the neural retina [44, 45]. The RPE is compared of a monolayer of highly specialized cuboidal cells located between the neural retina and the choroid [46]. It restricts the absorption and permeation of drugs from choroid to the retina, to its intercellular junctions it is considered to be a tight barrier [36].

RPE can easily be removed and its permeability function assessed by comparing tissue permeability values with and without removal of RPE [2, 47]. RPE permeability determines the transport of solute from the choroidal circulation to neural retina following systemic administration. Moreover, RPE permeability may also depend on drug binding to the melanin pigment or tissue proteins, active transport processes and metabolism [36, 48, 49]. In monkeys, the movement of horseradish peroxidase (44 kDa molecules) stopped at the tight RPE junctions [50, 51]. However, in another study following subconjunctival administration, it was observed that the fluorescein-conjugated pigment epithelium-derived factor (PEDF) and ovalbumin proteins permeated to the cultured RPE monolayer of monkey even in the presence of fully formed tight junction. This data suggests that subconjunctival protein delivery may be feasible for delivering of proteins like PEDF and ovalbumin [47].

With hydrophilic molecules and macromolecules, RPE may be the rate-limiting barrier for the retinal drug delivery. Permeability of bovine RPE for hydrophilic carboxyfluorescein and FITC-dextrans shows exponential decrease with increase in molecular radius. In addition, permeability of lipophilic compounds (metoprolol and atenolol) is significantly higher whereas scleral permeability is less sensitive to solute lipophilicity. Moreover, macromolecules (dextran) transported passively across the retina have shown similar permeability values in the outward (retina choroid) and inward directions. However, carboxyfluorescein active transport shows that difference in that outward permeability is higher than inward direction. It appears that the RPE is a tighter barrier than the sclera for hydrophilic small and large molecules and, therefore, scleral permeability alone is not sufficient to predict the drug delivery rate to the retina [2, 36].

Conjunctiva

The conjunctiva is a thin, mucus-secreting transparent epithelial barrier; relatively well vascularized tissue covering the anterior one-third of the globe. It consists of two layers: an outer epithelium and its underlying stroma (substantia propria). The epithelial cells connect with each other by tight junctions at the apical side and act as a permeability barrier. The conjunctiva acts as a simple protective role in the eye by functioning as a passive physical barrier. It also participates in the maintenance of tear film stability by secretion of electrolytes, fluid and mucins [52-54].

Paracellular transport, through the tight junctions of the conjunctival epithelial cells may be the rate-limiting step for diffusion of macromolecular drugs [52, 54]. Since hydrophilic drug penetrates occurs *via* paracellular pathway (between the cells through the tight junctions), the total penetration surface area for any hydrophilic drug is extremely small compared to the surface area offered by transcellular pathway for absorption of lipophilic drugs [52, 55, 56]. Hence paracellular pathway of epithelial barriers (like cornea and conjunctiva), where adjacent cells are held together at the apical membrane by tight junctions, can act as the rate-limiting step for diffusion of hydrophilic macromolecule drugs including peptides and proteins [52, 57, 58]. Data from equivalent pore analysis suggests that conjunctiva may allow the permeation of hydrophilic compounds having molecular weight less than 20 kDa. The theoretical radius of such equivalent pores is predicted to be ~5.5 nm [59]. Transport studies of a series of hydrophilic molecules *e.g.* D-mannitol (182 Da), 6-carboxyfluorescein (376 Da) and fluorescein isothiocyanate-labeled dextrans (FD-4400, 9400, 21300, 38600

Da) across the conjunctiva have shown a decline in permeability coefficients with increase in molecular weight of a solute. This results confirms that the conjunctiva may allow reasonable permeation of hydrophilic substances with a molecular weight less than 20 kDa, whereas cornea appears to offer significant resistance to inulin (5 kDa) and FD (20 kDa) solutes [58, 59]. Moreover, conjunctival surface area is larger (~9 and 17 times) than cornea in rabbits and human, respectively. This may be another contributing factor for greater absorption of hydrophilic drugs *via* conjunctival route, as conjunctiva is much leakier with less tight junctions than cornea [52, 60].

Tissue resistance is a good indicator of passive barrier properties of a given biological barrier. Kompella *et al.* have shown that the freshly excised pigmented rabbit conjunctiva portrays a moderately tight epithelium with a transepithelial electrical resistance (TEER) of~1.3 kU cm^2. The conjunctival tissues excised from pigmented rabbits have a lower TEER than the tighter rabbit cornea with a TEER value of ~7.0–9.0 kU cm^2 [61-63]. This data further explains that the rabbit conjunctiva in general is more permeable to hydrophilic solutes than cornea, as demonstrated earlier using *in vivo* study [64]. Thus, the conjunctival-scleral pathway is favored for delivery of hydrophilic drugs because this mode of administration may evade the anterior chamber and drug may get direct access to the intraocular tissues of the posterior segments [52].

In addition to structural barrier, the penetration of peptide drugs across the conjunctiva is also restricted by external enzymatic barrier [65]. For example, ocular delivery of enkephalins, substance P and insulin are significantly degraded due to enzymatic activity [65-67]. Co-administration of protease inhibitor(s) may be one of the approach to enhance absorption of peptide and protein drugs. The presence of camostat mesylate (an aminopeptidase inhibitor) and leupeptin (a serine protease inhibitor) in the mucosal fluid resulted in transport of intact arginine vasopressin across the pigmented rabbit conjunctiva [68].

DYNAMIC BARRIERS

Conjunctival Blood Flow

Tissues themselves (*i.e.* sclera, non-perfused choroid and retina) may not be the sole barrier to drug transport into the eye and other factors, such as lymph and blood circulation may play an important role in diminishing drug delivery to the posterior segment. The conjunctiva is well vascularized and several studies have reported that drug from conjunctival tissue may be cleared through blood and lymphatic vessels [35, 69].

Longer retention of subconjunctivally injected microparticles compared to nanoparticles and higher half-life of albumin compared to ^{22}Na in subconjunctival tissue suggest that molecular size may control the rate of conjunctival/episcleral clearance [70, 71]. The barrier location and clearance parameters of ocular tissue need to be considered when designing a transscleral drug delivery system. Rapid transscleral movement into the vitreous, under complete cessation of lymph and blood clearances following euthanasia, was demonstrated by hydrophilic contrast agents and magnetic resonance imaging (MRI) [72]. Robinson *et al.*, have also demonstrated that selective elimination of the conjunctival/episcleral clearance mechanisms results in higher amounts of intraocular drug penetration. Rabbits receiving a sub-tenon's injection of triamcinolone acetonide with an incised 'conjunctival window' inhibit local blood and lymphatic clearance in the conjunctiva. Under this condition higher drug levels in the vitreous were observed than rabbits that did not have the incision [2, 35].

Studies were also performed to compare the delivery of sodium fluorescien to the retina following periocular injection and a unidirectional episcleral exoplant. The exoplant allowed release of dye on the episcleral side but not on the conjunctival side. Higher amounts of sodium fluorescein were detected in the retina following a unidirectional episcleral explant than periocular injection. The results from these studies suggest that conjunctival/episcleral clearance mechanisms play a significant role in the reduction of intraocular drug penetration [2, 73].

Choroidal Blood Flow

Choroidal blood flow is among the highest per unit volume in the body. The choriocapillaris containing large fenestrations deliver oxygen and nutrients to the eye, suggesting that the choroidal blood flow could act as a sink for molecules and prevent therapeutic agents from reaching the target. A very few reports have been available in the literature showing effect of choroidal circulation on drug delivery to posterior segment tissues [74, 75]. Using episcleral implants on rabbits, Kim *et al.* have observed significant vitreous concentrations in *ex vivo* experiments but negligible vitreous concentrations during *in vivo* experiments. The authors had attributed the observed difference to the choroidal blood flow and assumed the choroid to be a complete sink in their computational model [72].

Robinson *et al.* have used cryotherapy as a method to eliminate choroidal blood flow locally. A single freeze-thaw cycle with cryotherapy forms a chorioretinal scar but leaves the conjunctiva and sclera intact. Results from this study showed that elimination *via* the conjunctival lymphatic/blood vessels was more effective in reducing vitreal concentrations than elimination by choroidal vessels. Hence, this study suggests that choroidal blood flow may not significantly contribute to drug elimination following transscleral delivery [35]. Balachandran *et al.* supports this finding with Thiele modulus that suggests that a large fraction of the dose diffuses through the choroid without being washed away by the blood flow. Hence, clearance by the blood flow is not as important factor for drug loss as previously thought. The results of the study show that a loss to choroidal circulation is not as important impeding factor as thought previously. In contrast, the mass transfer from the scleral surface was found to be significant and therefore, design of the drug vehicle to be placed on the episcleral region needs more attention [75].

Blood Retinal Barrier (BRB)

The integrity of the BRB has been recognized as an important component of normal vision. Disruption of this barrier may cause various retinal vascular diseases and macular pathologies, causing blindness. BRB serves as a selective partitioning barrier and restricts drug movement between the retina and blood circulation. It also maintains a highly specialized environment of the neural tight junction. BRB is located in the posterior part of the globe and is composed of two parts. The tight junctions of the retinal pigment epithelium serves as a outer part of the barrier while the endothelial cells and pericytes of the retinal blood vessels serve as a inner part of the barrier [76, 77]. Under normal pathological conditions, BRB serves as "non-leaky" firm tight junctions and restricts diffusion of various small molecules like glucose, amino acid [78], sodium ions and fluorescein into the retina [79, 80].

Inner Blood Retinal Barrier

The inner part of the BRB is similar to the blood-brain barrier except presence of higher density of interendothelial junctions and endothelial vesicles. In addition, it also possesses a slightly higher vascular permeability. Inner BRB also expresses about four times as many pericytes, which may limit leakiness of the vasculature despite a reduced transcellular resistance [81]. It has been suggested that pericytes can add to the tightness of the inner barrier. Lower pericyte density has been observed as one of pathological change in diabetic retinopathy where retinal vessels leak [82]. A break in the BRB at optic disc has been observed which may allow diffusion of hydrophilic substances from choroid into optic nerve head [79]. The barrier property of retinal vascular endothelium has been observed for fluorescein (376 Da) and also for larger molecules including thorium oxide, horseradish peroxidase (40 kDa) and microperoxidase (1.9 kDa) [77, 82, 83]. The significance of the BRB to retinal disease has been demonstrated by fluorescein angiography. Clinical investigation can detect relationships between the breakdown of the BRB and diverse retinal disease [84]. In a healthy eye, very small quantity of fluorescein or its metabolite fluorescein glucuronide transport is noted across the barrier. However, more fluorescein leakage occurs in diabetic retinopathy then in nonpathological state. Although fluorescein molecules in smaller diameter and eighteen times more lipid soluble then fluorescein glucuronide, the permeability of both molecules was found to be similar. This observation suggests that neither molecular dimension nor lipid solubility is the rate limiting factor for enhanced BRB transport in diabetic retinopathy. Rather, the leakiness appears across the water-filled pores in the barrier. Moreover ultrastructural changes can be seen in capillaries that invade the retina during phototoxic retinopathy [85, 86].

Outer Blood Retinal Barrier

It is comprised of junctions at apical border between adjacent retinal pigment epithelial cells. These tight junctions are composed of multiple layers of anastomosing strands. It has been reported that the BRB breakdown in diabetic RPE is due to alterations of plasma membrane permeability rather than a loss of tight junctions. In the dystrophic rat retina, there is no change in the plasma membrane permeability, rather there is a loss in the number of junction strands [77].

ROLE OF TRANSPORTERS IN OCULAR DRUG DELIVERY

Various influx and efflux transporters are located on the BRB. These transporters play a significant role in drug transport and disposition. Agents indicated in the treatment of posterior segment diseases may act as substrate or inhibitor of these transporters [87, 88]. Hence, it is imperative to understand their biological role while designing a drug delivery system. Influx transporters, also known as nutrient transporters, are mainly involved in the translocation of essential nutrients such as amino acids, glucose, vitamins, peptides, lactate *etc.* to the retina. Influx transporters present in posterior segment ocular tissues include peptide transporters, amino acid transporters, monocarboxylic acid transporters, nucleoside transporter, organic anion transporting peptide and organic cation transporters (Table **4**). Presence of efflux transporter such as P-glycoprotein (P-gp), multidrug-resistance-associated proteins (MRPs) and breast cancer resistance protein (BCRP) on BRB have also been reported. Efflux transporters play a critical role in eliminating neurotransmitter metabolites and toxins from the retina. Absorption and bioavailability of various active molecules within inner retinal tissues is limited by efflux pumps following transscleral or systemic administration (Table **5**) [89, 90].

Table 4: Expression of influx transporters in posterior segment of the eye

Transporter	Expression in retinal cell lines	Expression in retina/choroid tissues	References
Glutamate transporter	ARPE-19, D407, Y79	Bovine RPE	[106, 107]
Large amino acid transporter	TR-iBRB2,ARPE-19	Rabbit retina	[108-111]
Oligopeptide transporter	ARPE-19, primary mouse and human fetal RPE cells	Human (retina/choroid)	[89, 112]
Monocarboxylate transporter	ARPE-19, TR-iBRB2	Rat RPE, Human RPE	[113-116]
Nucleoside transporter	TR-iBRB2,ARPE-19	Rabbit retina	[117, 118]
Organic anion transporting peptide		Rat retina, Rat RPE, Rat RVECs, Human(retina/ choroid)	[89, 119-121]
Organic anion transporter		Rat RVECs	[122]

Table 4: contd...

Organic cation transporter	ARPE-19	Human(retina/choroid), Mouse RPE	[89, 123]
Folate transporter	ARPE-19	Mouse neural retina, Mouse RPE	[124-127]
Multivitamin transporter (SMVT)	Y79, ARPE-19		[91, 128]
Riboflavin transporter	Y79, ARPE-19	Rabbit Retina	[129, 130]

Abbreviations: Y79: Human retinoblastoma cell line; **ARPE-19:** Spontaneously arising retinal pigment epithelia (RPE) cell line; **h1RPE:** Immortalized human RPE cell line; **D407:** Human retinal pigment epithelial cell line; **TR-iBRB2:** Rat retinal capillary endothelial cell line; **Rat RVECs:** Retinal vascular endothelial cells; **HRPEpic:** Human retinal pigment epithelial cells

Table 5: Expression of efflux transporters in posterior segment of the eye

Transporter	Expression in retinal cell lines	Expression in tissues	References
P-gp	D407, h1RPE, TR-iBRB	Human(retina/ choroid), Human RPE, porcine RPE	[48, 90, 131-133]
MRP1	HRPEpic, ARPE-19, D407, Y79	Human(retina/ choroid), porcine RPE	[89, 90, 133, 134]
MRP2	D407, Y79 (low expression)	Human(retina/ choroid)	[89, 90, 134]
MRP3	ARPE- 19 (low expression), D407, HRPEpic	Human(retina/ choroid)	[89, 90]
MRP4	ARPE- 19, D407, HRPEpic, Y79	-	[90, 134]
MRP5	ARPE- 19, D407, HRPEpic	-	[90]
MRP6	Y79 (low expression)	-	[134]
BCRP	TR-iBRB, D407	Rat retina, Human(retina/ choroid)	[89, 90, 135]

Abbreviations: oBRB: Outer blood retinal barrier; **MRP1:** Multi drug resistance associated protein 1; **MRP2:** Multi drug resistance associated protein 2; **MRP3:** Multi drug resistance associated protein 3; **MRP4:** Multi drug resistance associated protein 4; **MRP5:** Multi drug resistance associated protein 5; **MRP6:** Multi drug resistance associated protein 6; **BCRP:** breast cancer resistance protein; **P-gp:** P-glycoprotein

Ocular drug bioavailability can be significantly enhanced by targeting therapeutic entities to influx transporters present on BRB. This approach is also known as a transporter targeted prodrug approach. It involves conjugating drug molecules with various nutrient moieties to generate prodrugs. A prodrug can act as a substrate for the influx transporter and hence can easily translocate across the epithelia. Further, it has been reported that a prodrug has lesser affinity towards efflux transporter relative to the parent drug. Hence transporter targeted prodrug approach (Fig. **1**) can also cause complete or partial evasion of efflux pump present on BRB. In addition to enhancement in ocular bioavailability, physicochemical properties of a drug such as solubility and stability can also be improved by prodrug derivatization. Ophthalmic drug delivery scientists and pharmacologist have utilized this approach for delivering various antivirals to the posterior segment ocular tissues following sub-conjunctival and intravitreous (IV) injection. Recently, Janoria *et al*. have synthesized biotin-ganciclovir (biotin-GCV) conjugate to target multivitamin transporter present on rabbit retina [91]. Biotin-GCV was recognized by SMVT system present on the ARPE-19 and rabbit retina. Animal studies have revealed no significant difference between vitreal pharmacokinetic parameters for GCV and biotin-GCV. However; with biotin-GCV, sustained levels of regenerated GCV was observed in vitreous. Oligopeptide transporter (OPT) targeted prodrugs of ganciclovir have also been reported for enhancing permeability of ganciclovir through RPE following transscleral administration. The synthesized dipeptide prodrugs (glycine-valine-GCV, valine-valine-GCV and tyrosine-valine-GCV) have shown two fold increment in permeability across rabbit RCS which was attributed to their higher lipophilicity as well as recognition by OPT [92].

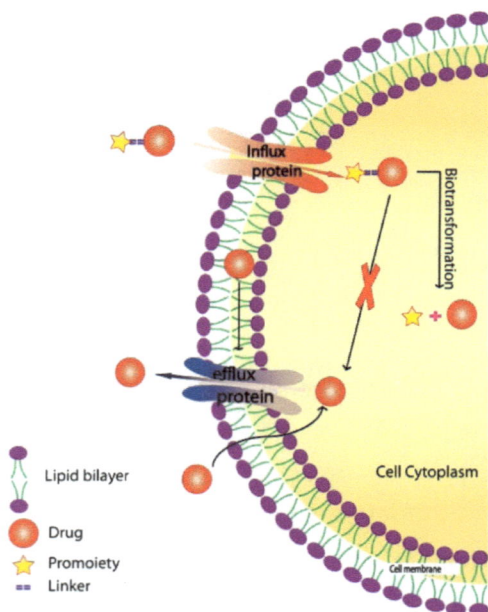

Figure 1: Transporter targeted prodrug approach.

ROLE OF METABOLISM IN OCULAR DRUG DELIVERY

Metabolism is a major drug elimination route and various metabolic enzymes are distributed in various tissues such as the liver, kidney, brain and in the eye. Studies regarding ocular distribution of metabolizing enzymes have shown excessive metabolizing activities in specific ocular structures which are adjacent to high uveal blood flow such as iris ciliary body and retina [93]. Knowledge of ocular metabolizing enzymes provides the impetus for the development of prodrug which can be specifically bio-activated in a desired ocular tissue. This approach may aid in improving efficacy and minimizing toxicity. In the present chapter, we have mainly focused on the metabolizing enzymes present in posterior ocular segment. Posterior segment of the eye includes retina, choroid, vitreous humor and blood retinal barriers. Both phase I and phase II metabolic enzymes are known to be expressed in the retina and RPE (Table **6**) [94]. In 1969, Shichi first identified the presence of microsomal electron transfer system in bovine retinal pigment epithelium [95]. Consequently, various members of CYP (Cytochrome P450) family and their isoforms have been identified in ocular tissues. Zhang *et al.* examined expression of various CYP enzymes at mRNA level in human ocular tissues [89]. The mRNA expression for CYP2C8, CYP2A6, CYP2D6 and CYP2E1 enzymes was observed in retina-choroid. However, the expression level is very low. Schwartzman *et al.* demonstrated the distribution of cytochrome P450 isozymes and their role in arachidonic acid metabolism in bovine ocular tissues. The investigators measured level of aryl hydrocarbon hydroxylase (AHH), 7-ethoxycoumarin- *O*-deethylase (ECOD) and benzphetamine demethylase (BPDM) in bovine ocular tissues and activities of all the three enzymes were found in retina and RPE. Activity of ECOD was highest in the retinal pigment epithelium compared to other ocular tissues. However, BPDM activity was detected only in RPE [96]. Various hydrolytic esterases such as acetylcholinesterase (AChE) and butyrylcholinesterase (BChE) are also distributed in ocular tissues [97]. Presence of phase II metabolizing enzymes in rabbit ocular tissues was studied by Watkins and co workers [98]. The rabbit ocular tissues including cornea, iris/ciliary body, choroid and retina exhibit significant phase II metabolizing enzyme activities such as p-aminobenzoic acid N-acetyltransferase, 2-naphthol sulfotransferase and 1-chloro-2,4-dinitrobenzene glutathione S-transferase.

Table 6: Expression of various metabolizing enzymes in posterior segment ocular tissues

Name of enzymes	Ocular Tissue	References
Phase I		
Oxidoreductases		
CYP2C	Mouse retina	[136]
CYP2C8	Human retina/choroid	[89]
CYP2A6	Human retina/choroid	[89]
CYP2D6	Human retina/choroid	[89]
CYP2E1	Human retina/choroid	[89]
Aryl hydrocarbon hydroxylase (AHH)	Bovine RPE, retina	[96]
Benzphetamine demethylase	Bovine RPE, retina	[96]
7-Ethoxycoumarin *O*-deethylase	Bovine RPE, retina	[96]
Catechol-O- methyl transferase(COMT)	Rabbit retina/choroid	[137]
Monoamine oxidase (MAO)	Rabbit retina/choroid	[137]
Hydrolytic Enzymes		
Peptidases	Rabbit vitreous humor, Rabbit retina	[93, 99]
Acetyl cholinesterase	Rat RPE, Rat retina	[97, 138, 139]
Butyrylcholinesterase	Rat RPE, Rat retina	[97, 138, 139]
Phase II		
Glutathione S-transferase	Bovine retina, Rabbit retina/choroid	[98, 140, 141]
N-acetyl transferase	Rabbit retina/choroid, Bovine retina	[98, 141]
2-naphthol sulfotransferase	Rabbit retina/choroid	[98]
γ-glutamyl transpeptidase	Bovine retina	[141]
Cysteinyl glycinase	Bovine retina	[141]

Vitreous humor is a semi solid fluid consisting of hyaluronic acid, collagen and water. It provides mechanical support to surrounding tissues by virtue of its viscoelastic properties. Metabolizing enzymes are not abundant in vitreous humor. However, presence of esterases and peptidases was observed in vitreous humor. Majumdar *et al.* reported vitreal pharmacokinetic of dipeptide prodrug of ganciclovir (Val-GCV, Val-Val- GCV, Gly-Val-GCV and Tyr-Val-GCV) in rabbit eye [99]. In the vitreous humor, all prodrugs were converted into their parent drugs *via* amino acid intermediate which established the presence of peptidase and esterases. Fig. **2** shows probable mechanism of hydrolysis of dipeptide prodrugs. Various enzymes involved in the production of hyaluronic acid and lipid metabolism were also identified in vitreous fluid [93, 100].

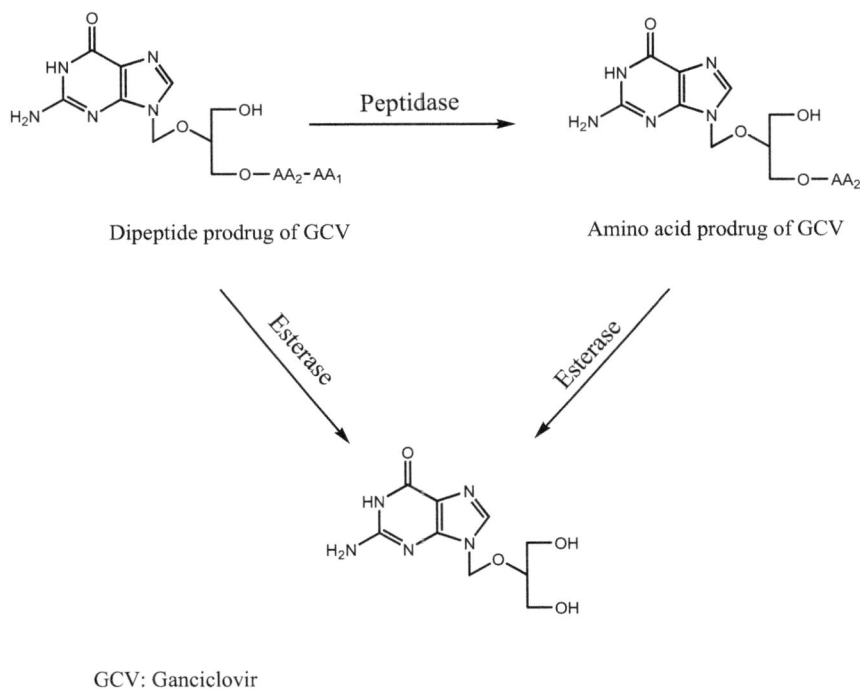

GCV: Ganciclovir

Figure 2: Bioconversion of peptide prodrug of ganciclovir in presence of peptidases and esterases.

FACTORS AFFECTING TRANSPORT OF DRUG MOLECULES IN SOLUTION OR IN COLLOIDAL DOSAGE FORM

Various factors such as molecular weight, radius, hydrophilicity and charge of the molecule play important role in transscleral permeability of a compound. Also, the size, dynamic barriers such as blood and lymphatic flows, affinity of the encapsulated drug towards melanin and surface conjugation of nanoparticles with various endogenous molecules determine the *in vivo* performance of a colloidal dosage form. Kompella *et al.* have studied the retention and ocular distribution of subconjunctivally administered nanoparticles and microparticles [70]. These researchers successfully detected 200 nm and 2 µm particles in the periocluar tissue at 60-days post administration while 20 nm particles were not retained in the periocular tissue due to rapid elimination. This report concluded that 20 nm periocular particles is an ineffective carrier for sustained transscleral drug delivery to the retina while 200-2000 nm periocular particles can serve as suitable carrier for sustained transscleral drug delivery to the retina. Kompella *et al.* also reported that transport of 20 nm nanoparticles across sclera was minimal due to periocular circulation (blood and lymphatic) [101]. This article also reported that smaller nanoparticles (20 nm) were capable of crossing static barrier (sclera) but are rapidly cleared away by periocular circulation. As a result such particles gain entry into spleen and liver (organs of reticulo-endothelial system). Csaky *et al.* investigated the movement of human serum albumin nanoparticles (HSA-NP) following intravitreal administration [102]. They reported that anionic nanoparticles diffused easily in comparison to cationic nanoparticles through the vitreal network of collagen fibrils. These investigators also reported that most of the intravitreally administered cationic nanoparticles bound and aggregated to vitreous whereas anionic nanoparticles diffused freely from the vitreous to retina. In the presence of vitreal hyaluronan (due to a negatively charged glycosaminoglycan), cationic molecules tend to aggregate in the vitreous humor where as anionic molecules are homogenously spread in vitreous humor. This kind of glycosaminoglycan interaction was first observed with polymeric and liposomal DNA complexes [103, 104]. Zeta potential of colloidal dosage form can be considered as a factor which can affect transport. Also, anionic nanoparticles can be selected as suitable carrier for administering drug or gene to the sub-retinal space and RPE. Domb *et al.* evaluated the delivery of charged fluorescent nanoparticles into rabbit eyes using hydrogel iontophoresis [105]. Positively charged nanoparticles have shown greater penetration than negatively charged nanoparticles. An increased fluorescence intensity of negatively charged particles was observed at the outer ocular tissues upto 4 hr following treatment. Whereas, upto 12 hr from treatment, an increased fluorescence intensity of positively charged nanoparticles was observed at the inner ocular tissues. This data clearly indicates the migration of particles to the inner ocular tissues (retina and choroid) from the outer tissues. It may be the result of electrostatic interaction between the positively charged nanoparticles and negatively charged corneal and conjunctival mucosa which eventually increases the concentration and residence time of drug. Peeters *et al.* reported how vitreous acts as a barrier to ocular drug delivery and how to overcome this barrier. Upon intravitreal administrations of DNA/cationic liposome complexes (LPXs) appear to adhere to the vitreal network of collagen fibrils. These LPXs aggregate in vitreous humor and hence results in a restricted mobility. It can be overcome by PEGylating the surface of nanosphers by hydrophilic chains of PEG and thus minimizing aggregation in the vitreous and binding to vitreal network of collagen fibrils. Thus LPXs obtained after PEGylation were shown to diffuse freely in the posterior direction from vitreous to retina after intravitreal injection. The authors concluded that modification of the surface of LPXs with hydrophilic PEG chains prevented their aggregation in vitreous [103].

CONCLUSION

Treatment of posterior segment ocular diseases is a major challenge due to a variety of reasons. These reasons include blood ocular barrier, efflux pumps, static and dynamic barriers. A detailed understanding of these barriers is necessary to design an effective drug delivery system. Adaption of a multidisciplinary approach has brought a great momentum in the development of delivery systems. New devices which can overcome various barriers are being developed. Current developments in the field hold a great promise for the future of posterior segment ocular drug therapy.

ACKNOWLEDGEMENTS

This work has been supported by NIH grants RO1 EY 09171 and RO1 EY 10659.

CONFLICT OF INTEREST

The author(s) confirm that this chapter content has no conflict of interest.

REFERENCES

[1]   Barar J, Javadzadeh AR, Omidi Y. Ocular novel drug delivery: impacts of membranes and barriers. Expert Opin Drug Deliv 2008; 5(5): 567-81.

[2]   Kim SH, Lutz RJ, Wang NS, Robinson MR. Transport barriers in transscleral drug delivery for retinal diseases. Ophthalmic Res 2007; 39(5): 244-54.

[3]   Kralinger MT, Kieselbach GF, Voigt M, *et al.* Experimental model for proliferative vitreoretinopathy by intravitreal dispase: limited by zonulolysis and cataract. Ophthalmologica 2006; 220(4): 211-6.

[4]   Ozkiris A, Erkilic K. Complications of intravitreal injection of triamcinolone acetonide. Can J Ophthalmol 2005; 40(1): 63-8.

[5]   Sutter FK, Gillies MC. Pseudo-endophthalmitis after intravitreal injection of triamcinolone. Br J Ophthalmol 2003; 87(8): 972-4.

[6]   Nelson ML, Tennant MT, Sivalingam A, *et al.* Infectious and presumed noninfectious endophthalmitis after intravitreal triamcinolone acetonide injection. Retina 2003; 23(5): 686-91.

[7]   Nicolo M, Ghiglione D, Calabria G. Retinal pigment epithelial tear following intravitreal injection of bevacizumab (Avastin). Eur J Ophthalmol 2006; 16(5): 770-3.

[8]   Lee SB, Geroski DH, Prausnitz MR, Edelhauser HF. Drug delivery through the sclera: effects of thickness, hydrationand sustained release systems. Exp Eye Res 2004; 78(3): 599-607.

[9]   Geroski DH, Edelhauser HF. Transscleral drug delivery for posterior segment disease. Adv Drug Deliv Rev 2001; 52(1): 37-48.

[10]   Ambati J, Adamis AP. Transscleral drug delivery to the retina and choroid. Prog Retin Eye Res 2002; 21(2): 145-51.

[11]   Olsen TW, Aaberg SY, Geroski DH, Edelhauser HF. Human sclera: thickness and surface area. Am J Ophthalmol 1998; 125(2): 237-41.

[12]   Friberg TR, Lace JW. A comparison of the elastic properties of human choroid and sclera. Exp Eye Res1988; 47(3): 429-36.

[13]   Boubriak OA, Urban JP, Bron AJ. Differential effects of aging on transport properties of anterior and posterior human sclera. Exp Eye Res 2003; 76(6): 701-13.

[14]   Jiang J, Geroski DH, Edelhauser HF, Prausnitz MR. Measurement and prediction of lateral diffusion within human sclera. Invest Ophthalmol Vis Sci 2006; 47(7): 3011-6.

[15]   Madhu C, Rix P, Nguyen T, *et al.* Penetration of natural prostaglandins and their ester prodrugs and analogs across human ocular tissues *in vitro*. J Ocul Pharmacol Ther 1998; 14(5): 389-99.

[16]   Edelhauser HF, Maren TH. Permeability of human cornea and sclera to sulfonamide carbonic anhydrase inhibitors. Arch Ophthalmol 1988; 106(8): 1110-5.

[17]   Hamalainen KM, Kananen K, Auriola S, Kontturi K, Urtti A. Characterization of paracellular and aqueous penetration routes in cornea, conjunctivaand sclera. Invest Ophthalmol Vis Sci 1997; 38(3): 627-34.

[18]   Unlu N, Robinson JR. Scleral permeability to hydrocortisone and mannitol in the albino rabbit eye. J Ocul Pharmacol Ther 1998; 14(3): 273-81.

[19]   Ahmed I, Patton TF. Importance of the noncorneal absorption route in topical ophthalmic drug delivery. Invest Ophthalmol Vis Sci 1985; 26(4): 584-7.

[20]   Boubriak OA, Urban JP, Akhtar S, Meek KM, Bron AJ. The effect of hydration and matrix composition on solute diffusion in rabbit sclera. Exp Eye Res 2000; 71(5): 503-14.

[21]   Ambati J, Canakis CS, Miller JW, *et al.* Diffusion of high molecular weight compounds through sclera. Invest Ophthalmol Vis Sci 2000; 41(5): 1181-5.

[22]   Olsen TW, Edelhauser HF, Lim JI, Geroski DH. Human scleral permeability. Effects of age, cryotherapy, transscleral diode laserand surgical thinning. Invest Ophthalmol Vis Sci 1995; 36(9): 1893-903.

[23]   Ambati J, Gragoudas ES, Miller JW, *et al.* Transscleral delivery of bioactive protein to the choroid and retina. Invest Ophthalmol Vis Sci 2000; 41(5): 1186-91.

[24]   Edwards A, Prausnitz MR. Fiber matrix model of sclera and corneal stroma for drug delivery to the eye. AIChE Journal 1998; 44(1): 214-225.

[25]   Kansara V, Mitra AK. Evaluation of an *ex vivo* model implication for carrier-mediated retinal drug delivery. Curr Eye Res 2006; 31(5): 415-26.

[26]   Cruysberg LP, Nuijts RM, Geroski DH, *et al. In vitro* human scleral permeability of fluorescein, dexamethasone-fluorescein, methotrexate-fluorescein and rhodamine 6G and the use of a coated coil as a new drug delivery system. J Ocul Pharmacol Ther 2002; 18(6): 559-69.

[27]   Chien DS, Homsy JJ, Gluchowski C, Tang-Liu DD. Corneal and conjunctival/scleral penetration of p-aminoclonidine, AGN 190342and clonidine in rabbit eyes. Curr Eye Res 1990; 9(11): 1051-9.

[28]   Ahmed I, Gokhale RD, Shah MV, Patton TF. Physicochemical determinants of drug diffusion across the conjunctiva, scleraand cornea. J Pharm Sci 1987; 76(8): 583-6.

[29]   Cheruvu NP, Kompella UB. Bovine and porcine transscleral solute transport: influence of lipophilicity and the Choroid-Bruch's layer. Invest Ophthalmol Vis Sci 2006; 47(10): 4513-22.

[30]   Church AL, Barza M, Baum J. An improved apparatus for transscleral iontophoresis of gentamicin. Invest Ophthalmol Vis Sci 1992; 33(13): 3543-5.

[31]   Yoshizumi MO, Cohen D, Verbukh I, Leinwand M, Kim J, Lee DA. Experimental transscleral iontophoresis of ciprofloxacin. J Ocul Pharmacol 1991; 7(2): 163-7.

[32]   Cruysberg LP, Nuijts RM, Geroski DH, *et al.* The influence of intraocular pressure on the transscleral diffusion of high-molecular-weight compounds. Invest Ophthalmol Vis Sci 2005; 46(10): 3790-4.

[33]   Rudnick DE, Noonan JS, Geroski DH, Prausnitz MR, Edelhauser HF. The effect of intraocular pressure on human and rabbit scleral permeability. Invest Ophthalmol Vis Sci 1999; 40(12): 3054-8.

[34]   Hogan J. Histology of the Human Eye. Philadelphia 1971.

[35]   Robinson MR, Lee SS, Kim H, *et al.* A rabbit model for assessing the ocular barriers to the transscleral delivery of triamcinolone acetonide. Exp Eye Res 2006; 82(3): 479-87.

[36]   Pitkanen L, Ranta VP, Moilanen H, Urtti A. Permeability of retinal pigment epithelium: effects of permeant molecular weight and lipophilicity. Invest Ophthalmol Vis Sci 2005; 46(2): 641-6.

[37]   Kadam RS, Kompella UB. Influence of lipophilicity on drug partitioning into sclera, choroid-retinal pigment epithelium, retina, trabecular meshworkand optic nerve. J Pharmacol Exp Ther 2010; 332(3): 1107-20.

[38]   Maurice DM, Polgar J. Diffusion across the sclera. Exp Eye Res 1977; 25(6): 577-82.

[39]   Hillenkamp J, Hussain AA, Jackson TL, Cunningham JR, Marshall J. The influence of path length and matrix components on ageing characteristics of transport between the choroid and the outer retina. Invest Ophthalmol Vis Sci 2004; 45(5): 1493-8.

[40]   Ramrattan RS, van der Schaft TL, Mooy CM, *et al.* Morphometric analysis of Bruch's membrane, the choriocapillarisand the choroid in aging. Invest Ophthalmol Vis Sci 1994; 35(6): 2857-64.

[41]   Hussain AA, Rowe L, Marshall J. Age-related alterations in the diffusional transport of amino acids across the human Bruch's-choroid complex. J Opt Soc Am A Opt Image Sci Vis 2002; 19(1): 166-72.

[42]   Moore DJ, Hussain AA, Marshall J. Age-related variation in the hydraulic conductivity of Bruch's membrane. Invest Ophthalmol Vis Sci 1995; 36(7): 1290-7.

[43] Moore DJ, Clover GM. The effect of age on the macromolecular permeability of human Bruch's membrane. Invest Ophthalmol Vis Sci 2001; 42(12): 2970-5.

[44] Cunha-Vaz JG. The blood-retinal barriers. Doc Ophthalmol 1976; 41(2): 287-327.

[45] Gunda S HS, Mandava N, Mitra AK. Barriers in Ocular Drug Delivery. In: Tombran-Tink J, Barnstable CJ, Eds. Ocular Transporters, Ophthalmic Diseases and Drug Delivery. New Jersey, Humana Press, 2008; pp. 399-414.

[46] Zinn KM, Benjamin-Henkind J. Retinal Pigment Epithelium. In: Tasman W, Ed. Duane's Foundations of Clinical Ophthalmology Vol. 1. Philadelphia, Lippincott-Raven, 1995; pp. 1–20.

[47] Amaral J, Fariss RN, Campos MM, *et al.* Transscleral-RPE permeability of PEDF and ovalbumin proteins: implications for subconjunctival protein delivery. Invest Ophthalmol Vis Sci 2005; 46(12): 4383-92.

[48] Kennedy BG, Mangini NJ. P-glycoprotein expression in human retinal pigment epithelium. Mol Vis 2002; 8: 422-30.

[49] Maurice DM, Mishima S. Ocular Pharmacokinetics. In: Sears ML, Ed. Pharmacology of the Eye. Berlin, Springler-Verlag, 1984; pp. 19–116.

[50] Peyman GA, Bok D. Peroxidase diffusion in the normal and laser-coagulated primate retina. Invest Ophthalmol 1972; 11(1): 35-45.

[51] Toris CB, Pederson JE. Experimental retinal detachment. VII. Intravenous horseradish peroxidase diffusion across the blood-retinal barrier. Arch Ophthalmol 1984; 102(5): 752-6.

[52] Hosoya K, Lee VH, Kim KJ. Roles of the conjunctiva in ocular drug delivery: a review of conjunctival transport mechanisms and their regulation. Eur J Pharm Biopharm 2005; 60(2): 227-40.

[53] Dartt DA. Regulation of mucin and fluid secretion by conjunctival epithelial cells. Prog Retin Eye Res 2002; 21(6): 555-76.

[54] Gukasyan HJ, Kim KJ, Lee VH. The Conjunctival Barrier in Ocular Drug Delivery. In: Ehrhardt C, Kim KJ, Eds. Drug Absorption Studies. New York, Springer, 2008; pp. 307-20.

[55] Adson A, Raub TJ, Burton PS, *et al.* Quantitative approaches to delineate paracellular diffusion in cultured epithelial cell monolayers. J Pharm Sci 1994; 83(11): 1529-36.

[56] Burton PS, Conradi RA, Hilgers AR. Mechanisms of peptide and protein absorption: transcellular mechanism of peptide and protein absorption: passive aspects. Adv Drug Deliv Rev 1991; 7: 365-86.

[57] Gumbiner B. Structure, biochemistryand assembly of epithelial tight junctions. Am J Physiol 1987; 253(6 Pt 1): C749-58.

[58] Huang AJ, Tseng SC, Kenyon KR. Paracellular permeability of corneal and conjunctival epithelia. Invest Ophthalmol Vis Sci 1989; 30(4): 684-9.

[59] Horibe Y, Hosoya K, Kim KJ, Ogiso T, Lee VH. Polar solute transport across the pigmented rabbit conjunctiva: size dependence and the influence of 8-bromo cyclic adenosine monophosphate. Pharm Res 1997; 14(9): 1246-51.

[60] Watsky MA, Jablonski MM, Edelhauser HF. Comparison of conjunctival and corneal surface areas in rabbit and human. Curr Eye Res 1988; 7(5): 483-6.

[61] Crosson CE, Beuerman RW, Klyce SD. Dopamine modulation of active ion transport in rabbit corneal epithelium. Invest Ophthalmol Vis Sci 1984; 25(11): 1240-5.

[62] Klyce SD. Electrical profiles in the corneal epithelium. J Physiol 1972; 226(2): 407-29.

[63]   Kompella UB, Kim KJ, Lee VH. Active chloride transport in the pigmented rabbit conjunctiva. Curr Eye Res 1993; 12(12): 1041-8.

[64]   Maurice DM. Electrical potential and ion transport across the conjunctiva. Exp Eye Res 1973; 15(5): 527-32.

[65]   Lee VH, Carson LW, Kashi SD, Stratford RE Jr. *et al.* Metabolic and permeation barriers to the ocular absorption of topically applied enkephalins in albino rabbits. J Ocul Pharmacol 1986; 2(4): 345-52.

[66]   Hayakawa E, Chien DS, Inagaki K, *et al.* Conjunctival penetration of insulin and peptide drugs in the albino rabbit. Pharm Res 1992; 9(6): 769-75.

[67]   Stratford RE, Jr., Carson LW, Dodda-Kashi S, Lee VH. Systemic absorption of ocularly administered enkephalinamide and inulin in the albino rabbit: extent, pathwaysand vehicle effects. J Pharm Sci 1988; 77(10): 838-42.

[68]   Sun L, Basu SK, Kim KJ, Lee VH. Arginine vasopressin transport and metabolism in the pigmented rabbit conjunctiva. Eur J Pharm Sci 1998; 6(1): 47-52.

[69]   Prince JH DC, Eglitis I, Ruskell GL. The Rabbit. In: Prince JH, Ed. Anatomy and Histology of the Eye and Orbit in Domestic Animals. Springfield, Charles c Thomas, 1960; pp. 268.

[70]   Amrite AC, Kompella UB. Size-dependent disposition of nanoparticles and microparticles following subconjunctival administration. J Pharm Pharmacol 2005; 57(12): 1555-63.

[71]   Maurice DM, Ota Y. The kinetics of subconjunctival injections. Jpn J Ophthalmol 1978; 22: 95-100.

[72]   Kim H, Robinson MR, Lizak MJ, *et al.* Controlled drug release from an ocular implant: an evaluation using dynamic three-dimensional magnetic resonance imaging. Invest Ophthalmol Vis Sci 2004; 45(8): 2722-31.

[73]   Pontes de Carvalho RA, Krausse ML, Murphree AL, *et al.* Delivery from episcleral exoplants. Invest Ophthalmol Vis Sci 2006; 47(10): 4532-9.

[74]   Bill A, Tornquist P, Alm A. Permeability of the intraocular blood vessels. Trans Ophthalmol Soc U K. 1980; 100(3): 332-6.

[75]   Balachandran RK, Barocas VH. Computer modeling of drug delivery to the posterior eye: effect of active transport and loss to choroidal blood flow. Pharm Res 2008; 25(11): 2685-96.

[76]   Gardner TW, Antonetti DA, Barber AJ, Lieth E, Tarbell JA. The molecular structure and function of the inner blood-retinal barrier. Penn State Retina Research Group. Doc Ophthalmol 1999; 97(3-4): 229-37.

[77]   Lang JC, Stiemke MM. Biological Barriers to Ocular Delivery. In: Reddy IK, Ed. Ocular Therapeutics and Drug Delivery: A Multidisciplinary Approach. Pennsylvania, Technomic Publishing Company, Inc. 1996; pp. 85-88.

[78]   Miller S, Steinberg RH. L-methionine and 3-o-methyl-D-glucose across frog retinal pigment epithelium. Exp Eye Res 1976; 2: 177-89.

[79]   Tornquist P, Alm A, Bill A. Studies on ocular blood flow and retinal capillary permeability to sodium in pigs. Acta Physiol Scand 1979; 106(3): 343-50.

[80]   Grayson MC, Laties AM. Ocular localization of sodium fluorescein. Effects of administration in rabbit and monkey. Arch Ophthalmol 1971; 85(5): 600-3.

[81]   Stewart PA, Tuor UI. Blood-eye barriers in the rat: correlation of ultrastructure with function. J Comp Neurol 1994; 340(4): 566-76.

[82]   de Oliveira F. Pericytes in diabetic retincpathy. Br J Ophthalmol 1966; 50(3): 134-43.

[83]   Larsen M. Ocular fluorometry methodological improvements and clinical studies--with special reference to the blood-retina barrier permeability to fluorescein and fluorescein glucuronide. Acta Ophthalmol Suppl 1993; (211): 1-52.

[84]   Cumha-Vaz JG. The blood-ocular barriers. Invest Ophthalmol Vis Sci 1978; 17(11): 1037-9.

[85]   Korte GE, Bellhorn RW, Burns MS. Ultrastructure of blood-retinal barrier permeability in rat phototoxic retinopathy. Invest Ophthalmol Vis Sci 1983; 24(7): 962-71.

[86]   Bellhorn RW, Burns MS, Benjamin JV. Retinal vessel abnormalities of phototoxic retinopathy in rats. Invest Ophthalmol Vis Sci 1980; 19(6): 584-95.

[87]   Gaudana R, Ananthula HK, Parenky A, Mitra AK. Ocular drug delivery. AAPS J 2010; 12(3): 348-60.

[88]   Mannermaa E, Vellonen KS, Urtti A. Drug transport in corneal epithelium and blood-retina barrier: emerging role of transporters in ocular pharmacokinetics. Adv Drug Deliv Rev 2006; 58(11): 1136-63.

[89]   Zhang T, Xiang CD, Gale D, et al. Drug transporter and cytochrome P450 mRNA expression in human ocular barriers: implications for ocular drug disposition. Drug Metab Dispos 2008; 36(7): 1300-7.

[90]   Mannermaa E, Vellonen KS, Ryhanen T, et al. Efflux protein expression in human retinal pigment epithelium cell lines. Pharm Res 2009; 26(7): 1785-91.

[91]   Janoria KG, Boddu SH, Wang Z, et al. Vitreal pharmacokinetics of biotinylated ganciclovir: role of sodium-dependent multivitamin transporter expressed on retina. J Ocul Pharmacol Ther 2009; 25(1): 39-49.

[92]   Kansara V, Hao Y, Mitra AK. Dipeptide monoester ganciclovir prodrugs for transscleral drug delivery: targeting the oligopeptide transporter on rabbit retina. J Ocul Pharmacol Ther 2007; 23(4): 321-34.

[93]   Duvvuri S, Majumdar S, Mitra AK. Role of metabolism in ocular drug delivery. Curr Drug Metab 2004; 5(6): 507-15.

[94]   Al-Ghananeem AM, Crooks PA. Phase I and phase II ocular metabolic activities and the role of metabolism in ophthalmic prodrug and codrug design and delivery. Molecules 2007; 12(3): 373-88.

[95]   Shichi H. Microsomal electron transfer system of bovine retinal pigment epithelium. Exp Eye Res 1969; 8(1): 60-8.

[96]   Schwartzman ML, Masferrer J, Dunn MW, Abraham NG. Cytochrome P450, drug metabolizing enzymes and arachidonic acid metabolism in bovine ocular tissues. Curr Eye Res 1987; 6(4): 623-30.

[97]   Sanchez-Chavez G, Vidal CJ, Salceda R. Acetyl- and butyrylcholinesterase activities in the rat retina and retinal pigment epithelium. J Neurosci Res 1995; 41(5): 655-62.

[98]   Watkins JB, 3rd, Wirthwein DP, Sanders RA. Comparative study of phase II biotransformation in rabbit ocular tissues. Drug Metab Dispos 1991; 19(3): 708-13.

[99]   Majumdar S, Kansara V, Mitra AK. Vitreal pharmacokinetics of dipeptide monoester prodrugs of ganciclovir. J Ocul Pharmacol Ther 2006; 22(4): 231-41.

[100] Berman ER. Biochemistry of the Eye. New York PP, 1991; pp. 291-305.

[101] Amrite AC, Edelhauser HF, Singh SR, Kompella UB. Effect of circulation on the disposition and ocular tissue distribution of 20 nm nanoparticles after periocular administration. Mol Vis 2008; 14: 150-60.

[102] Kim H, Robinson SB, Csaky KG. Investigating the movement of intravitreal human serum albumin nanoparticles in the vitreous and retina. Pharm Res 2009; 26(2): 329-37.

[103] Peeters L, Sanders NN, Braeckmans K, *et al*. Vitreous: a barrier to nonviral ocular gene therapy. Invest Ophthalmol Vis Sci 2005; 46(10): 3553-61.

[104] Ruponen M, Yla-Herttuala S, Urtti A. Interactions of polymeric and liposomal gene delivery systems with extracellular glycosaminoglycans: physicochemical and transfection studies. Biochim Biophys Acta 1999; 14:5(2): 331-41.

[105] Eljarrat-Binstock E, Orucov F, Aldouby Y, *et al*. Charged nanoparticles delivery to the eye using hydrogel iontophoresis. J Control Release 2008; 126(2): 156-61.

[106] Maenpaa H, Gegelashvili G, Tahti H. Expression of glutamate transporter subtypes in cultured retinal pigment epithelial and retinoblastoma cells. Curr Eye Res 2004; 28(3): 159-65.

[107] Pautler EL, Tengerdy C. Transport of acidic amino acids by the bovine pigment epithelium. Exp Eye Res 1986; 43(2): 207-14.

[108] Gandhi MD, Pal D, Mitra AK. Identification and functional characterization of a Na(+)-independent large neutral amino acid transporter (LAT2) on ARPE-19 cells. Int J Pharm 2004; 275(1-2): 189-200.

[109] Atluri H, Talluri RS, Mitra AK. Functional activity of a large neutral amino acid transporter (LAT) in rabbit retina: a study involving the *in vivo* retinal uptake and vitreal pharmacokinetics of L-phenyl alanine. Int J Pharm 2008; 347(1-2): 23-30.

[110] Tomi M, Mori M, Tachikawa M, *et al*. L-type amino acid transporter 1-mediated L-leucine transport at the inner blood-retinal barrier. Invest Ophthalmol Vis Sci 2005; 46(7): 2522-30.

[111] Yamamoto A, Akanuma S, Tachikawa M, Hosoya K. Involvement of LAT1 and LAT2 in the high- and low-affinity transport of L-leucine in human retinal pigment epithelial cells (ARPE-19 cells). J Pharm Sci 2010; 99(5): 2475-82.

[112] Chothe PP, Thakkar SV, Gnana-Prakasam JP, *et al*. Identification of a novel sodium-coupled oligopeptide transporter (SOPT2) in mouse and human retinal pigment epithelial cells. Invest Ophthalmol Vis Sci 2010; 51(1): 413-20.

[113] Majumdar S, Gunda S, Pal D, Mitra AK. Functional activity of a monocarboxylate transporter, MCT1, in the human retinal pigmented epithelium cell line, ARPE-19. Mol Pharm 2005; 2(2): 109-17.

[114] Philp NJ, Wang D, Yoon H, Hjelmeland LM. Polarized expression of monocarboxylate transporters in human retinal pigment epithelium and ARPE-19 cells. Invest Ophthalmol Vis Sci 2003; 44(4): 1716-21.

[115] Hosoya K, Kondo T, Tomi M, *et al*. MCT1-mediated transport of L-lactic acid at the inner blood-retinal barrier: a possible route for delivery of monocarboxylic acid drugs to the retina. Pharm Res 2001; 18(12): 1669-76.

[116] Philp NJ, Yoon H, Grollman EF. Monocarboxylate transporter MCT1 is located in the apical membrane and MCT3 in the basal membrane of rat RPE. Am J Physiol 1998; 274(6 Pt 2): R1824-8.

[117] Nagase K, Tomi M, Tachikawa M, Hosoya K. Functional and molecular characterization of adenosine transport at the rat inner blood-retinal barrier. Biochim Biophys Acta 2006; 1758(1): 13-9.

[118] Majumdar S, Macha S, Pal D, Mitra AK. Mechanism of ganciclovir uptake by rabbit retina and human retinal pigmented epithelium cell line ARPE-19. Curr Eye Res 2004; 29(2-3): 127-36.

[119] Gao B, Wenzel A, Grimm C, *et al*. Localization of organic anion transport protein 2 in the apical region of rat retinal pigment epithelium. Invest Ophthalmol Vis Sci 2002; 43(2): 510-4.

[120] Ito A, Yamaguchi K, Onogawa T, *et al*. Distribution of organic anion-transporting polypeptide 2 (oatp2) and oatp3 in the rat retina. Invest Ophthalmol Vis Sci 2002; 43(3): 858-63.

[121] Tomi M, Hosoya K. Application of magnetically isolated rat retinal vascular endothelial cells for the determination of transporter gene expression levels at the inner blood-retinal barrier. J Neurochem 2004; 91(5): 1244-8.

[122] Hosoya K, Makihara A, Tsujikawa Y, *et al*. Roles of inner blood-retinal barrier organic anion transporter 3 in the vitreous/retina-to-blood efflux transport of p-aminohippuric acid, benzylpenicillinand 6-mercaptopurine. J Pharmacol Exp Ther 2009; 329(1): 87-93.

[123] Rajan PD, Kekuda R, Chancy CD, *et al*. Expression of the extraneuronal monoamine transporter in RPE and neural retina. Curr Eye Res 2000; 20(3): 195-204.

[124] Umapathy NS, Gnana-Prakasam JP, Martin PM, *et al*. Cloning and functional characterization of the proton-coupled electrogenic folate transporter and analysis of its expression in retinal cell types. Invest Ophthalmol Vis Sci 2007; 48(11): 5299-305.

[125] Chancy CD, Kekuda R, Huang W, *et al*. Expression and differential polarization of the reduced-folate transporter-1 and the folate receptor alpha in mammalian retinal pigment epithelium. J Biol Chem 2000; 275(27): 20676-84.

[126] Bridges CC, El-Sherbeny A, Ola MS, *et al*. Transcellular transfer of folate across the retinal pigment epithelium. Curr Eye Res 2002; 24(2): 129-38.

[127] Naggar H, Van Ells TK, Ganapathy V, Smith SB. Regulation of reduced-folate transporter-1 in retinal pigment epithelial cells by folate. Curr Eye Res 2005; 30(1): 35-44.

[128] Kansara V, Luo S, Balasubrahmanyam B, *et al*. Biotin uptake and cellular translocation in human derived retinoblastoma cell line (Y-79): a role of hSMVT system. Int J Pharm 2006; 312(1-2): 43-52.

[129] Kansara V, Pal D, Jain R, *et al*. Identification and functional characterization of riboflavin transporter in human-derived retinoblastoma cell line (Y-79): mechanisms of cellular uptake and translocation. J Ocul Pharmacol Ther 2005; 21(4): 275-87.

[130] Patel K TS, Pal D, Mitra AK. Identification and characterization of Riboflavin transport system in rabbit retina and ARPE-19 cell line, AAPS-2005.

[131] Shen J, Cross ST, Tang-Liu DD, Welty DF. Evaluation of an immortalized retinal endothelial cell line as an *in vitro* model for drug transport studies across the blood-retinal barrier. Pharm Res 2003; 20(9): 1357-63.

[132] Constable PA, Lawrenson JG, Dolman DE, *et al*. P-Glycoprotein expression in human retinal pigment epithelium cell lines. Exp Eye Res 2006; 83(1): 24-30.

[133] Steuer H, Jaworski A, Elger B, *et al*. Functional characterization and comparison of the outer blood-retina barrier and the blood-brain barrier. Invest Ophthalmol Vis Sci 2005; 46(3): 1047-53.

[134] Hendig D, Langmann T, Zarbock R, *et al*. Characterization of the ATP-binding cassette transporter gene expression profile in Y79: a retinoblastoma cell line. Mol Cell Biochem 2009; 328(1-2): 85-92.

[135] Asashima T, Hori S, Ohtsuki S, *et al*. ATP-binding cassette transporter G2 mediates the efflux of phototoxins on the luminal membrane of retinal capillary endothelial cells. Pharm Res 2006; 23(6): 1235-42.

[136] Tsao CC, Coulter SJ, Chien A, *et al.* Identification and localization of five CYP2Cs in murine extrahepatic tissues and their metabolism of arachidonic acid to regio- and stereoselective products. J Pharmacol Exp Ther 2001; 299(1): 39-47.

[137] Waltman S, Sears M. Catechol-O-Methyl Transferase and Monoamine Oxidase Activity in the Ocular Tissues of Albino Rabbits. Invest Ophthalmol 1964; 3: 601-5.

[138] Sanchez-Chavez G, Salceda R. Acetyl- and butyrylcholinesterase in normal and diabetic rat retina. Neurochem Res 2001; 26(2): 153-9.

[139] Sanchez-Chavez G, Salceda R. Acetyl- and butyrylcholinesterase molecular forms in normal and streptozotocin-diabetic rat retinal pigment epithelium. Neurochem Int. 2001; 39(3): 209-15.

[140] Saneto RP, Awasthi YC, Srivastava SK. Glutathione S-transferases of the bovine retina. Evidence that glutathione peroxidase activity is the result of glutathione S-transferase. Biochem J 1982; 205(1): 213-7.

[141] Saneto RP, Awasthi YC, Srivastava SK. Mercapturic acid pathway enzymes in bovine ocular lens, cornea, retina and retinal pigmented epithelium. Exp Eye Res 1982; 35(2): 107-11.

Send Orders of Reprints at reprints@benthamscience.net

CHAPTER 5

Biodegradable Polymers for Ophthalmic Applications

Viral Tamboli[#], Sulabh Patel[#], Gyan P. Mishra[#] and Ashim K. Mitra[*]

Division of Pharmaceutical Sciences, School of Pharmacy, University of Missouri-Kansas City, 2464 Charlotte Street, Kansas City, MO 64108-2718, USA

Abstract: Biodegradable polymers (both synthetic and natural) have been extensively explored for ophthalmic applications. These biomaterials are mainly biocompatible and biodegradable in nature. Moreover, different biodegradable polymers have different physico-chemical properties which can further be modulated to formulate desirable drug products. A wide range of ocular drug delivery systems such as implants, inserts, corneal shields, contact lenses, micelles, nanoparticles, microparticles, liposomes, dendrimers and stimuli sensitive hydrogels can be formulated with biodegradable polymers. Moreover, controlled drug delivery systems made up of biodegradable polymers can deliver a variety of therapeutic molecules including hydrophilic and hydrophobic small and macromolecules for prolonged periods to the targeted ocular tissues. In this chapter, we reviewed various synthetic and natural biodegradable polymers applied to ocular drug delivery.

Keywords: Alginates, biodegradable polymers, chitosan, collagen, fibrin, gelatin, hyaluronic acid, poly alkyl cyanoacrylates, poly amino acids, poly anhydrides, poly caprolactone, polyester, polyglycolide, polylactide, poly (lactide-co-glycolide), polysaccharides.

INTRODUCTION

Biodegradable polymers appear to have numerous applications in the field of ocular drug delivery and can be classified as natural or synthetic polymers. Applications of polyglycolide (PGA) as suture material in late 1960 provided an impetus for the design and development of novel synthetic biodegradable polymers. Synthetic biodegradable polymers can be tailored to various compositions and molecular weights which can regulate degradation of polymer.

*Address correspondence to Ashim K. Mitra: University of Missouri Curators' Professor of Pharmacy, Chairman, Division of Pharmaceutical Sciences, Vice-Provost for Interdisciplinary Research, University of Missouri - Kansas City, School of Pharmacy, 2464 Charlotte Street, Kansas City, MO 64108, USA; Tel: 816-235-1615: Fax: 816-235-5779; E-mail: mitraa@umkc.edu
[#]All authors have contributed equally in this work.

Biodegradable polymers generally undergo homogenous or heterogeneous erosion. Homogenous erosion, commonly referred as bulk erosion, involves hydrolytic cleavage of complete cross-section of polymer matrix. Degradation rate of bulk eroding polymers is slower and varies from several weeks to years. Polymers of poly (α-hydroxyl esters) usually undergo bulk erosion and follow first order degradation kinetics. Polyesters show complex patterns of no significant degradation in initial phase followed by rapid mass loss [1, 2]. Hydrolytic degradation rate of polyesters depends on their molecular weight and crystallinity. Low molecular weight poly- (lactic-co-glycolic acid) (PLGA) degrades at a faster rate than high molecular weight PLGA [3]. Heterogeneous degradation is generally referred to as surface erosion. This process is much more rapid than homogenous degradation due to slower diffusion of water molecules into polymer matrix. Drug release from a bulk eroding polymer depends upon swelling, diffusion and hydrolytic degradation in contrast to surface eroding polymers, which primarily depend on hydrolytic degradation. Heterogeneous erosion occurs primarily in faster degrading polymers such as polyanhydrides and poly-(ortho esters) [4].

SYNTHETIC BIODEGRADABLE POLYMERS

Polyesters

Polyesters are biodegradable polymers with short aliphatic ester linked backbone. These classes of polymers are generally produced by either ring opening or condensation polymerization. Ring opening polymerization (ROP) is preferred over condensation to produce high molecular weight polyesters. Homo or co-polymers of cyclic lactones and anhydrides having narrow molecular weight distribution can be produced *via* ROP. The molecular weight of final polymer can be controlled by varying the ratio of monomers. The molecular weight of the polyesters regulates the hydrolytic cleavage that follows bulk erosion kinetics to produce metabolic products which are eliminated through normal metabolic and renal pathways [5]. The hydrolytic degradation rate of the polymers can be altered by adjusting the molecular weight, crystallinity and structure of the polymeric chains. Among polyesters, poly-α-hydroxy esters are the most broadly investigated class of polymers for ocular drug delivery applications. This mainly includes poly (glycolic acid) (PGA), poly (lactic acid) (PLA) and their copolymers.

Polyglycolide (PGA)

PGA (Fig. **1**) is a relatively hydrophilic polymer compared to other polyesters with high crystallinity and low solubility in organic solvents. PGA can easily be synthesized *via* ring opening polymerization (Fig. **2**). Low solubility in organic solvent is attributed to higher tensile modulus. The polymer has a high melting point of 225 °C and glass transition temperature of 36 °C. It has a comparatively faster degradation rate than other polyesters and this polymer generates glycine upon degradation, which eventually eliminates through the citric acid cycle. Major loss in mechanical strength of PGA usually occurs in one to two months. However the polymer completely degrades within six to twelve months. PGA was initially explored for developing sutures because of their fiber-forming properties and excellent mechanical strength. However, it has limited role in ocular drug delivery due to faster degradation rate and higher crystallinity. PGA implants can easily be fabricated by widely applicable processing techniques such as solvent casting, compression and extrusion techniques. Processing technique utilized for the production of implant regulates the degradation properties of implant [6].

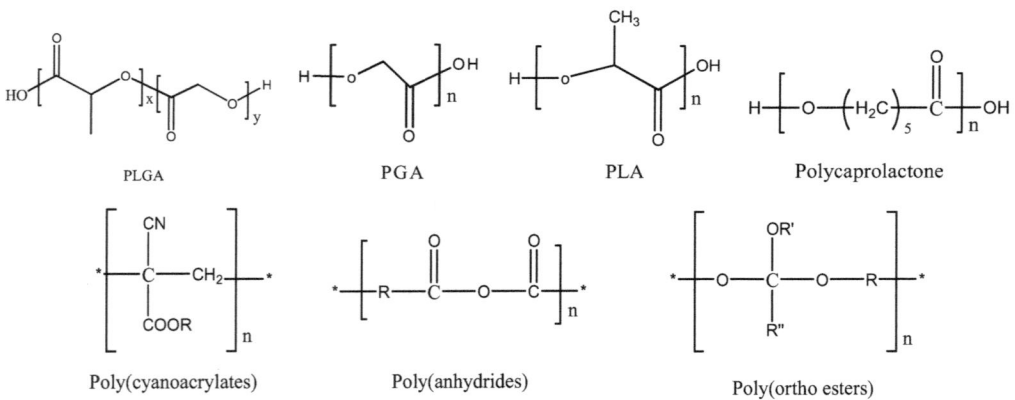

Figure 1: Structures of different synthetic biodegradable polymers.

Polylactide (PLA)

PLA is comparatively more hydrophobic than PGA due to the presence of additional methyl group (Fig. **1**). It is chiral in nature and commonly exists in three isomeric forms D (-), L (+) and racemic (D, L) lactide. The crystalline nature of PLA depends upon the isomeric forms and molecular weight of the polymer. Poly (L-lactide) (PLLA) is crystalline in nature and hydrolyzed through normal metabolic pathway due to the presence of naturally occurring isomer (L-lactide). It has a melting point of 175 °C and glass transition temperature of 60–65 °C. The polymer also possesses a good tensile strength of 50–70 MPa and a high modulus of 4.8 GPa. On the other hand, poly (DL-lactide) (PDLLA) is amorphous in nature due to racemic mixture. It has glass transition temperature of 55-60 °C and comparatively faster degradation rate than PLLA. All isomeric forms of PLA follow bulk erosion kinetics and generate lactic acid upon hydrolytic cleavage [7]. PLA has been selected in some cases for ocular drug delivery applications. Bourges *et al.* evaluated the ocular kinetics of PLA nanoparticles loaded with Rh-6G (Rh) after intravitreal injection. The PLA nanoparticles found to be localized in RPE cells and released the encapsulated die for more than 4 months [8].

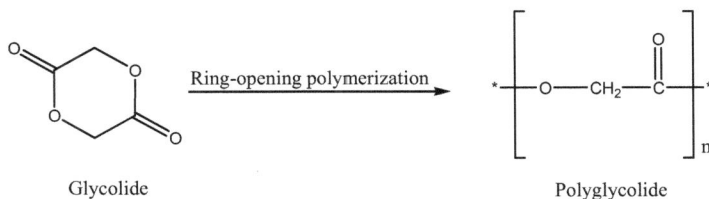

Glycolide   Ring-opening polymerization   Polyglycolide

Figure 2: Synthetic scheme of Polyglycolide.

Poly (Lactide-co-Glycolide) (PLGA)

Poly-lactide-co-glycolide, commonly known as PLGA is obtained by copolymerization of lactide and glycolide. This copolymer is hydrolytically less stable than the homopolymers, PLA or PGA. Extensive research on full range of these copolymers suggests their implication in drug delivery. These copolymers are divided into two main compositions, lactide and glycolide. PLGA follows bulk erosion kinetics and degradation depending on molecular weight and lactide to glycolide ratio. As the ratio of glycolide in copolymer decreases hydrolytic degradation rate also slows down. The intermediate PLGA *i.e.* 50:50 hydrolyses faster relative to PLGA 75:25 and PLGA 85:15. This polymer has been approved by FDA for human applications because of its excellent biocompatibility and controlled degradation profiles [9]. PLGA carries a overall negative charge and thus has non-mucoadhesive nature. Studies by Gupta *et al.* on sparfloxacin loaded PLGA nanoparticles suggest that smaller size nanoparticles improve spreading coefficient and retention time of the formulation [10]. PLGA was also utilized for the production of a drug eluting contact lens. Ciolino *et al.* investigated the role of pHEMA (poly [hydroxyethyl methacrylate]) coated PLGA films for the delivery of ciprofloxacin in the treatment of *staphylococcus aureus* associated ocular infections. This article reported zero-order release kinetics for a period of 4 weeks and concluded that PLGA derived contact lens could serve as a platform for ocular drug delivery [11]. PLGA based drug delivery systems are biodegradable in nature and do not require surgical removal, therefore provide better patient compliance. Post-operative inflammation and rise in intraocular pressure were observed following the application of triamcinolone loaded PLGA drug delivery systems [12].

Polycaprolactone (PCL)

PCL is a semicyrstalline polymer synthesized by ring opening polymerization of ε-caprolactone. It has a glass transition temperature of -60 °C and a melting temperature in the range of 59-64 °C. PCL was investigated for long term delivery due to higher drug permeability, excellent biocompatibility and extremely slow hydrolytic cleavage of polyester backbone. The PCL based Capronor® implant was developed for controlled delivery of levonorgestrel. It has a low tensile strength of 23 MPa and an extremely high elongation (more than 700%). Numerous attempts were made to improve slower degradation rate of PCL. Copolymers of ε-caprolactone with lactide or glycolide exhibit remarkably better degradation profile. Ocular bioavailability of cyclosporine A (Cy A) loaded PCL nanoparticles alone and coated with hyaluronic acid (HA) was evaluated. The investigators observed Cy A concentration of 5.9 - 15.5 ng/mg and 11.4-23.0 ng/mg in corneal tissues following administration of PCL nanoparticles and HA-coated PCL nanoparticles, respectively. Significantly higher Cy A levels were achieved in ocular tissues following application of nanoparticles relative to conventional eye drops, indicating significance of nanoparticles in the treatment of immune mediated corneal diseases [13]. Beeley *et al.* designed a triamcinolone acetonide (TA) loaded PCL implant for the treatment of retinal diseases. PCL implant was well tolerated in the sub-retinal space of rabbit eyes and TA release was observed for a period of four weeks [14].

Poly (Alkyl Cyanoacrylates) (PACA)

Poly (Alkyl Cyanoacrylates) PACA belongs to the class of acrylate polymers synthesized from alkyl cyanoacrylic monomers through anionic polymerization. Faster degradation rate of PACA was attributed to instability of carbon-carbon sigma bond and the presence of electron withdrawing neighboring groups. It has shown remarkable applicability as surgical glue and skin adhesive. PACA was also explored for the development of nanoparticles. PACA degradation rate varies from hours to days depends on the length of alkyl side chain. For example PACA having shorter alkyl chain length such as poly-methyl cyanoacrlates degrades in a few hours whereas higher alkyl chain length derivatives such as octyl and isobutylcyanoacrylates degrade slowly over days and months. Nanoparticles composed of PACA are advantageous in terms of fabrication and in drug delivery [15, 16]. Ocular tolerability and *in vivo* ocular bioavailability of PEG coated polyethyl-2-cyanoacrylate nanospheres loaded with ACV have been examined. PEG lowers the zeta potential of nanospheres from -25.9 mv to -12.2 mv. PEG coated nanospheres are well tolerated by ocular tissues and the study reported 25 fold raise in ocular bioavailability in comparison to drug alone [17]. Desai *et al*. fabricated pilocarpine loaded polyisobutyl cyanoacrylate (PIBCA) nanocapsules with drug loading of 13.5 % and size of 370 to 460 nm. This study reported that incorporation of 1.1 % pilocarpine nanocapsules in pluronic F127 gel generated higher mitotic response in albino rabbit eyes than the nanocapsules alone [18].

Polyanhydrides

Numerous studies elucidated the role of polyanhydrides (POA) for ocular drug delivery applications. These polymers exhibit faster degradation and limited mechanical strength, which render these compounds ideal candidates for fabrication of sustained release devices. Low molecular weight polyanhydrides were synthesized through dehydrative coupling and dehydrochlorination whereas melt polycondensation polymerization was employed for synthesis of high molecular weight polymers. Degradation rate of polyanhydrides can easily be modulated by changing the polymer composition depending upon the crystallinity and hydrophilicity of the polymer. These polymers undergo surface erosion and generate monomeric acid which is non toxic nature. Homo polyanhydrides have limited application in controlled drug delivery due to their crystalline nature. In contrast, copolymers such as poly [(carboxyphenoxy)propane–sebacic acid (PCPP-SA) demonstrated controlled degradation rate [19]. This polymer was approved by FDA for human applications for the delivery of carmustine in the treatment of brain cancer [20]. Other approaches based on aromatic co-monomers composed of hydrophobic aliphatic liner fatty acid were also investigated for drug delivery applications [21].

Poly (Ortho Esters)

Poly (ortho ester) (POE) is a hydrophobic polymer composed of hydrolytically unstable polyester linkage. However, these polymers exhibit slower degradation due to surface erosion. Such degradation kinetics is ideal for designing sustained release devices. Polymer degradation profile can easily be adjusted by varying diols for polymerization [22]. POE is hydrolytically unstable in acidic conditions and requires basic additives to inhibit autocatalysis. The first generation POE was developed by ALZA Corporation. This polymer was synthesized by trans-esterification reaction of diol with diethoxytetrahydrofuran [23]. Degradation profile of POE II can easily be altered by incorporation of acidic additives such as adipic acid. POE III upon hydrolysis generates diol and pentaerythriol dipropionate, which subsequently generate proponic acid and pentaerythriol. This class of polymers is biocompatible and follows pH dependent degradation kinetics. The polymers do not require organic solvent for drug incorporation due to semisolid nature. However, difficulties in scale up process limit its application in drug delivery. Modification of second generation polyester (POE II) with smaller chain of lactic or glycolic acid leads to the development of POE IV. This polymer upon hydrolysis liberates acids which further catalyzes polymer degradation. Physical form and degradation rate of the polymer can be easily altered by changing diols and acid segment respectively. POE IV demonstrated excellent biocompatibility for controlled delivery application [24-26]. In a recent study by Polak *et al.* controlled delivery of 5- flurouracil and 5-chlorouracil was attempted utilizing POE in the treatment of glaucoma filtration surgery. The researchers observed rise in intraocular pressure and bulb persistence after injecting the POE formulation into subconjunctival space. In addition, histological analysis revealed functioning bulb and no damage to the conjunctival epithelium. Investigators concluded that POE formulation is effective in patients undergoes glaucoma filtration surgery [27]. Einmahl *et al.* suggested POE IV biocompatibility after intraocular administrations through various routes such as subconjunctival, intracaramel and intravitreal injections [28, 29].

NATURAL BIODEGRADABLE POLYMERS

Proteins and Poly (Amino Acids)

Proteins/amino acid polymers are arranged in a three-dimensional folded structure. These biomaterials (a pharmacologically and systematically inert substance designed to incorporate with or within the living systems) constitute major components of natural tissues. Therefore these polymers are widely investigated for the development of delivery systems and also for biomedical applications such as sutures, haemostatic agents and scaffolds. Protein based biomaterials are known to possess low antigenicity, good biocompatibility and excellent biodegradability. Protein and polypeptides such as collagen, gelatin and fibrin are widely explored in the development of ophthalmic drug delivery systems.

Collagen

Among all vertebral proteins, approximately 30% is collagen. It is a major component of skin and musculoskeletal tissues, consisting of more than 50% of the extracellular skin proteins and 90% in the tendon and bones. It is a rod like polymer structure, with 2600 – 26000Å in length and 15Å in diameter [30]. Twenty two different types of collagen have been identified in the human body. These polymers are varying in compositions and size of the helix as well as non helical portions. In general, collagen is comprised of a unique triple-helix structure of three polypeptide subunits, which are commonly known as α chain. Out of twenty two different collagens, Types I – IV are the most commonly used. Type I collagen is composed of three polypeptide chains and each chain carries 1050 amino acids. These polypeptide subunits are composed of similar repeating amino acids *i.e.*, proline (25%), hydroxylproline (25%), glycine (33%) and comparable amounts of lysine. Collagen is resistant to neutral protease, which might be due to its role as structural protein in the body. At neutral pH, it undergoes enzymatic degradation *via* metalloproteinase and collagenases [31].

Collagen is the most extensively studied natural polymer in biomedical applications because of its biodegradability, high mechanical strength, low antigenicity and good physicochemical properties. Mechanical, biological and degradation properties can be easily tailored by enzymatic pretreatment or cross linking with different cross linkers [32]. Many attempts have been made to develop this polymer as a drug carrier system in a number of biomedical applications such as, tumor treatment [33-35], tissue engineering [36-38], ophthalmology, wound treatment and burn dressings [39].

Collagen is the most widely studied natural polymer for ophthalmic applications such as grafts for corneal replacement, suture materials, bandage lenses, punctual plugs and viscous solutions for the replacement of vitreous [31]. It is also explored for the formulation of inserts, shields, particles and gels. Concept of ocular drug delivery using collagen inserts was initiated in early 1970s. Studies were conducted to fabricate drug loaded inserts prepared from an air dried mixture of drug and collagen. Pilocarpine loaded inserts demonstrated delayed release of pilocarpine with no inflammatory responses even after complete degradation of collagen [40]. After ocular administration of collagen inserts loaded with gentamicin, maximum drug concentration was observed in tear film and other ocular tissues relative to topical drops, ointment and subconjunctival administration of gentamicin [41]. In the 1980's, collagen shields had been introduced as an ocular delivery system for antibiotics. Collagen films are very thin and can take the shape of the cornea. It allows oxygen perfusion for regular corneal metabolism and also acts as a corneal bandage [42, 43]. Collagen shields are often studied with antibiotics such as tobramycin [42,44,45], polymyxin B sulfate [46], trimethoprim [46], amphotericin B [47], vancomycin [48] and gentamicin [41,48,49]. Moreover steroids [49], pilocarpine [50] and flurbiprofen sodium [50] have also been formulated with collagen shields.

Gelatin

Gelatin is collagen derived non-antigenic, biodegradable and biocompatible natural polymer with numerous pharmaceutical and biomedical applications. It contains large amounts of glycine, proline and 4 hydroxyproline residues [51]. Gelatin is a denatured protein, which can be obtained by acid or alkali pretreatment of collagen. Two types of gelatin are commercially available, type A and type B. Type A gelatin is derived by acid treatment of collagen while type B is derived by alkali treatment and therefore the isoelectric point of type A gelatin lies between 7-9 and for gelatin type B it is within 4-5 [51]. Hori *et al.*, have investigated the ability of gelatin hydrogel to deliver growth factors in the conjunctival sac of mice. This study also examined the release profile of growth factors [52]. Results showed that gelatin hydrogel undergoes slow biodegradation and controls the release of growth factors for upto 7 days. Applications of gelatin as hydrogel, nanoparticles and lyophilisates have indicated its ability to deliver a wide variety of small (hydrophilic and hydrophobic) and large molecules (epidermal growth factors, proteins) in ocular diseases.

Fibrin

Fibrinogen is plasma soluble protein, which releases insoluble fibrin peptides after degradation in the presence of thrombin. The fibrin peptides aggregate to produce insoluble meshwork of fibrin, which is capable of entrapping drug or any biological molecules. Ionic strength, pH and concentrations of calcium, fibrinogen and thrombin are important factors that alter the properties of fibrin meshwork. Fibrin sealant is a FDA approved biodegradable surgical adhesive and it has been investigated as an ocular drug delivery device [53]. Carboplatin loaded fibrin sealant was evaluated for the targeted and sustained ocular delivery [54]. Properties of fibrin can be easily tailored by changing the concentration of thrombin and fibrinogen. It is constituted from human proteins and therefore it is associated with very low immunogenicity and foreign matter reactions. Nevertheless, it can incorporate drug concentration above its solubility levels, as well as it can control and target drug release. These advantages render this material a more promising natural polymer for ocular delivery.

Polysaccharides

Many monosaccharide units joined together by glycosidic linkages produce polysaccharides. Polysaccharides are generating interest as biomaterials due to unique biological functions ranging from immune recognition to cell signaling. In addition, their biodegradability, physicochemical properties, commercial availability and mechanical ability to fabricate in appropriate structure render this polymer group one of the most significant natural polymers. Polysaccharides from the non-human (chitosan and alginic acid) and human origins (hyaluronic acid) are one of the most widely explored material as ocular drug delivery carriers (Fig. **3**).

Chitosan

Chitosan is a deacetylated form of chitin, composed of α (1-4)-2-amino-2deoxy β-D-glucan (Fig. **3**). Chitin is the second most abundant natural polymer. It is biodegradable, biocompatible, non-antigenic, non-toxic and bifunctional in nature, which make chitosan a very interesting biomaterial for application in ophthalmic drug delivery. The degree of deacetylation for commercially available chitosan usually ranges between 70% to 95% and molecular weight ranges within 10 to 1000 kDa [55]. Chitosan is a cationic polysaccharide with pseudoplastic and viscoelastic properties [56]. It facilitates retention and permits easy spreading of the solution with blinking. Because of its cationic nature, the polymer strongly interacts with negatively charged ophthalmic fluid (mucin)and increases precorneal retention. However, besides the electrostatic and hydrophobic interactions, hydrogen bonding also plays a critical role in this process [57, 58]. Chitosan can improve permeability of therapeutic agents through paracellular route by opening tight junctions located between epithelial cells [59, 60]. Some authors have also reported the role of intracellular routes in the enhancement of cellular permeability [61]. Chitosan is a good emulsifier, which not only stabilizes the emulsion but also prevents coalescence by stearic and electrostatic repulsions [62].

Incorporation of biomaterials into chitosan leads to the development of nanostructures with improved property. A rational mixture of chitosan with phospholipids not only increases the stability of nanostructure in biological fluids but it is also suitable for entrapment of labile macromolecules [63]. Chitosan-lipid complexes can efficiently interact with ocular tissues, without compromising the integrity of membrane structure [63]. This liposome system has excellent transfection efficiency and has already yielded promising results in ocular gene therapy. Chitosan is widely explored as a potential gene carrier for ocular delivery because of its ability to complex with negatively charged nucleic acids. Hybrid nanostructure of chitosan with hyaluronic acid was also investigated for ocular delivery of macromolecules [64]. Recently, Motwani *et al.* have reported application of gatifloxacin loaded alginate-chitosan nanoparticles in the treatment of ocular infections [65].

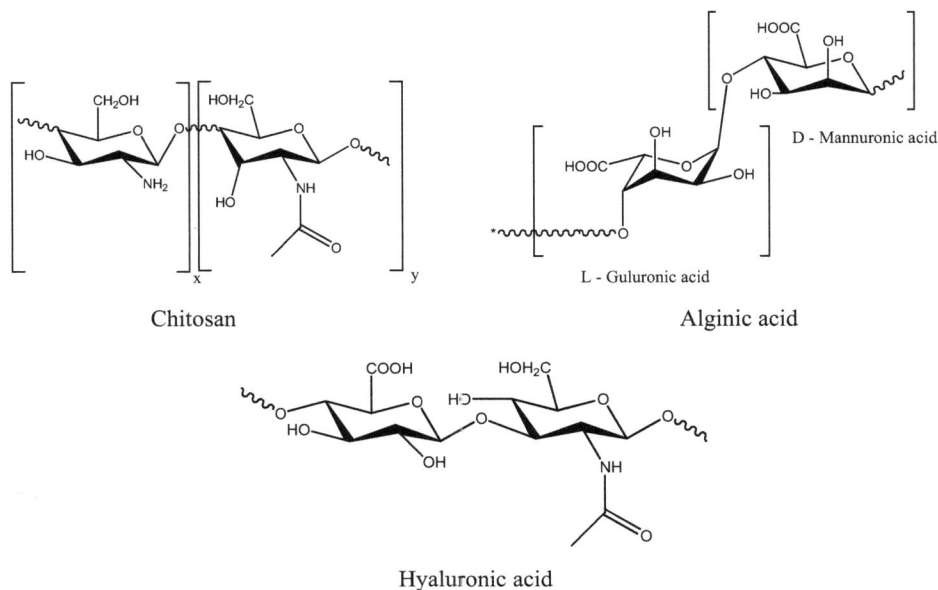

Figure 3: Chemical structures of natural biodegradable polymers.

Alginates

Alginate is one of the most studied polysaccharide in tissue engineering and drug delivery. Laminaria hyperborean, Ascophyllumnodosum and Macrocystispyrifera are the main sources of alginates. Sodium alginate is a water soluble linear block copolymer (Fig. **3**) of β-D mannuronic acid monomers (M block) and α-L guluronic acid (G block) [55]. Most interestingly, alginate can form gels by interacting with divalent cations such as Ca^{++}, Sr^{++} or Ba^{++}. Tear fluid is full of ions and therefore *in situ* gelling may be possible by the application of drug loaded sodium alginate solution to the eye [66]. Koelwel *et al.* have examined different alginate inserts containing epidermal growth factor in human [67]. Abraham *et al.* have prepared *in situ* gelling formulation of ofloxacin containing sodium alginate solution [68]. The formulation controlled the release of ofloxacin upto 8 hours. Carteolol is a β adrenoceptor antagonist, which is prescribed for twice a day application (topical eye drops) to reduce intra ocular pressure associated with glaucoma. Alginate solution (1%) containing carteolol sustained drug release and reduced dosing frequency to once a day. Investigators have reported that newly formulated alginate carteolol solution was effective in maintaining therapeutic levels upto 24 h, with no side effects [69].

Hyaluronic Acid

Hyaluronic acid (HA) exists as a polyanion under physiological conditions and thus it is referred as hyaluronan. It was first discovered in bovine vitreous humor by Meyer and Palmer in 1934. Weissman and Meyer reported precise structure of HA, which consists of repeating units of N-acetyl-D-glucosamine and D-glucoronic acid (Fig. **3**) [70]. The molecular weight of HA mainly depends on the source. Refinement of isolation processes produce several grades of HA with molecular weights upto 5,000 kDa [71]. HA has been studied more extensively for its chemical, physiological and biological properties. It has a wide range of cosmetic, medical and pharmaceutical applications, due to its biocompatible, biodegradable, non-immunogenic and viscoelastic nature. HA has been extensively investigated for the development of drug carrier systems in dermal, nasal, pulmonary, parenteral, ophthalmic and gene delivery [70]. Viscoelestic and mucoadhesive nature make HA an excellent vehicle in ophthalmic drug delivery [72, 73]. It enhances viscosity of formulation and prolongs precorneal residence time and improves ocular bioavailability. Numerous studies reported that incorporation of pilocarpine in HA formulation had significantly improved ocular bioavailability [74-77]. Saettone *et al.* and Harrero-vanrell *et al.* indicated higher bioavailability of tropicamide when formulated with HA as an ophthalmic vehicle [78]. Similarly, enhanced bioavailability of gentamicin [79,80], tobramycin [81] and timolol [81] has also been reported in various studies.

CONCLUSIONS

During the last two decades biodegradable polymeric materials have been explored for the development of various controlled drug delivery systems in the ophthalmology. Various polymeric drug delivery systems have been explored for anterior and posterior chamber diseases such as liposomes, nanoparticles, dendrimers, microparticles, environment sensitive gels (temperature, pH and ionic strength), implants, inserts, shields, nanosuspensions and nanoemulsions. An efficient drug delivery system requires biomaterials with specific chemical, physical, biomechanical, biological and biodegradation properties along with very high biocompatibility. Development of various novel biodegradable polymers is now possible due to advancement in bioprocesses and synthetic organic chemistry. The success of novel ocular drug delivery systems lies in the ability of scientists to design of biomaterials with appropriate biological and pharmacological responses.

ACKNOWLEDGEMENTS

We would like to acknowledge NIH grants R01EY09171-16 and R01EY010659-14 for financial support.

CONFLICT OF INTEREST

The author(s) confirm that this chapter content has no conflict of interest.

REFERENCES

[1]   Pulapura S, Kohn J. Trends in the development of bioresorbable polymers for medical applications. J Biomater Appl. 1992; 6(3): 216-50.
[2]   Lee KB, Yoon KR, Woo SI, Choi IS. Surface modification of poly(glycolic acid) (PGA) for biomedical applications. J Pharm Sci 2003; 92(5): 933-7.
[3]   Lu L, Peter SJ, Lyman MD, Lai HL, Leite SM, Tamada JA. *In vitro* and *in vivo* degradation of porous poly(DL-lactic-co-glycolic acid) foams. Biomaterials 2000; 21(18): 1837-45.
[4]   Jain JP, Chitkara D, Kumar N. Polyanhydrides as localized drug delivery carrier: an update. Expert Opin Drug Deliv 2008; 5(8): 889-907.
[5]   Middleton JC, Tipton AJ. Synthetic biodegradable polymers as orthopedic devices. Biomaterials 2000; 21(23): 2335-46.
[6]   Jain R, Shah NH, Malick AW, Rhodes CT. Controlled drug delivery by biodegradable poly(ester) devices: different preparative approaches. Drug Dev Ind Pharm 1998; 24(8): 703-27.
[7]   Hyon SH, Jamshidi K, Ikada Y. Synthesis of polylactides with different molecular weights. Biomaterials 1997; 18(22): 1503-8.
[8]   Bourges JL, Gautier SE, Delie F, Bejjani RA, Jeanny JC, Gurny R. Ocular drug delivery targeting the retina and retinal pigment epithelium using polylactide nanoparticles. Invest Ophthalmol Vis Sci 2003; 44(8): 3562-9.

[9]   Lu JM, Wang X, Marin-Muller C, *et al.* Current advances in research and clinical applications of PLGA-based nanotechnology. Expert Rev Mol Diagn 2009; 9(4): 325-41.

[10]   Gupta H, Aqil M, Khar RK, Ali A, Bhatnagar A, Mittal G. Sparfloxacin-loaded PLGA nanoparticles for sustained ocular drug delivery. Nanomedicine 2010; 6(2): 324-33.

[11]   Ciolino JB, Hoare TR, Iwata NG, Behlau I, Dohlman CH, Langer R. A drug-eluting contact lens. Invest Ophthalmol Vis Sci 2009; 50(7): 3346-52.

[12]   Eperon S, Bossy-Nobs L, Petropoulos IK, Gurny R, Guex-Crosier Y. A biodegradable drug delivery system for the treatment of postoperative inflammation. Int J Pharm 2008; 352(1-2): 240-7.

[13]   Yenice I, Mocan MC, Palaska E, Bochot A, Bilensoy E, Vural I. Hyaluronic acid coated poly-epsilon-caprolactone nanospheres deliver high concentrations of cyclosporine A into the cornea. Exp Eye Res 2008; 87(3): 162-7.

[14]   Beeley NR, Rossi JV, Mello-Filho PA, Mahmoud MI, Fujii GY, de Juan E, Jr. Fabrication, implantation, elution and retrieval of a steroid-loaded polycaprolactone subretinal implant. J Biomed Mater Res A 2005; 73(4): 437-44.

[15]   Arias JL, Ruiz MA, Lopez-Viota M, Delgado AV. Poly(alkylcyanoacrylate) colloidal particles as vehicles for antitumour drug delivery: a comparative study. Colloids Surf B Biointerfaces 2008; 62(1): 64-70.

[16]   Arias JL, Gallardo V, Ruiz MA, Delgado AV. Magnetite/poly(alkylcyanoacrylate) (core/shell) nanoparticles as 5-Fluorouracil delivery systems for active targeting. Eur J Pharm Biopharm 2008; 69(1): 54-63.

[17]   Fresta M, Fontana G, Bucolo C, Cavallaro G, Giammona G, Puglisi G. Ocular tolerability and *in vivo* bioavailability of poly(ethylene glycol) (PEG)-coated polyethyl-2-cyanoacrylate nanosphere-encapsulated acyclovir. J Pharm Sci 2001; 90(3): 288-97.

[18]   Desai SD, Blanchard J. Pluronic F127-based ocular delivery system containing biodegradable polyisobutylcyanoacrylate nanocapsules of pilocarpine. Drug Deliv 2000; 7(4): 201-7.

[19]   Tamargo RJ, Epstein JI, Reinhard CS, Chasin M, Brem H. Brain biocompatibility of a biodegradable, controlled-release polymer in rats. J Biomed Mater Res 1989; 23(2): 253-66.

[20]   Brem H. Polymers to treat brain tumours. Biomaterials 1990; 11(9): 699-701.

[21]   Kumar N, Langer RS, Domb AJ. Polyanhydrides: an overview. Adv Drug Deliv Rev 2002; 54(7): 889-910.

[22]   Tang R, Palumbo RN, Ji W, Wang C. Poly(ortho ester amides): acid-labile temperature-responsive copolymers for potential biomedical applications. Biomacromolecules 2009; 10(4): 722-7.

[23]   Heller J, Barr J, Ng SY, Abdellauoi KS, Gurny R. Poly(ortho esters): synthesis, characterization, properties and uses. Adv Drug Deliv Rev 2002; 54(7): 1015-39.

[24]   Einmahl S, Capancioni S, Schwach-Abdellaoui K, Moeller M, Behar-Cohen F, Gurny R. Therapeutic applications of viscous and injectable poly(ortho esters). Adv Drug Deliv Rev 2001; 53(1): 45-73.

[25]   Heller J, Barr J, Ng SY, Shen HR, Schwach-Abdellaoui K, Einmahl S. Poly(ortho esters) - their development and some recent applications. Eur J Pharm Biopharm 2000; 50(1): 121-8.

[26]   Heller J. Ocular delivery using poly(ortho esters). Adv Drug Deliv Rev 2005; 57(14): 2053-62.

[27]   Polak MB, Valamanesh F, Felt O, *et al.* Controlled delivery of 5-chlorouracil using poly(ortho esters) in filtering surgery for glaucoma. Invest Ophthalmol Vis Sci 2008; 49(7): 2993-3003.

[28]   Einmahl S, Behar-Cohen F, D'Hermies F, *et al.* A new poly(ortho ester)-based drug delivery system as an adjunct treatment in filtering surgery. Invest Ophthalmol Vis Sci 2001; 42(3): 695-700.

[29]   Einmahl S, Ponsart S, Bejjani RA, *et al.* Ocular biocompatibility of a poly(ortho ester) characterized by autocatalyzed degradation. J Biomed Mater Res A 2003; 67(1): 44-53.

[30]   Chvapil M, Kronenthal L, Van Winkle W, Jr. Medical and surgical applications of collagen. Int Rev Connect Tissue Res 1973; 6: 1-61.

[31]   Friess W. Collagen--biomaterial for drug delivery. Eur J Pharm Biopharm 1998; 45(2): 113-36.

[32]   Kuwano M, Horibe Y, Kawashima Y. Effect of collagen cross-linking in collagen corneal shields on ocular drug delivery. J Ocul Pharmacol Ther 1997; 13(1): 31-40.

[33]   Sutton R, Yu N, Luck E, Brown D, Conley F. Reduction of vinblastine neurotoxicity in mice utilizing a collagen matrix carrier. Sel Cancer Ther 1990; 6(1): 35-49.

[34]   Davidson BS, Izzo F, Cromeens DM, Stephens LC, Siddik ZH, Curley SA. Collagen matrix cisplatin prevents local tumor growth after margin-positive resection. J Surg Res 1995; 58(6): 618-24.

[35]   Ning S, Trisler K, Brown DM, *et al.* Intratumoral radioimmunotherapy of a human colon cancer xenograft using a sustained-release gel. Radiother Oncol 1996; 39(2): 179-89.

[36]   Royce PM, Kato T, Ohsaki K, Miura A. The enhancement of cellular infiltration and vascularisation of a collagenous dermal implant in the rat by platelet-derived growth factor BB. J Dermatol Sci 1995; 10(1): 42-52.

[37]   Lepisto J, Kujari H, Niinikoski J, Laato M. Effects of heterodimeric isoform of platelet-derived growth factor PDGF-AB on wound healing in the rat. Eur Surg Res 1994; 26(5): 267-72.

[38]   Tweden KS, Spadone DP, Terranova VP. Neovascularization of surface demineralized dentin. J Periodontol 1989; 60(8): 460-6.

[39]   Slavin J, Nash JR, Kingsnorth AN. Effect of transforming growth factor beta and basic fibroblast growth factor on steroid-impaired healing intestinal wounds. Br J Surg 1992; 79(1): 69-72.

[40]   Rubin AL, Stenzel KH, Miyata T, White MJ, Dunn M. Collagen as a vehicle for drug delivery. Preliminary report. J Clin Pharmacol 1973;13(8): 309-12.

[41]   Bloomfield SE, Miyata T, Dunn MW, Bueser N, Stenzel KH, Rubin AL. Soluble gentamicin ophthalmic inserts as a drug delivery system. Arch Ophthalmol 1978; 96(5): 885-7.

[42]   Poland DE, Kaufman HE. Clinical uses of collagen shields. J Cataract Refract Surg 1988; 14(5): 489-91.

[43]   Robin JB, Keys CL, Kaminski LA, Viana MA. The effect of collagen shields on rabbit corneal reepithelialization after chemical debridement. Invest Ophthalmol Vis Sci 1990; 31(7): 1294-300.

[44]   Unterman SR, Rootman DS, Hill JM, Parelman JJ, Thompson HW, Kaufman HE. Collagen shield drug delivery: therapeutic concentrations of tobramycin in the rabbit cornea and aqueous humor. J Cataract Refract Surg 1988; 14(5): 500-4.

[45] O'Brien TP, Sawusch MR, Dick JD, Hamburg TR, Gottsch JD. Use of collagen corneal shields *vs.* soft contact lenses to enhance penetration of topical tobramycin. J Cataract Refract Surg 1988; 14(5): 505-7.

[46] Palmer RM, McDonald MB. A corneal lens/shield system to promote postoperative corneal epithelial healing. J Cataract Refract Surg 1995; 21(2): 125-6.

[47] Schwartz SD, Harrison SA, Engstrom RE, Jr., Bawdon RE, Lee DA, Mondino BJ. Collagen shield delivery of amphotericin B. Am J Ophthalmol 1990; 109(6): 701-4.

[48] Phinney RB, Schwartz SD, Lee DA, Mondino BJ. Collagen-shield delivery of gentamicin and vancomycin. Arch Ophthalmol 1988; 106(11): 1599-604.

[49] Milani JK, Verbukh I, Pleyer U, *et al.* Collagen shields impregnated with gentamicin-dexamethasone as a potential drug delivery device. Am J Ophthalmol 1993; 116(5): 622-7.

[50] Aquavella JV, Ruffini JJ, LoCascio JA. Use of collagen shields as a surgical adjunct. J Cataract Refract Surg 1988; 14(5): 492-5.

[51] Malafaya PB, Silva GA, Reis RL. Natural-origin polymers as carriers and scaffolds for biomolecules and cell delivery in tissue engineering applications. Adv Drug Deliv Rev 2007; 59(4-5): 207-33.

[52] Hori K, Sotozono C, Hamuro J, *et al.* Controlled-release of epidermal growth factor from cationized gelatin hydrogel enhances corneal epithelial wound healing. J Control Release 2007; 118(2): 169-76.

[53] Tsui JY, Dalgard C, Van Quill KR, *et al.* Subconjunctival topotecan in fibrin sealant in the treatment of transgenic murine retinoblastoma. Invest Ophthalmol Vis Sci 2008; 49(2): 490-6.

[54] Pardue MT, Hejny C, Gilbert JA, *et al.* Retinal function after subconjunctival injection of carboplatin in fibrin sealant. Retina 2004; 24(5): 776-82.

[55] George M, Abraham TE. Polyionic hydrocolloids for the intestinal delivery of protein drugs: alginate and chitosan--a review. J Control Release 2006; 114(1): 1-14.

[56] Wang W, Xu D. Viscosity and flow properties of concentrated solutions of chitosan with different degrees of deacetylation. Int J Biol Macromol 1994; 16(3): 149-52.

[57] Hassan EE, Gallo JM. A simple rheological method for the *in vitro* assessment of mucin-polymer bioadhesive bond strength. Pharm Res 1990; 7(5): 491-5.

[58] Sogias IA, Williams AC, Khutoryanskiy VV. Why is chitosan mucoadhesive? Biomacromolecules 2008; 9(7): 1837-42.

[59] van der Merwe SM, Verhoef JC, Verheijden JH, Kotze AF, Junginger HE. Trimethylated chitosan as polymeric absorption enhancer for improved peroral delivery of peptide drugs. Eur J Pharm Biopharm 2004; 58(2): 225-35.

[60] Artursson P, Lindmark T, Davis SS, Illum L. Effect of chitosan on the permeability of monolayers of intestinal epithelial cells (Caco-2). Pharm Res 1994; 11(9): 1358-61.

[61] Dodane V, Amin Khan M, Merwin JR. Effect of chitosan on epithelial permeability and structure. Int J Pharm 1999; 182(1): 21-32.

[62] Payet L, Terentjev EM. Emulsification and stabilization mechanisms of o/w emulsions in the presence of chitosan. Langmuir 2008; 24(21): 12247-52.

[63] Diebold Y, Jarrin M, Saez V, *et al.* Ocular drug delivery by liposome-chitosan nanoparticle complexes (LCS-NP). Biomaterials 2007; 28(8): 1553-64.

[64] de la Fuente M, Seijo B, Alonso MJ. Bioadhesive hyaluronan-chitosan nanoparticles can transport genes across the ocular mucosa and transfect ocular tissue. Gene Ther 2008; 15(9): 668-76.

[65]   Motwani SK, Chopra S, Talegaonkar S, *et al.* Chitosan-sodium alginate nanoparticles as submicroscopic reservoirs for ocular delivery: formulation, optimisation and *in vitro* characterisation. Eur J Pharm Biopharm 2008; 68(3): 513-25.

[66]   Ludwig A. The use of mucoadhesive polymers in ocular drug delivery. Adv Drug Deliv Rev 2005; 57(11): 1595-639.

[67]   Koelwel C, Rothschenk S, Fuchs-Koelwel B, Gabler B, Lohmann C, Gopferich A. Alginate inserts loaded with epidermal growth factor for the treatment of keratoconjunctivitis sicca. Pharm Dev Technol 2008; 13(3): 221-31.

[68]   Abraham S, Furtado S, Bharath S, *et al.* Sustained ophthalmic delivery of ofloxacin from an ion-activated *in situ* gelling system. Pak J Pharm Sci 2009; 22(2): 175-9.

[69]   Demailly P, Allaire C, Trinquand C. Ocular hypotensive efficacy and safety of once daily carteolol alginate. Br J Ophthalmol 2001; 85(8): 921-4.

[70]   Liao YH, Jones SA, Forbes B, Martin GP, Brown MB. Hyaluronan: pharmaceutical characterization and drug delivery. Drug Deliv 2005; 12(6): 327-42.

[71]   Milas M, Rinaudo M, Roure I, Al-Assaf S, Phillips GO, Williams PA. Comparative rheological behavior of hyaluronan from bacterial and animal sources with cross-linked hyaluronan (hylan) in aqueous solution. Biopolymers 2001; 59(4): 191-204.

[72]   Lapcik L, Jr., Lapcik L, De Smedt S, Demeester J, Chabrecek P. Hyaluronan: Preparation, Structure, Properties and Applications. Chem Rev 1998; 98(8): 2663-84.

[73]   Kaur IP, Smitha R. Penetration enhancers and ocular bioadhesives: two new avenues for ophthalmic drug delivery. Drug Dev Ind Pharm 2002; 28(4): 353-69.

[74]   Bucolo C, Mangiafico P. Pharmacological profile of a new topical pilocarpine formulation. J Ocul Pharmacol Ther 1999; 15(6): 567-73.

[75]   Bucolo C, Spadaro A, Mangiafico S. Pharmacological evaluation of a new timolol/pilocarpine formulation. Ophthalmic Res 1998; 30(2): 101-6.

[76]   Camber O, Edman P. Sodium hyaluronate as an ophthalmic vehicle: some factors governing its effect on the ocular absorption of pilocarpine. Curr Eye Res 1989; 8(6): 563-7.

[77]   Camber O, Edman P, Gurny R. Influence of sodium hyaluronate on the meiotic effect of pilocarpine in rabbits. Curr Eye Res 1987; 6(6): 779-84.

[78]   Saettone MF, Chetoni P, Torracca MT, Burgalassi S, Giannaccini B. Evaluation of muco-adhesive properties and *in vivo* activity of ophthalmic vehicles based on hyaluronic-acid. Int J Pharm 1989; 51: 203-12.

[79]   Moreira CA, Jr., Armstrong DK, Jelliffe RW, *et al.* Sodium hyaluronate as a carrier for intravitreal gentamicin. An experimental study. Acta Ophthalmol (Copenh) 1991; 69(1): 45-9.

[80]   Moreira CA, Jr., Moreira AT, Armstrong DK, *et al. In vitro* and *in vivo* studies with sodium hyaluronate as a carrier for intraocular gentamicin. Acta Ophthalmol (Copenh) 1991; 69(1): 50-6.

[81]   Gandolfi SA, Massari A, Orsoni JG. Low-molecular-weight sodium hyaluronate in the treatment of bacterial corneal ulcers. Graefes Arch Clin Exp Ophthalmol 1992; 230(1): 20-3.

Send Orders of Reprints at reprints@benthamscience.net

CHAPTER 6

Drug Delivery Systems for Diseases of the Back of the Eye

Ashish Thakur[1,2] and Uday B. Kompella[1,2] *

[1]*Department of Pharmaceutical Sciences and Department of Ophthalmology, University of Colorado Anschutz Medical Campus, Aurora, CO 80045, USA and* [2]*Department of Pharmaceutical Sciences, University of Nebraska Medical Center, Omaha, NE 68198, USA*

Abstract: Drug delivery to the back of the eye currently relies largely on localized drug delivery systems. These systems provide high drug concentrations at the target sites and low concentrations in the systemic circulation, thereby improving the risk: benefit ratio of the therapeutic agent. Since localized drug delivery requires either a surgical procedure or an injection in or around the eye, drug delivery systems developed for the back of the eye are either self-sustaining or slow release systems. In this chapter, various drug delivery systems including non-degradable implants, biodegradable implants, encapsulated cell technology based implants, microparticles, nanoparticles, liposomes, micelles and hydrogels suitable for localized drug delivery to the back of the eye are discussed. Further, iontophoretic approaches are also briefly addressed.

Keywords: Drug delivery systems, Implants, Microparticles, Nanoparticles, Liposomes, Micelles, Hydrogels, Iontophoresis, Posterior eye.

INTRODUCTION

Drug delivery to the posterior segment of the eye for a variety of chorioretinal disorders such as age related macular degeneration (AMD), diabetic retinopathy, retinitis pigmentosa and uveitis is a challenge [1-3]. This task becomes more difficult when drug effects are desired for prolonged periods of time ranging from weeks to months. Traditional routes of administration do not typically achieve the necessary therapeutic drug levels for posterior eye segment diseases. For example, to attain therapeutic concentrations in the back of the eye, systemic routes require high doses that might lead to systemic toxicity. The topical ocular route, although

***Address correspondence to Uday B. Kompella:** Skaggs School of Pharmacy and Pharmaceutical Sciences, University of Colorado Anschutz Medical Campus, Aurora, CO 80045; Tel: (303) 724-4028; Fax: (303) 724-4666. E-mail: Uday.Kompella@ucdenver.edu

Ashim K. Mitra (Ed)

most used in treating ophthalmic diseases, is inefficient in delivering adequate therapeutic drug levels to the posterior segment of the eye [4]. It is limited by tear fluid drainage and turnover, significant permeability barriers imposed by the corneal epithelium and rapid clearance of drug by the conjunctival and episcleral blood circulation prior to entry into the back of the eye. Topical formulations have been developed with the intent of enhancing retention and penetration across the corneal surface. These developments make use of viscosity and permeability enhancers, microemulsions and vesicular systems. Unfortunately, none of these attempts have successfully been used to treat chronic posterior ocular segment diseases. In light of this, intraocular (*e.g.*, intravitreal, subretinal, suprachoroidal and intrascleral) and periocular (*e.g.*, subconjunctival, sub-Tenon, retrobulbar, peribulbar and posterior juxtascleral) routes of administration (Fig. **1**) are opening new avenues for research and products based on some of these routes (*e.g.*, intravitreal) have been approved by the FDA.

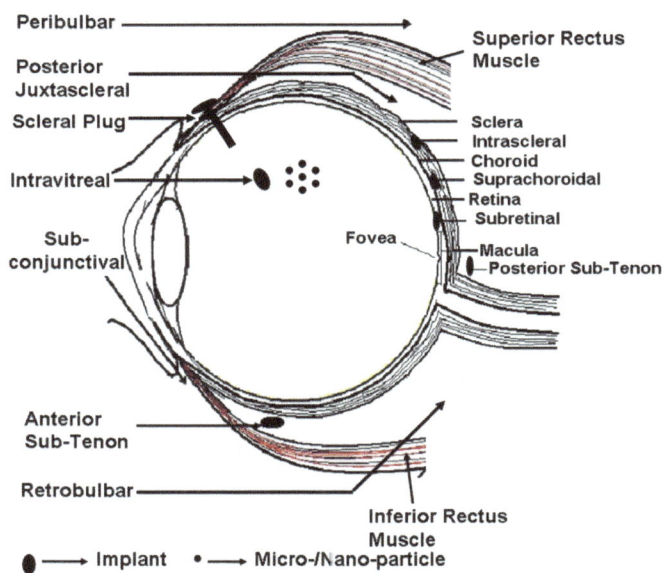

Figure 1: Schematic representation of the eye with various routes of drug administration for treating diseases of the back of the eye.

The above invasive routes of administration allow drug delivery directly into the globe or around the globe near the target site. Of the above routes, intravitreal administration is well accepted in clinical practice. However, there are some complications associated with repeated administrations *via* this route including retinal detachment, hemorrhage, endophthalmitis and cataracts. In spite of this, intraocular and periocular routes [5,6] deliver adequate drug levels to the retina, therefore, researchers worldwide are concentrating their efforts towards developing systems which will retain the beneficial effects of these routes while reducing/eliminating the adverse effects [7,8].

Solutions, emulsions, suspensions and implants are dosage forms that can potentially be administered for treating back of the eye disorders, with the solid dosage forms typically sustaining drug delivery for the longest period. Solid ocular drug delivery systems for the back of the eye can generally be categorized [9] as implant and non-implant systems depending upon their physical forms. Implant systems are typically based on a polymer. The polymers used in the preparation of such systems/devices can either be biodegradable or non-biodegradable. Usually, non-biodegradable reservoir type implants provide greater drug persistence. Non-implant systems include conventional dosage forms such as plain drug solutions, emulsions, or suspensions as well as novel delivery systems. Non-implant novel delivery systems include polymeric nano-/micro-particles, liposomes, micelles and gels (Fig. **2**). Depending on their size, drug containing particles can be grouped as nanoparticles (few nm – 1 μm) or microparticles (> 1 μm). Liposomes are vesicular delivery systems based on lipidic material, with diameters ranging from nanometers to micrometers. Micellar systems are usually made of amphiphilic polymers or surfactants [10]. When the constituent materials are present above their critical micellar concentration (CMC), micelles are formed. Micelles with a hydrophobic core and a hydrophilic corona in aqueous medium can solubilize water insoluble drugs in the hydrophobic core. Gel based systems are crosslinked hydrophilic homopolymers or copolymers, which forms gels at room temperature or remain in solution form at room temperature and turn into gels at physiological temperatures.

Polymeric controlled release delivery systems can be classified as matrix and reservoir systems. In a matrix system, the drug is distributed throughout the polymeric matrix. In a reservoir system on the other hand, the drug is present in a core, surrounded by a polymeric film that is rate-limiting. Reservoir systems can easily be manufactured for large implant devices but not particulate systems. Reservoir systems typically allow zero-order or constant drug release.

Table 1: Some drug delivery systems for treating diseases of the back of the eye

Registered name	Manufacturer (~ Release date), Place	Type (Route)	Material	Active substance	Indication	Delivery period	Current status
Non-biodegradable reservoir implants							
Vitrasert®	Bausch and Lomb (1996), USA	Reservoir implant (intravitreal)	EVA/PVA	Ganciclovir	CMV	~6 months	Clinical use
Retisert®	Bausch and Lomb (2005), USA	Reservoir implant (intravitreal)	Silicone/PVA	Fluocinolone acetonide	Uveitis	~2.5 years	Clinical use
Medidur®	Psivida Corp./Pfizer, USA	Reservoir implant (intravitreal)	Silicone/PVA	Fluocinolone acetonide	DME/AMD	~1.5-3 years	Additional data requested by FDA after Phase III trials for DME/Under Phase II trials for AMD
NT-501	Neurotech Pharm Inc. USA	Reservoir implant (intravitreal)	Hollow fibre membrane/ Poly(ethylene terephthalate)	Ciliary Neurotropic Factor (encapsulated cell technology)	AMD/Retinitis pigmentosa	> 1 year	Phase III
Non-biodegradable matrix implant							
I-vation™	Surmodics and Merck and Co. Inc. USA	Matrix implant (scleral plug)	Nonferrous alloy	Variety of drugs, *e.g.*, triamcinolone acetonide	DME	> 1 year	Clinical trial incomplete
Biodegradable matrix implant							
Ozurdex®	Allergan, USA	Matrix implant (intravitreal)	PLGA	Dexamethasone	Macular Edema/Noninfectious uveitis	6 months	Clinical use
Surodex®	Oculex Pharm Inc.(1999), USA	Matrix implant (intravitreal)	PLGA	Dexamethasone	Inflammation following cataract surgery	1-2 weeks	Inactive
Liposomes							
Visudyne®	Novartis, USA	Intravenous liposomal formulation	Phosphatidyl glycerol	Verteporfin	Choroidal neovascularization	1-4 weeks	Clinical use

EVA: Ethylene vinyl acetate; PVA: Polyvinyl alcohol; CMV: Cytomegalovirus retinitis; AMD: Age-related macular degeneration; DME: Diabetic macular edema; PLGA: Poly(lactic-co-glycolic acid)

The purpose of this chapter is to discuss a variety of implantable and non-implantable drug delivery systems for the treatment of posterior ocular segment disorders along with their limitations. In addition, iontophoretic drug delivery is also discussed. A scheme representing various drug delivery systems for posterior ocular segment disorders with their approximate duration of action is shown in (Fig. **2**). Table **1** summarizes various delivery systems that are either approved or assessed in clinical trials for drug delivery to the back of the eye. These systems are further discussed in subsequent sections.

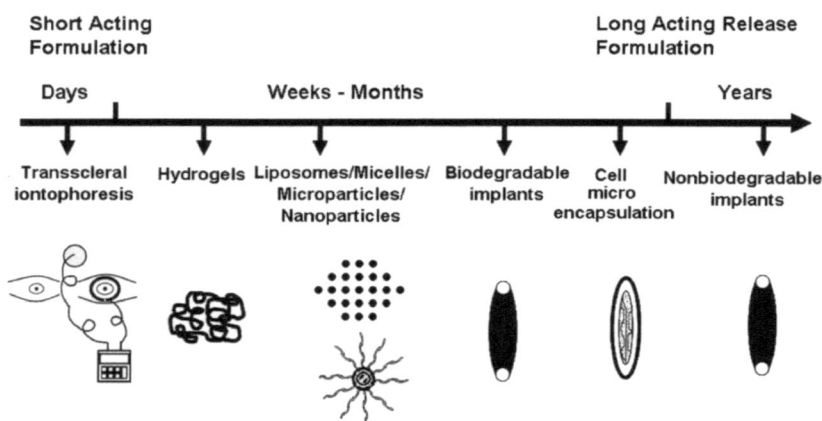

Figure 2: Drug delivery systems for posterior ocular segment disorders with their approximate duration of action. Figure based on [11].

DRUG DELIVERY DEVICES FOR POSTERIOR OCULAR DISORDERS

Ocular Implants

Ocular implants are drug loaded polymeric sustained release systems placed either inside the eye or around the globe. These systems can be non-degradable or degradable in the body. Ocular implants efficiently place the drug near the target, thereby allowing a reduction in dose as well as systemic side effects. For non-biodegradable implants, a combination of ethylene vinyl acetate (EVA) and polyvinyl alcohol (PVA) is commonly used [9]. Systems based on non-degradable membranes are reservoir type drug delivery systems and typically allow zero-order drug release. For biodegradable implants, polylactic acid (PLA), poly(lactic-co-glycolic) acid (PLGA), polycaprolactone (PCL) and polyanhydrides are most commonly used. From biodegradable implants, although near zero-order release is theoretically feasible, the drug is generally released in three phases: an initial burst phase, a diffusive phase and a final burst phase. These systems might be more suitable for conditions where an initial rapid release or loading dose of the drug followed by slow release or maintenance dose is desirable. An advantage of biodegradable implants is that there is no surgical procedure required to remove these devices since they are degraded and eliminated from the body. Non-biodegradable implants are either surgically removed or left to remain inside the body once the therapy is complete. The advantage of non-biodegradable implants is that they offer zero-order drug release over prolonged periods of time (*e.g.*, up to about 2.5 years with Retisert®, a fluocinolone acetonide implant), when compared to biodegradable implants [11]. A detailed discussion of biodegradable and non-biodegradable implants either in clinical or preclinical phases is presented below.

Non-Biodegradable (Reservoir) Implants

Vitrasert®, Retisert® (Bausch and Lomb, USA), Iluvien®/Medidur® (Psivida Corp./Pfizer, USA) and NT-501 (Neurotech Pharmaceuticals Inc., USA) are examples of non-biodegradable implants intended for placement into the vitreous cavity. While the first two implants are in clinical use, additional clinical studies based on phase III data have been requested by the FDA in support of Iluvien®/Medidur® safety and efficacy and NT-501 is currently in phase III clinical trials.

Vitrasert® is the first non-biodegradable (reservoir) implant for the back of the eye to gain approval by the FDA in 1996. The implant contains about 4.5 mg of ganciclovir in the form of a tablet along with magnesium stearate as an inactive ingredient. The tablet has polymeric coats of EVA and PVA encapsulating ganciclovir to control the drug release for a period of 6-8 months in the treatment of cytomegalovirus retinitis (CMV) associated with acquired immunodeficiency syndrome (AIDS) [12]. EVA is an impermeable polymer and PVA is a permeable polymer, both are used to control drug permeation through the device [12]. The mean value of the *in vivo* release rate of ganciclovir from this implant was found to be 1.40 µg/h. The median effective inhibitory doses (ED$_{50}$) of ganciclovir for human CMV isolates ranged from 0.2-3.0 µg/ml [13]. This device requires a 4-5 mm sclerotomy at the pars plana for vitreal implantation and the device needs to be replaced surgically with another implant as required. Phase III clinical trials conducted by Bausch and Lomb indicated that the implant significantly delayed the progression to CMV associated with AIDS as compared to patients who received intravenous ganciclovir. However, disadvantages of Vitrasert® include its relatively large size and complications associated with its use such as endophthalmitis and increased rate of retinal detachment.

Retisert® is a reservoir type non-biodegradable implant of fluocinolone acetonide approved by the FDA in 2005 for the treatment of chronic non-infectious uveitis. The implant was designed based on the success of Vitrasert® and is more refined with respect to device size and its ability to control drug release for about 2.5 years. The implant contains 0.59 mg tablet of fluocinolone acetonide as the active drug substance. PVA, microcrystalline cellulose and magnesium stearate are present as inactive ingredients. PVA and silicone elastomer form the polymer coating around the tablet. The fluocinolone acetonide tablet is encased in the silicone elastomer cup containing a release orifice and PVA membrane positioned between the orifice and the tablet [14]. The device is usually placed in the inferior quadrant after conjunctival peritomy. The implant is designed to release fluocinolone acetonide at a nominal initial rate of 0.6 µg/day, decreasing over the first month to a steady state between 0.3-0.4 µg/day over ~30 months [12,15,16]. Pharmacokinetics of Retisert® (0.5 mg and 2 mg implant) in pigmented rabbits in a study period of one year resulted in nearly constant vitreous levels from first time point till the end of the study [17]. Also, the drug levels in different ocular tissues were higher for the 2 mg implant when compared to the 0.5 mg implant (Fig. **3**). Within the same treatment group, vitreal as well as retinal drug levels were found to be higher than aqueous humor levels. However, the clinical use of the implant should be carefully considered based on the risk-benefit ratio of corticosteroids for ocular purposes. Despite its benefits, Retisert® was found to increase the occurrence of glaucoma by 50 % in diabetic macular edema patients [12]. Additionally, cataracts developed in almost every case after 3 years of treatment using Retisert® [12,16].

Medidur®/Iluvien® is a tube-shaped reservoir-type non-biodegradable implant (3.5 X 0.37 mm) of fluocinolone acetonide designed to provide an initial release rate of 0.5 or 0.2 µg/day of the drug followed by slow release at near zero order kinetics for 2-3 years [18]. Phase III studies (Fluocinolone Acetonide in Diabetic Macular Edema or FAME study) conducted by Psivida Corp. and Alimera Sciences Inc. have shown positive results with respect to visual improvement in DME patients. However, patients experienced adverse effects such as accelerated cataract formation and intraocular pressure elevation. FDA requested additional clinical trials in support of product safety and efficacy. Both companies together are also conducting phase II clinical trials with Medidur®/Iluvien® in wet and dry age-related macular degeneration (AMD) and Retinal Vein Occlusion [19]. The advantage with this implant is that it is much smaller compared to Vitrasert® and Retisert® and can be placed in the vitreous using a 25G needle during an office visit without the need of special surgical procedure [12,19]. Thus, for Iluvien®, there is no need to suture the implant to the eye wall and it is administered as an intravitreal injection. The implant has been shown to successfully control the release of the drug for a period of time ranging from 1.5 to 3 years [12]. Medidur® results in far fewer side effects when compared to Retisert®.

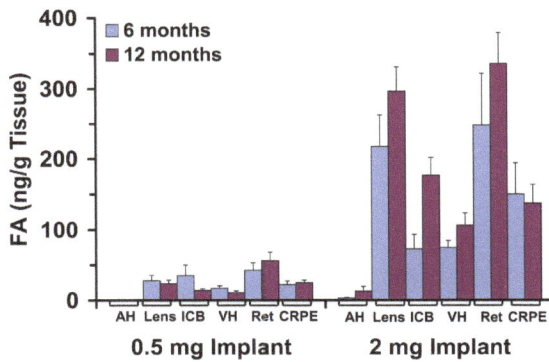

Figure 3: Mean fluocinolone acetonide concentrations at 6 months and 12 months in rabbit ocular tissues (ng/g) after 0.5 mg and 2 mg intravitreal implant (Retisert®). Plot was made from the data provided in the publication by Driot *et al.* [17]. Error bars represent standard error of mean. AH: aqueous humor, ICB: iris-ciliary body, VH: vitreous humor, Ret: retina and CRPE: choroid-RPE.

Encapsulated Cell Technology Implant

Another key advance in the field of implants is in "Encapsulated Cell Technology". This technology exploits the use of genetically modified cells to ensure the release of a therapeutic protein. NT501 implant [9, 20] is an example of this technology. NT501 is currently in phase III clinical trials for the treatment of age-related macular degeneration and retinitis pigmentosa. Results of phase II clinical studies demonstrated significant positive outcomes without any serious adverse effects. The implant holds genetically engineered human retinal pigment epithelial cells that release ciliary neurotrophic factor for over 12 months in the vitreous humor. The implant is 6 mm in length and 1 mm in diameter, roughly similar in size to a rice grain. It consists of an outer sealed semi-permeable outer capsule with about 15 nm pores [21]. The capsule contains internal scaffold of six strands of polyethylene terephthalate yarn loaded with cells [22]. The device is designed to promote long-term survival of the genetically engineered cells by allowing the influx of oxygen and nutrients.

Biodegradable (Matrix) Implants

Biodegradable implants currently marketed are matrix type delivery systems. For such biodegradable implants (Table **1**), the drug release generally follows first order kinetics [23], releasing high concentrations initially followed by lower concentrations with an increase in time [24]. The implants are usually made of poly(lactide) (PLA) and/or poly(lactide-co-glycolide) (PLGA). The rate of drug release can be controlled by (1) altering the lactide to glycolide ratio, with higher lactide content resulting in slower drug release; (2) use of high molecular weight polymers, with drug release declining with an increase in molecular weight; and (3) using hydrophobic drugs, which tend to remain with the polymer due to their greater affinity for the polymer. Apart from the other forces, basic or acidic drugs may catalyze the degradation of the polymer. The benefit of biodegradable implants is that they may be tailored for both short (weeks) as well as long term treatment (year) depending upon the polymer ratios used in engineering the device [23]. Surodex® [25] and Ozurdex® [26] (Allergan, USA) are PLGA based implants. Surodex® contains 60 µg of dexamethasone, whereas Ozurdex® contains 700 µg of the same corticosteroid. Surodex® is designed to control the post operative inflammation following cataract surgery; however, no further development of this implant is currently taking place [9]. Ozurdex® is in clinical use for the treatment of macular edema arising from branch or central retinal vein occlusion and has been shown to maintain drug effects for about 6 months. In addition, Ozurdex® is under phase II clinical investigation for the treatment of macular edema secondary to diabetic retinopathy.

Scleral Plugs

A scleral plug [27] is a device made of drug loaded biodegradable polymers typically consisting of a cap and a shaft. The device can be implanted at the pars plana using a simple procedure. In order to anchor the plug, sclera is exposed followed by 1 mm sclerotomy about 3.5 mm from the limbus. Depending upon the type (*e.g.*, PLA/PLGA) and molecular weight of the polymer as well as the amount of drug used in fabricating a scleral plug, release of the effective doses of drug can be controlled over several months. Scleral plug can be of various dimensions, however, an increase in the total surface area of the device may increase the release rate. To make scleral plugs, the polymer and drug are dissolved in a medium which is a good solvent for both. The resultant solution on lyophilization results in a homogeneous cake. Using the compression-molding technique, the homogeneous cake can be fabricated into scleral plugs on a hot plate. Therefore, in general, drugs that do not degrade upon heating in the range of 80-100 °C must be chosen since such high temperatures are necessary for fabricating the scleral plugs. Drug release profiles from scleral plug devices generally have a triphasic release pattern [28-31]: an initial burst phase, a diffusional release phase and a final burst phase. PLA or PLGA can be used to formulate biodegradable scleral plugs. For instance, ganciclovir loaded PLA or PLGA scleral plugs have been assessed for their *in vitro* as well as *in vivo* release profiles in the treatment of cytomegalovirus (CMV) retinitis [28, 32]. The results demonstrate that higher the GCV loading (for example, 40 % *vs.* 10 %) in the PLGA scleral plug, faster the release. In comparison to PLGA, PLA scleral plugs with molecular weights approximately the same as PLGA resulted in a more sustained release profiles. Furthermore, blending of PLA of various molecular weights (PLA-70 000 and 5000, 80/20) prolongs the linear release period for GCV.

Another example of scleral plug type implant is based on I-vation® technology [16] from Surmodics Ltd. (Eden Prairie, MN, USA). In this technology, a nonferrous alloy helix coated with drug-containing (*e.g.*, triamcinolone acetonide) polymer has been assessed in phase I clinical trials with positive outcomes for the treatment of diabetic macular edema. The drug delivery period was found to be > 12 months. However, further efficacy trials (phase IIb) were stopped possibly due to the reports that laser treatment may be more effective than triamcinolone acetonide [9].

Nano-/Micro-Particles

Nano-/micro-particle systems are advantageous in that they require less invasive procedures for administration when compared to most implants. These systems can be administered as suspensions and possess higher drug loading capacity and stability in biological fluids as compared to other colloidal systems such as liposomes and micelles [33,34] which are discussed later in this chapter.

Understanding the physicochemical properties of the drug as well as the polymer is of the utmost importance prior to formulating the nano-/micro-particulate systems. Physicochemical properties of the drug govern the selection of the encapsulation technique used for nano-/micro-particle formation. Readers are encouraged to refer to the review by Wischke and Schwendeman for further discussion on principles of drug encapsulation in nano-/micro-particles [35]. Polymers assessed for ophthalmic nanoparticle preparations include PLA/PLGA, hyaluronic acid, polycaprolactone, poly(methyl) methacrylate, poly(alkyl) cyanoacrylate, albumin, gelatin, chitosanand eudragit [33], Biocompatibility of the polymer, drug loading capacity and drug release rate are key parameters to be considered when preparing nano-/micro-particle systems. There are a number of microparticulate depot formulations, that have entered into the market but no such system is in clinical use for back of the eye diseases [35]. Studies from the literature which demonstrate the potential of intravitreal, transscleral, or intravenous delivery of nano-/micro-particlulate formulations for posterior ocular disorders are listed below in some detail and are briefly summarized in Table **2**.

Table 2: Literature reports related to micro-/nano-particulate systems used for posterior segment disorders

Material	Active substance	Evaluation	Results	References
Microparticles				
PLGA	Macugen®	Transscleral delivery in rabbits	*In vitro* delivery for a period of 20 days at an average rate of 2 µg/day. *In vivo* transscleral delivery for 6 days in rabbits.	Adamis *et al.* [36]
PLGA	PKC 412	Periocularly in laser-induced CNV pigs	Significant levels in choroid, retina and vitreous detected after 20 days of periocular injection	Campochiaro *et al.* [37]
PLGA	Anti-TGFβ2	Subconjunctival injection	Microspheres prevent post surgical fibrosis in rabbits for 42 days after glaucoma filtering surgery	Gomes dos Santos *et al.* [38]
PLGA	Celecoxib	Subconjunctival injection for retinal disorder in SD rats	Celecoxib-PLGA microparticles sustain retinal celecoxib delivery and inhibit diabetes-induced retinal oxidative damage	Kompella *et al.* [39]
PLGA	Celecoxib	Subconjunctival injection for safety study in SD rats	Celecoxib-PLGA microparticles are safe and do not cause any damage to the retina. Microparticles sustain the drug effects for 2 months in diabetes-induced rat model	Kompella *et al.* [40]
PLA	Budesonide	Subconjunctival injection in SD rats	Budesonide PLA microparticles have much greater sustain release *in vitro* as well as *in vivo* as compared to nanoparticles and plain solution	Kompella *et al.* [41]

Table 2: contd….

PLA	Doxorubicin	Intravitreal injection in rabbits	Microspheres reduce the occurrence of tractional retinal detachment from 50 % to 10% after 28 days in a rabbit model of experimental proliferative vitreal retinopathy whereas free drug could not prevent retinal necrosis and detachment	Moritera *et al.* [42]
Nanoparticles				
PLGA - surface functionalized	Anti-VEGF Intraceptor plasmid	Intravenously in laser-induced CNV rats	Surface functionalized nanoparticles either with transferring or RGD peptide or both show much higher delivery as well as efficacy in the treatment of CNV	Kompella *et al.* [43]
PLGA	VEGF antisense oligonucleotide	ARPE-19 cells	Nanoparticles enhance cellular uptake of antisense oligonucleotide and inhibit VEGF secretion and mRNA expression in ARPE-19 cells	Kompella *et al.* [44]
PLA	Rhodamine 6G Nile red	Intravitreal injection in rats	Nanoparticles could be seen within the RPE cells after 4 months of single intravitreal injection	Bourges *et al.* [45]
PLA	Betamethasone phosphate	Intravenous injection in rats	Nanoparticles accumulate in the choroids and retina within 3 h and reduce the EAU score of rats within one day. The effect is maintained up to 14 days.	Sakai *et al.* [46]
Poly styrene	Bodipy-loaded fluorescent particles	Subconjunctival injection in SD rats	200 nm or larger particles retain at the site of injection even after 2 months whereas 20 nm particles do not. Periocular circulation plays an important role in clearance of 20 nm particles.	Kompella *et al.* [47,48]
Gelatin	bFGF	Intravitreal injection in rats	Nanoparticles prevent photoreceptor degeneration for 6 weeks	Sakai *et al.* [49]
Albumin	Ganciclovir	Intravitreal injection in rats	Nanoparticles localize in the vitreal cavity for 2 weeks and show control release for the treatment of CMV	Irache *et al.* [50]
PEG	Tamoxifen	Intravitreal injection in rats	Drug loaded nanoparticles significantly inhibit the onset of EAU whereas free tamoxifen does not.	De Kozak *et al.* [51]

It is well known that vascular endothelial growth factor (VEGF) induces vascular permeability and angiogenesis; its elevated expression is directly related to ocular neovascularization which can lead to severe vision loss. Therefore, anti-VEGF therapeutic agents have been of value in treating disorders associated with angiogenesis. Macugen® (anti-VEGF aptamer) and Lucentis® (anti-VEGF antibody fragment) are examples of intravitreally injected anti-VEGF agents currently approved by the FDA for clinical use. These macromolecules persist at or above therapeutic levels for a few weeks and require repeated dosing every few weeks. For the purpose of long term inhibition of VEGF, pegylated Macugen®, with a dosing frequency of every 6 weeks (better than unmodified aptamer), was encapsulated into biodegradable PLGA microparticles [48,49]. The *in vitro* release studies at 37 °C assessed that the aptamer was chemically stable in PLGA microparticles over several months and retained its full biological activity. Therapeutically effective levels in the rabbit vitreous were detected up to 4 months following intravitreal administration. Upon extrapolation of these results for human application, the estimated release time was found to be approximately 6 months. Intravitreal injection of PLA microparticles containing doxorubicin have been shown to reduce the rate of retinal detachment in the treatment of proliferative vitreoretinopathy (PVR) in rabbits [42]. Doxorubicin loaded microparticles were found be non toxic to the retina whereas similar amounts of the free drug caused retinal necrosis and detachment.

Bourges *et al.* reported that after a single intravitreal injection in rats, PLA nanoparticles diffused through the retina and localized in the cytoplasm of RPE cells for 4 months [45]. This may probably be due to the phagocytic activity of RPE cells which can be utilized for specific delivery of drugs for retinal disorders. Aukunuru *et al.* [44] demonstrated that PLGA nanoparticles enhance retinal pigment epithelial cell uptake and efficacy of a VEGF antisense oligonucleotide. Intravitreally injected gelatin nanoparticles containing human basic fibroblast growth factor (bFGF) could be localized to the retina [49]. These nanoparticles prevented photoreceptor degeneration for 6 weeks by targeted and sustained release of bFGF. Albumin nanoparticles encapsulating anticytomegaloviral drugs (*e.g.*, ganciclovir) have proved to be an effective and safe delivery system for intravitreal drug administration [50]. These nanoparticles showed controlled drug release and were well tolerated. Ocular disposition studies of these nanoparticles in rats demonstrated their localization in the vitreal cavity for two weeks after single intravitreal injection. Mo *et al.* demonstrated that intravitreally injected nanoparticles enhance Cu, Zn superoxide dismutase gene delivery to the retina [52]. Efficiency of tamoxifen, a non-steroidal estrogen receptor modulator, incorporated into polyethylene glycol coated nanoparticles was assessed for the treatment of EAU in rats [51]. Tamoxifen loaded nanoparticles injected into the vitreous significantly inhibited the onset of EAU whereas free tamoxifen did not alter the course of EAU.

Following periocular injection, PLGA microparticles of PKC412, an inhibitor of protein kinase C and receptors for VEGF, significantly suppressed choroidal neovascularization (CNV) in young domestic pig eyes equivalent in size to human eyes [37]. Moreover, PKC412 levels could be detected in vitreous, retina and choroid even at 20 days after periocular injection. PLGA microparticles encapsulating celecoxib increase the retinal delivery of celecoxib by several fold following subconjunctival administration in rats compared to systemic administration and were capable of inhibiting diabetes-induced retinal oxidative damage, vascular leakage and VEGF expression [6,39,40]. A single subconjunctival injection of carboplatin loaded in poly (amido amine) dendrimer nanoparticles was shown to treat transgenic murine retinoblastoma [53]. The treatment did not result in any toxic effects.

Clearance of nanoparticles from the site of administration even before the drug is released can be a challenge [54]. Kompella *et al.* showed that the size of the nanoparticles is particularly important; while 20 nm particles are cleared rapidly within a few hours from the periocular space, 200 nm particles remain almost completely intact for at least 2 months following periocular injection [47,48,55]. This group also showed that surface modification of nanoparticles by conjugating a luteinizing hormone-releasing hormone (LHRH) agonist or transferrin is a useful approach that provides rapid, efficient delivery of intact nanoparticles into and/or across the cornea and conjunctiva after topical application [56].

Single intravenous injection of PLA nanoparticles loaded with betamethasone phosphate targeted a specific lesion and sustained the release of the therapeutic agent for the treatment of experimental autoimmune uveoretinitis (EAU) [46]. Nanoparticles accumulated in the retina and choroid of rats with EAU within 3 h and remained over the succeeding 7-day period. Singh *et al.* showed that nanoparticles functionalized with transferrin or an RGD peptide can enhance retinal delivery and efficacy of VEGF intraceptor gene [43].

Liposomes

When phospholipids are hydrated, they spontaneously form closed structures with an internal aqueous environment bound by phospholipid bilayer membranes; the resulting vesicular system is called as liposome [57]. In other words, liposomes are lipid bilayer enclosed vesicles composed of one or more phospholipids. Like nano/microparticles, liposomes can be used to entrap hydrophilic as well as lipophilic drugs. There are different methods of classifications of liposomes [57]. Based on their structures/number of lipid bilayers, liposomes can be classified as (i) unilamellar (one lipid bilayer) vesicle (diameter size: all size range), (ii) small unilamellar vesicle (20-100 nm), (iii) medium/large unilamellar vesicle (> 100 nm), (iv) giant unilamellar vesicle (> 1 μm), (v) oligolamellar vesicle (0.1-1 μm, ~ 5 lipid bilayers), (vi) multilamellar vesicle (> 0.5 μm, 5-25 lipid bilayers) or (vii) multivesicular vesicle (> 1 μm, multicompartmental structure). Factors which affect the suitability of liposomes as ocular drug delivery systems include size, drug encapsulation efficiency, stability of the preparation and liposomal surface charge [58]. Charge is important because positively charged preparations will preferentially bind with the negatively charged ocular surface and will be better adsorbed. However, the lack of cytotoxicity of positively charged liposomes has to be ensured. One potential limitation of liposomes, as drug delivery systems for the posterior eye segment, is the disruption of liposomal membrane components after interaction with other proteins, lipids, or cellular components. This may lead to a burst release of the drug. Light induced systems for retinal diseases which have been developed based on liposome technology (for example Visudyne®) are discussed below.

Verteporfin (Visudyne®, Novartis Pharmaceuticals, USA) is the only liposomal drug currently in clinical use for the treatment of choroidal neovascularization and age-related macular degeneration (AMD) [59,60]. It works as a photodynamic therapy, where a non-thermal red laser (wavelength 693 nm) is applied to the retina to activate verteporfin after the liposomal preparation is intravenously infused. Upon activation, verteporfin produces reactive oxygen radicals that cause local damage to the neovascular endothelium, resulting in blockage of the abnormal blood vessels. Patient follow up is done every 3 months and retreatment is considered in only those cases with persistent leakage from the CNV areas. However, in some cases, Visudyne® produces insufficient effects [11,59] because of the increased production of VEGF as a result of photodynamic therapy. Rostaporfin (Photrex®, Miravant Medical Technologies, USA) is another example of light activated (red light with a wavelength of 664 nm) cytotoxic agent for the treatment of AMD [60]. It binds with the lipoproteins, which are produced in high concentrations by the hyper proliferating cells and upon activation selectively kills those cells. In case of rostaporfin, the frequency of required treatments is significantly lower than verteporfin. After initial treatment, depending on the disease severity during subsequent visits, the drug administration is repeated. The frequency of retreatment was at the most three times during a 2 year follow-up period in phase III clinical trials [61]. FDA approval of rostaporfin is currently pending.

In addition to the above examples, some literature reports on the potential use of liposomes for posterior ocular delivery are listed below. Liposomes composed of soybean phospholipids (PC), cholesterol (CHOL) and 1,2-Distearoyl-*sn*-glycero-3 phosphatidylethanolamine-*N*-[poly(ethyleneglycol)-2000] (PEG-DSPE) encapsulated with phosphodiester oligonucleotide resulted in sustained release of the oligonucleotide into the vitreous and retina-choroid after single intravitreal injection for the treatment of retinal diseases [38]. Moreover, concentrations in the ocular tissues were significantly higher following liposomal injection compared to simple solution of oligonucleotide. Liposomes protected phosphodiester oligonucleotide from degradation. In another study, liposomes encapsulated ganciclovir were proved to be more effective in the management of retinal detachment in cytomegalovirus (CMV) retinitis in AIDS patients compared to free ganciclovir [62]. Liposomes encapsulated ganciclovir reduced the number of intravitreal injections in stabilizing CMV retinitis.

Micelles

A polymer micelle is composed of amphiphilic surfactants or block copolymers [11]. These materials have a critical micelle concentration (CMC) which is defined as the lowest concentration at which these materials form a micelle structure with a hydrophilic corona and a hydrophobic core in aqueous medium. In polymeric micelles, polyethylene glycol (PEG) is the most commonly used hydrophilic block and polyesters such as poly(lactic acid, PLA), poly(ε-caprolactone, PCL) and poly(glycolic acid, PGA) are commonly used hydrophobic blocks [63]. A balance between hydrophilic and hydrophobic blocks (hydrophilic-lipophilic balance, HLB) in aqueous medium controls various micellar properties such as CMC and drug loading capacity. Hydrophobic drug loading is typically higher when a long hydrophobic block is present in the polymer.

Another variation of micelle like structures is poly-ion complexes. Typically these complexes are formed with a core based on charge interactions and a corona based on a hydrophilic segment [64,65]. The polymers used for this purpose typically contain a hydrophilic, uncharged region and a charged region. While PEG is commonly used as the hydrophilic region, blocks such as polyethyleneimine (PEI), poly(aspartic acid, PAsP) or poly(L-lysine, PLL) are used as ionic blocks [66,67]. A polyion-complex micelle system composed of PEG-PLL encapsulated with a dendritic photosensitizer (DP) has been tested in CNV-induced rats for its efficacy in photodynamic therapy [68]. The results demonstrate that upon administration of DP loaded micelles, the levels of DP in the CNV lesions were higher and more prolonged as compared to administration of free DP, proving that DP loaded micelles result in pronounced photodynamic effects [68,69].

In general, micelles are relatively less stable under *in vivo* conditions that limited applications of these systems for sustained delivery purposes. There are a few PEG-PLA, PEG-PAsP and Pluronic based micelle formulations which are either in phase I or II clinical trials for tumor treatment [64]. Efforts are currently underway to develop slow release micellar delivery systems that are more stable [10].

Hydrogels

Hydrogels are polymers that are capable of holding high quantities of water. Hydrogels are made of hydrophilic homopolymers or coplymers which are either crosslinked chemically (*e.g.*, covalent bonds) or physically (*e.g.*, chain entanglement, H-bonding or hydrophobic forces) [70]. Chemically bonded hydrogels are also called permanent, whereas physically crosslinked hydrogels are called reversible hydrogels. Many natural and synthetic polymers/proteins can be used in the preparation of hydrogels: methyl cellulose, chitosan, dextran, xyloglucan, gelatin, hyaluronic acid, polyvinyl alcohol, carbomer, pluronic and *N*-Isopropylacrylamide (NIPAAm) based systems are good examples. Hydrogels may have different physical forms [70], including (a) solid molded forms (*e.g.*, soft contact lenses), (b) liquids (*e.g.*, liquids that forms gels on heating or cooling), or (c) membranes or sheets (*e.g.*, as a reservoir in a transdermal drug delivery patch). Soft contact lens based ophthalmic drug delivery systems [71] have been used to improve the bioavailability of ophthalmic drugs in different ways. Examples of this technique include surface modification of a polymeric hydrogel used to immobilize the drug on the surface of the hydrogel or by inclusion of drugs in a colloidal structure which is then dispersed into a polymeric hydrogel. Such systems have found ocular applications with respect to directing and prolonging the drug action in the anterior segment. Timoptic-XE® (Merck and Co. Inc., USA), Pilogel® (Alcon Inc., Switzerland) and Azasite® (Insite Vision, USA) are examples of gel forming solutions for topical use in clinics [11] .

Some materials can change their gelling properties depending on temperature or other stimuli. Polymers that exhibit sharp changes in gelling behavior as a function of temperature are called as thermoresponsive hydrogels [72]. There is a threshold temperature called lower critical solution temperature (LCST) below which some thermoresponsive polymers remain in solution. Above this temperature they become increasingly hydrophobic and insoluble, resulting in gel formation. Contrarily, hydrogels that are formed from a decrease in temperature have a upper critical solution temperature. Similarly, pH sensitive hydrogels utilize changes in the pH of the surrounding medium for their sol-gel behavior.

Derwent and Mieler assessed a thermoresponsive hydrogel based on PNIPAAm crosslinked with poly(ethylene glycol) diacrylate as intravitreal injection in a rodent model for the delivery of bovine serum albumin (BSA) and immunoglobulin G (IgG) [73]. They demonstrated that after 2 months there was no change in the location of the hydrogel in the vitreal cavity and fluorescence could be seen from these FITC labeled hydrogels.

Smart stimuli responsive hydrogels are of particular interest. One early example of a feedback control mechanism modulating drug release from the imprinted polymeric hydrogel with a sensor is the release of insulin from the hydrogels as blood glucose level rises [74]. Acrylic hydrogels with amine functionality then immobilized with glucose oxidase produce enough glucuronic acid once the blood glucose level reaches a critical value. The acid produced causes ionization of the amine groups resulting in swelling of the hydrogel thereby causing a release of insulin. Upon recovery of base glucose levels, glucuronic acid production is halted, pH inside the hydrogel returns to initial value resulting in shrinkage of the hydrogel and blockade of the insulin release.

Molecularly imprinted hydrogels are currently gaining considerable attention as a drug delivery vehicle [75]. These systems are also recognized as intelligent or smart drug delivery systems because they can modulate the drug release as a function of specific stimuli [75,76]. The fundamental principle governing the function of these systems is similar to the feedback mechanism that we all studied in general biology; the level of one substance influences the level of the other. This type of system requires molecular recognition properties so that it is able to bind and release only specific molecular species under conditions where equilibrium concentrations are critical [75]. Molecularly imprinted polymers with or without a specific sensor of the triggering molecule are used for fabrication of such hydrogels. There are some specialized requirements for synthesis of molecularly imprinted polymers used in the preparation of hydrogels. One major requirement is a high degree of cross linking in order to fix the spatial orientation of the functional groups in the polymeric chains to maintain the molecular recognition capabilities [75]. Under the influence of an external stimulus, there is a change in the degree of swelling that modulates the capture and release (reversible reaction) of the imprinted template molecule (drug). These systems act as sustain release reservoir for low molecular weight species as they potentially increase the residence time of the drug inside the body. Imprinting of a drug molecule onto the polymer can be non covalent or covalent with the former being the more preferred approach because of the favorable binding and release kinetics. Unfortunately, the technology has been marginally successful in prolonging the drug effects by a few days in the case of imprinted soft contact lenses. Timolol imprinted soft contact lenses [77] made from N,N-diethylacrylamide (DEAA; main component of the matrix), methacrylic acid (MAA; functional monomer) and ethylene glycol dimethacrylate (EGDMA; crosslinker) showed greater and more sustained drug concentrations (2-3 fold) in the tear fluid in rabbits as compared to conventional lenses and eye drops. In another study, release of ketotifen fumarate from molecularly imprinted hydrogel showed zero order kinetics/concentration independent kinetics, a highly desirable feature for drug delivery [78]. However, *in vitro* release studies of the imprinted hydrogel demonstrated sustain release for only 5 days with three distinct rates of release. This may not be suitable for posterior segment ocular disorders. To date, no report has been published on the usefulness of molecularly imprinted hydrogels as intraocular delivery system for posterior segment ocular disorders.

Iontophoresis

Iontophoresis is a non-invasive technique for enhancing the penetration of ionic drugs through tissues, using a low electric current [33]. The technique is based on the concept of repulsive electromotive forces where the donor electrode (for example, anode) containing the drug with the same charge as the electrode (positive) is placed on the eye and the return electrode is placed on another body surface. Upon application of the current, the electrode repels the similarly charged molecules through the ocular tissues, thus enhancing their penetration. In general, iontophoresis enhances the drug penetration by three mechanisms [33]: electrophoresis, electroosmosis and electroporation. Electrophoresis utilizes the application of an electric field for enhanced movement of ionic drugs. Electroosmosis utilizes electric field-induced convective solvent flow for the enhanced movement of both neutral and charged drug molecules. Electroporation on the other hand enhances the intrinsic permeability of the membrane by altering the tissue barrier. Ocular iontophoresis can be either transcorneal or transscleral [11,79]. Since sclera has a larger surface area than the cornea, high degree of hydration, low number of cells and permeable to large molecular weight compounds [80], transscleral iontophoresis is an interesting option.

Ocuphor® (Iomed Inc., USA) [81,82], Eyegate II Delivery System® (EyeGate Pharma, USA) [83] and Visulex® (Aciont Inc., USA) [84] are examples of non-invasive transscleral iontophoretic ocular drug delivery devices. These devices are expected to be beneficial specifically in those cases where patients do not prefer invasive intraocular surgery (example, intravitreal or periocular implantation) for the treatment of disorders of back of the eye. These patients generally prefer disease progression over invasive treatment. The OcuPhor® system consists of a drug reservoir/applicator, iontophoretic electrode and an electronic drug delivery controller. The drug applicator consists of patented silver-silver chloride ink conductive element encased in a small silicone shell which is connected through a small flexible wire to the conductive element of the dose controller. The other end of the dose controller is connected to a drug dispersive pad. that can be placed on patients skin to complete the electrical circuit [33]. Immediately before using the device, drug pad is always hydrated with drug solution. The Visulex® system claims an easy to use drug applicator, drug delivery controller and connective wires. The system has been tested for delivery as well as efficacy of triamcinolone acetonide phosphate (TAP) in normal and endotoxin-induced posterior uveitis rabbit models [12,51,85]. Results demonstrate a significant improvement in the uveitis score of the eyes treated with TAP-loaded Visulex®. However, the drug actions with iontophoretic device are less prolonged as compared to other systems such as implants and particulate delivery systems. Eyegate II Delivery System® infused with a corticosteroid derivative is the first iontophoretic system that is being assessed in human clinical trials for eye diseases [83].

CONCLUSION

Engineering of ocular drug delivery systems is an important field of ophthalmic research. Patient compliance, biocompatibility and safety of these systems are of paramount importance prior to clinical use. Once validated, systems with sustained and controlled release properties will provide clinicians with more appropriate treatment options for posterior ocular segment disorders. Delivery systems can be selected on the basis of disease and patient needs. These systems will allow flexibility in terms of selecting long acting or short acting formulations depending upon the patient's disease state. For example, treatments for very long durations with a constant drug release, moderate durations and short durations would be feasible by applying non-degradable implants, biodegradable implants and encapsulated cell technologies and iontophoresis, respectively.

ACKNOWLEDGEMENT

Declared none.

CONFLICT OF INTEREST

The author(s) confirm that this chapter content has no conflict of interest.

REFERENCES

[1]   Marra M, Gukasyan HJ, Raghava S, Kompella UB. 2nd Ophthalmic Drug Development and Delivery Summit San Diego, CA, USA, 19 - 20 September 2006. Expert Opin Drug Deliv 2007; 4(1): 77-85.

[2]   Kompella UB. Drug delivery to the back of the eye. Arch Soc Esp Oftalmol 2007; 82(11): 667-70.

[3]   Ghate D, Edelhauser HF. Ocular drug delivery. Expert Opin Drug Deliv 2006; 3(2): 275-87.

[4]   Jarvinen KJ, T. & Urtti, A. Ocular absorption following topical delivery. Advanced Drug Delivery Reviews 1995; 16 3-19.

[5]   Maurice D. Review: practical issues in intravitreal drug delivery. J Ocul Pharmacol Ther 2001; 17(4): 393-401.

[6]   Ayalasomayajula SP, Kompella UB. Retinal delivery of celecoxib is several-fold higher following subconjunctival administration compared to systemic administration. Pharm Res 2004; 21(10): 1797-804.

[7]   Raghava S, Hammond M, Kompella UB. Periocular routes for retinal drug delivery. Expert Opin Drug Deliv 2004; 1(1): 99-114.

[8]   Geroski DH, Edelhauser HF. Transscleral drug delivery for posterior segment disease. Adv Drug Deliv Rev 2001; 52(1): 37-48.

[9]   Kearns VR, Williams RL. Drug delivery systems for the eye. Expert Rev Med Devices 2009; 6(3): 277-90.

[10]   Trivedi R, Kompella UB. Nanomicellar formulations for sustained drug delivery: strategies and underlying principles. Nanomedicine (Lond) 2010; 5(3): 485-505.

[11]   Del Amo EM, Urtti A. Current and future ophthalmic drug delivery systems. A shift to the posterior segment. Drug Discov Today 2008; 13(3-4): 135-43.

[12]   Choonara YE, Pillay V, Danckwerts MP, Carmichael TR, du Toit LC. A review of implantable intravitreal drug delivery technologies for the treatment of posterior segment eye diseases. J Pharm Sci 2009; 99(5): 2219-39.

[13]   http://www.bausch.com/en_US/package_insert/surgical/vitrasert_pkg_insert.pdf.

[14]   http://www.bausch.com/en_US/downloads/ecp/pharma/general/retisert_prescinfopdf.pdf.

[15]   http://www.bausch.com/en_US/downloads/ecp/pharma/general/retisert_pkginsert.pdf.

[16]   Kuppermann BD. Implant delivery of corticosteroids and other pharmacologic agents. Presented at Retina 2006: Emerging New Concepts. Held in conjunction with the American Academy of Ophthalmology 2006 Annual Meeting, November 10-11, 2006, Las vegas.

[17]   Driot JY, Novack GD, Rittenhouse KD, Milazzo C, Pearson PA. Ocular pharmacokinetics of fluocinolone acetonide after Retisert intravitreal implantation in rabbits over a 1-year period. J Ocul Pharmacol Ther 2004; 20(3): 269-75.

[18]   Campochiaro PA, Hafiz G, Shah SM, *et al.* Sustained Ocular Delivery of Fluocinolone Acetonide by an Intravitreal Insert. Ophthalmology 2010; 117(7): 1393-9.

[19]   http://www.psivida.com/products-medidur.html.

[20]   Emerich DF, Thanos CG. NT-501: an ophthalmic implant of polymer-encapsulated ciliary neurotrophic factor-producing cells. Curr Opin Mol Ther 2008; 10(5): 506-15.

[21]   Sieving PA, Caruso RC, Tao W, *et al*. Ciliary neurotrophic factor (CNTF) for human retinal degeneration: phase I trial of CNTF delivered by encapsulated cell intraocular implants. Proc Natl Acad Sci U S A 2006; 103(10): 3896-901.

[22]   Kuno N, Fujii S. Biodegradable intraocular therapies for retinal disorders: progress to date. Drugs Aging 2010; 27(2): 117-34.

[23]   Short BG. Safety evaluation of ocular drug delivery formulations: techniques and practical considerations. Toxicol Pathol 2008; 36(1): 49-62.

[24]   Davis JL, Gilger BC, Robinson MR. Novel approaches to ocular drug delivery. Curr Opin Mol Ther 2004; 6(2): 195-205.

[25]   Seah SK, Husain R, Gazzard G, *et al*. Use of surodex in phacotrabeculectomy surgery. Am J Ophthalmol 2005; 139(5): 927-8.

[26]   Kuppermann BD, Blumenkranz MS, Haller JA, *et al*. Randomized controlled study of an intravitreous dexamethasone drug delivery system in patients with persistent macular edema. Arch Ophthalmol 2007; 125(3): 309-17.

[27]   Yasukawa T, Kimura H, Tabata Y, Ogura Y. Biodegradable scleral plugs for vitreoretinal drug delivery. Adv Drug Deliv Rev 2001; 52(1): 25-36.

[28]   Kunou N, Ogura Y, Hashizoe M, Honda Y, Hyon SH, Ikada Y. Controlled intraocular delivery of ganciclovir with use of biodegradable scleral implant in rabbits. J Control Release 1995; 37: 143-50.

[29]   Pitt CG, Gratzl MM, Jeffcoat AR, Zweidinger R, Schindler A. Sustained drug delivery systems II: Factors affecting release rates from poly(epsilon-caprolactone) and related biodegradable polyesters. J Pharm Sci 1979; 68(12): 1534-8.

[30]   Hora MS, Rana RK, Nunberg JH, Tice TR, Gilley RM, Hudson ME. Release of human serum albumin from poly(lactide-co-glycolide) microspheres. Pharm Res 1990; 7(11): 1190-4.

[31]   Sanders LM, Kent JS, McRae GI, Vickery BH, Tice TR, Lewis DH. Controlled release of a luteinizing hormone-releasing hormone analogue from poly(d,l-lactide-co-glycolide) microspheres. J Pharm Sci 1984; 73(9): 1294-7.

[32]   Yasukawa T, Kimura H, Kunou N, *et al*. Biodegradable scleral implant for intravitreal controlled release of ganciclovir. Graefes Arch Clin Exp Ophthalmol 2000; 238(2): 186-90.

[33]   Eljarrat-Binstock E, Pe'er J, Domb AJ. New techniques for drug delivery to the posterior eye segment. Pharm Res 2010; 27(4): 530-43.

[34]   Kothuri MK, Pinnamaneni S, Das NG, D.S.K. Microparticles and nanoparticles in ocular drug delivery. In: Mitra AK, editor. Ophthalmic drug delivery systems NY: Marcel Dekker, Inc. 2003: 437-66.

[35]   Wischke C, Schwendeman SP. Principles of encapsulating hydrophobic drugs in PLA/PLGA microparticles. Int J Pharm 2008; 364(2): 298-327.

[36]   Carrasquillo KG, Ricker JA, Rigas IK, Miller JW, Gragoudas ES, Adamis AP. Controlled delivery of the anti-VEGF aptamer EYE001 with poly(lactic-co-glycolic)acid microspheres. Invest Ophthalmol Vis Sci 2003; 44(1): 290-9.

[37]   Saishin Y, Silva RL, Saishin Y, *et al*. Periocular injection of microspheres containing PKC412 inhibits choroidal neovascularization in a porcine model. Invest Ophthalmol Vis Sci 2003; 44(11): 4989-93.

[38]   Gomes dos Santos AL, Bochot A, Doyle A, *et al*. Sustained release of nanosized complexes of polyethylenimine and anti-TGF-beta 2 oligonucleotide improves the outcome of glaucoma surgery. J Control Release 2006; 112(3): 369-81.

[39]   Ayalasomayajula SP, Kompella UB. Subconjunctivally administered celecoxib-PLGA microparticles sustain retinal drug levels and alleviate diabetes-induced oxidative stress in a rat model. Eur J Pharmacol 2005; 511(2-3): 191-8.

[40]   Amrite AC, Ayalasomayajula SP, Cheruvu NP, Kompella UB. Single periocular injection of celecoxib-PLGA microparticles inhibits diabetes-induced elevations in retinal PGE2, VEGFand vascular leakage. Invest Ophthalmol Vis Sci 2006; 47(3): 1149-60.

[41]   Kompella UB, Bandi N, Ayalasomayajula SP. Subconjunctival nano- and microparticles sustain retinal delivery of budesonide, a corticosteroid capable of inhibiting VEGF expression. Invest Ophthalmol Vis Sci 2003; 44(3): 1192-201.

[42]   Moritera T, Ogura Y, Yoshimura N, *et al*. Biodegradable microspheres containing adriamycin in the treatment of proliferative vitreoretinopathy. Invest Ophthalmol Vis Sci 1992; 33(11): 3125-30.

[43]   Singh SR, Grossniklaus HE, Kang SJ, Edelhauser HF, Ambati BK, Kompella UB. Intravenous transferrin, RGD peptide and dual-targeted nanoparticles enhance anti-VEGF intraceptor gene delivery to laser-induced CNV. Gene Ther 2009; 16(5): 645-59.

[44]   Aukunuru JV, Ayalasomayajula SP, Kompella UB. Nanoparticle formulation enhances the delivery and activity of a vascular endothelial growth factor antisense oligonucleotide in human retinal pigment epithelial cells. J Pharm Pharmacol 2003; 55(9): 1199-206.

[45]   Bourges JL, Gautier SE, Delie F, *et al*. Ocular drug delivery targeting the retina and retinal pigment epithelium using polylactide nanoparticles. Invest Ophthalmol Vis Sci. 2003; 44(8): 3562-9.

[46]   Sakai T, Kohno H, Ishihara T, *et al*. Treatment of experimental autoimmune uveoretinitis with poly(lactic acid) nanoparticles encapsulating betamethasone phosphate. Exp Eye Res 2006; 82(4): 657-63.

[47]   Amrite AC, Kompella UB. Size-dependent disposition of nanoparticles and microparticles following subconjunctival administration. J Pharm Pharmacol 2005; 57(12): 1555-63.

[48]   Amrite AC, Edelhauser HF, Singh SR, Kompella UB. Effect of circulation on the disposition and ocular tissue distribution of 20 nm nanoparticles after periocular administration. Mol Vis 2008; 14: 150-60.

[49]   Sakai T, Kuno N, Takamatsu F, *et al*. Prolonged protective effect of basic fibroblast growth factor-impregnated nanoparticles in royal college of surgeons rats. Invest Ophthalmol Vis Sci 2007; 48(7): 3381-7.

[50]   Irache JM, Merodio M, Arnedo A, Camapanero MA, Mirshahi M, Espuelas S. Albumin nanoparticles for the intravitreal delivery of anticytomegaloviral drugs. Mini Rev Med Chem 2005; 5(3): 293-305.

[51]   de Kozak Yandrieux K, Villarroya H, *et al*. Intraocular injection of tamoxifen-loaded nanoparticles: a new treatment of experimental autoimmune uveoretinitis. Eur J Immunol 2004; 34(12): 3702-12.

[52]   Mo Y, Barnett ME, Takemoto D, Davidson H, Kompella UB. Human serum albumin nanoparticles for efficient delivery of Cu, Zn superoxide dismutase gene. Mol Vis 2007; 13: 746-57.

[53]   Kang SJ, Durairaj C, Kompella UB, O'Brien JM, Grossniklaus HE. Subconjunctival nanoparticle carboplatin in the treatment of murine retinoblastoma. Arch Ophthalmol 2009; 127(8): 1043-7.

[54]   Amrite AC, Kompella UB. Nanoparticles for ocular drug delivery. In: Gupta RB, Kompella UB, editors. Nanoparticle Technology for Drug Delivery. New York: Marcel Dekker, Inc.; 2006. p. 319-60.

[55] Cheruvu NP, Amrite AC, Kompella UB. Effect of eye pigmentation on transscleral drug delivery. Invest Ophthalmol Vis Sci 2008; 49(1): 333-41.

[56] Kompella UB, Sundaram S, Raghava S, Escobar ER. Luteinizing hormone-releasing hormone agonist and transferrin functionalizations enhance nanoparticle delivery in a novel bovine *ex vivo* eye model. Mol Vis 2006; 12: 1185-98.

[57] Samad A, Sultana Y, Aqil M. Liposomal drug delivery systems: an update review. Curr Drug Deliv 2007; 4(4): 297-305.

[58] Mainardes RM, Urban MC, Cinto PO, *et al.* Colloidal carriers for ophthalmic drug delivery. Curr Drug Targets 2005; 6(3): 363-71.

[59] Ruiz-Moreno JM, Montero JA. Photodynamic therapy in macular diseases. Expert Rev Ophthalmol 2006; 1: 97-112.

[60] Woodburn KW, Engelman CJ, Blumenkranz MS. Photodynamic therapy for choroidal neovascularization: a review. Retina 2002; 22(4): 391-405; quiz 527-8.

[61] Rostaporfin: PhotoPoint SnET2, Purlytin, Sn(IV) etiopurpurin, SnET2, tin ethyl etiopurpurin. Drugs in R & D 2004; 5: 58-61.

[62] Akula SK, Ma PE, Peyman GA, Rahimy MH, Hyslop NE, Jr., Janney A, *et al.* Treatment of cytomegalovirus retinitis with intravitreal injection of liposome encapsulated ganciclovir in a patient with AIDS. Br J Ophthalmol 1994; 78(9): 677-80.

[63] Attwood D, Booth C, Yeates SG, Chaibundit C, Ricardo NM. Block copolymers for drug solubilisation: relative hydrophobicities of polyether and polyester micelle-core-forming blocks. Int J Pharm 2007; 345(1-2): 35-41.

[64] Kim S, Shi Y, Kim JY, Park K, Cheng JX. Overcoming the barriers in micellar drug delivery: loading efficiency, *in vivo* stabilityand micelle-cell interaction. Expert Opin Drug Deliv 2010; 7(1): 49-62.

[65] Gaucher G, Dufresne MH, Sant VP, Kang N, Maysinger D, Leroux JC. Block copolymer micelles: preparation, characterization and application in drug delivery. J Control Release 2005; 109(1-3): 169-88.

[66] Oishi M, Hayama T, Akiyama Y, *et al.* Supramolecular assemblies for the cytoplasmic delivery of antisense oligodeoxynucleotide: polyion complex (PIC) micelles based on poly(ethylene glycol)-SS-oligodeoxynucleotide conjugate. Biomacromolecules 2005; 6(5): 2449-54.

[67] Tian HY, Deng C, Lin H, *et al.* Biodegradable cationic PEG-PEI-PBLG hyperbranched block copolymer: synthesis and micelle characterization. Biomaterials 2005; 26(20): 4209-17.

[68] Jang WD, Nakagishi Y, Nishiyama N, *et al.* Polyion complex micelles for photodynamic therapy: incorporation of dendritic photosensitizer excitable at long wavelength relevant to improved tissue-penetrating property. J Control Release 2006; 113(1): 73-9.

[69] Ideta R, Tasaka F, Jang WD, *et al.* Nanotechnology-based photodynamic therapy for neovascular disease using a supramolecular nanocarrier loaded with a dendritic photosensitizer. Nano Lett 2005; 5(12): 2426-31.

[70] Hoffman AS. Hydrogels for biomedical applications. Adv Drug Deliv Rev 2002; 54(1): 3-12.

[71] Xinming L, Yingde C, Lloyd AW, *et al.* Polymeric hydrogels for novel contact lens-based ophthalmic drug delivery systems: a review. Cont Lens Anterior Eye 2008; 31(2): 57-64.

[72] Klouda L, Mikos AG. Thermoresponsive hydrogels in biomedical applications. Eur J Pharm Biopharm. 2008; 68(1): 34-45.

[73]   Kang Derwent JJ, Mieler WF. Thermoresponsive hydrogels as a new ocular drug delivery platform to the posterior segment of the eye. Trans Am Ophthalmol Soc 2008; 106: 206-13; discussion 13-4.

[74]   Peppas NA. J Drug Del Sci Technol. 2004; 14: 214.

[75]   Cunliffe D, Kirby A, Alexander C. Molecularly imprinted drug delivery systems. Adv Drug Deliv Rev 2005; 57(12): 1836-53.

[76]   Alvarez-Lorenzo C, Concheiro A. Intelligent drug delivery systems: polymeric micelles and hydrogels. Mini Rev Med Chem 2008; 8(11): 1065-74.

[77]   Hiratani H, Fujiwara A, Tamiya Y, Mizutani Y, Alvarez-Lorenzo C. Ocular release of timolol from molecularly imprinted soft contact lenses. Biomaterials 2005; 26(11): 1293-8.

[78]   Ali M, Horikawa S, Venkatesh S, Saha J, Hong JW, Byrne ME. Zero-order therapeutic release from imprinted hydrogel contact lenses within *in vitro* physiological ocular tear flow. J Control Release 2007; 124(3): 154-62.

[79]   Bejjani RAandrieu C, Bloquel C, Berdugo M, BenEzra D, Behar-Cohen F. Electrically assisted ocular gene therapy. Surv Ophthalmol 2007; 52(2): 196-208.

[80]   Pitkanen L, Ranta VP, Moilanen H, Urtti A. Permeability of retinal pigment epithelium: effects of permeant molecular weight and lipophilicity. Invest Ophthalmol Vis Sci 2005; 46(2): 641-6.

[81]   Parkinson TM, Ferguson E, Febbraro S, Bakhtyari A, King M, Mundasad M. Tolerance of ocular iontophoresis in healthy volunteers. J Ocul Pharmacol Ther 2003; 19(2): 145-51.

[82]   Fischer GA, Parkinson TM, Szlek MA. OcuPhor - The future of ocular drug delivery. Drug Delivery Tech 2002; 2: 50-2.

[83]   Halhal M, Renard G, Courtois Y, BenEzra D, Behar-Cohen F. Iontophoresis: from the lab to the bed side. Exp Eye Res 2004; 78(3): 751-7.

[84]   Hastings MS, Li SK, Miller DJ, Bernstein PS, Mufson D. Visulex: advancing iontophoresis for the effective noninvasive back-to-the-eye therapeutics. Drug Delivery Tech 2004; 4: 53-7.

[85]   Csaky KG. New developments in the transscleral delivery of ophthalmic agents. The profile of the drug being delivered is as important as the delivery method. Retina Today 2007; 32-3.

Send Orders of Reprints at reprints@benthamscience.net

CHAPTER 7

Novel Strategies to Enhance Ocular Bioavailability

Pradeep K. Karla[1], Sai HS. Boddu[2], Ashaben Patel[3], Ann-Marie Ako-Adouno[1] and Ashim K. Mitra[3],*

[1]*Division of Pharmaceutical Sciences, School of Pharmacy, Howard University, 2300 4th St NW, Washington D.C. 20059, USA;* [2]*Department of Pharmacy Practice, College of Pharmacy and Pharmaceutical Sciences, The University of Toledo, Ohio, USA – 43614 and* [3]*Division of Pharmaceutical Sciences, School of Pharmacy, University of Missouri-Kansas City, 2464 Charlotte Street, Kansas City, MO 64108-2718, USA*

Abstract: Drug delivery to the eye is highly challenging due to the existence of protective anatomical barriers. Numerous vision threatening diseases affect the anterior and posterior segments of the eye. The topical route is the most common mode of drug administration for the treatment of eye diseases. Following topical administration, less than 5% of instilled dose may be absorbed primarily by corneal and secondarily by conjunctival pathway. However, the remaining portion of the drug is washed out by pre-corneal mechanisms such as tear turnover, nasolachrymal drainage and blink reflex. In addition, the physicochemical properties of the drug and lipoidal nature of the cornea limit ocular absorption. Various therapeutic strategies such as ultrasound, microneedle and prodrug modification are known to enhance drug concentrations at the target tissues. In this chapter, we made an attempt to discuss briefly these strategies and their role in enhancing bioavailability in the anterior and posterior ocular segments.

Keywords: Eye, bioavailability, efflux transporter, prodrugs, microneedles.

INTRODUCTION

The eye is primarily divided into anterior and posterior segments [1]. Both the compartments are protected by various anatomical and biological barriers. These barriers along with the complex structure of the globe result in poor ocular bioavailability [2]. The topical route is the most common mode of drug administration for targeting the anterior segment [2,3]. However, following

---

*Address correspondence to Ashim K. Mitra: University of Missouri Curators' Professor of Pharmacy, Chairman, Division of Pharmaceutical Sciences, Vice-Provost for Interdisciplinary Research, University of Missouri - Kansas City, School of Pharmacy, 2464 Charlotte Street, Kansas City, MO 64108, USA; Tel: 816-235-1615: Fax: 816-235-5779; E-mail: mitraa@umkc.edu

topical administration, a large fraction cf the instilled dose is washed away due to tear turn over (0.5-2.2 μL/min) and rapid blinking (6-15times/min) within 2-5 minutes. These non productive processes result in poor ocular bioavailability, generally less than 5% [4-6]. Anterior segment bioavailability is further diminished by the presence of various barriers such as nasolachryimal drainage, impermeable corneal epithelium and blood ocular barriers. The cornea is primarily composed of five different layers, *i.e.*, epithelium, Bowman's membrane, stroma, Descemet's membrane and endothelium (Fig. **1**) [7].

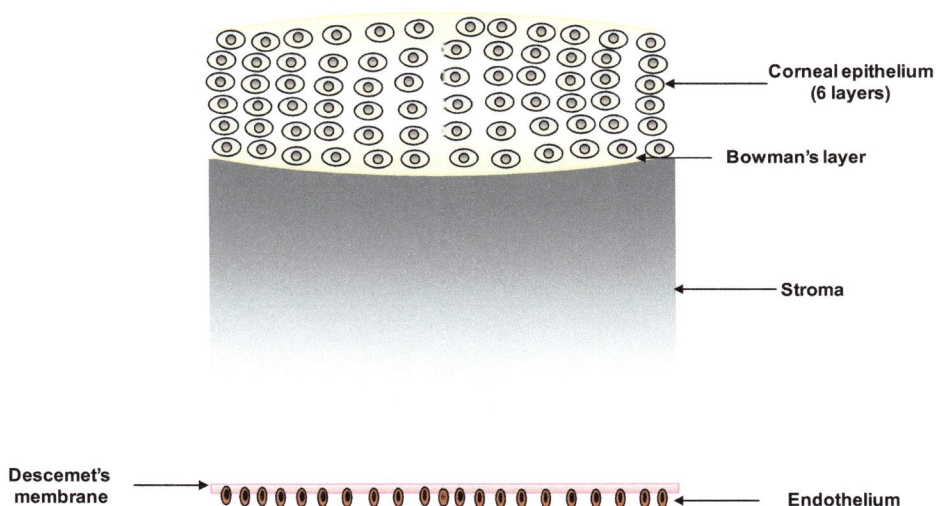

Figure 1: Structure of human cornea – A major barrier for anterior segment drug delivery.

The corneal epithelium acts as a barrier to the absorption of hydrophilic drugs while the stroma acts as a barrier for the passage of hydrophobic drugs [8,9]. Therefore compounds with an optimum oil to water partition will exhibit maximum corneal penetration [8]. Topical formulations consisting of penetration enhancers and mucoadhesives can also significantly enhance the ocular bioavailability. Incorporation of mucoadhesive and viscosity enhancers such as carbopols, polyacrylic acids and chitosan in the topical formulations helps to prolong drug residence time in the cul-de-sac and thereby improving ocular absorption [10]. Penetration enhancers (surfactants, calcium chelators) disrupt tight epithelial junctions on the cornea in a reversible manner and thereby facilitating drug penetration [11,12]. Karla *et al.* [13] identified a wide array of efflux transporters (MRPs) on human corneal epithelium and demonstrated that these transporters can significantly lower permeability of anti-glaucoma and anti-viral agents.

Drug delivery to the posterior segment is challenging due to the presence of unique anatomical and physiological barriers [14]. Intravitreal injection is primarily employed as a drug delivery strategy for the treatment of posterior segment disorders as age related macular degeneration, proliferative vitreoretinopathy, diabetic retinopathy, retinoblastoma and cytomegalovirus retinitis [4]. Although intravitreal injections deliver molecules directly to the neural retina; adverse effects such as endophthalmitis, retinal detachment and hemorrhage, often result in poor patient compliance [15,16]. Entry of xenobiotics following systemic or periocular (subconjunctival, retrobulbar, peribulbar and sub-tenon) administration is hindered by the blood aqueous barrier (BAB) and blood retinal barrier (BRB) [17]. Various ocular barriers associated with the anterior and posterior segment delivery are illustrated in Fig. **2**.

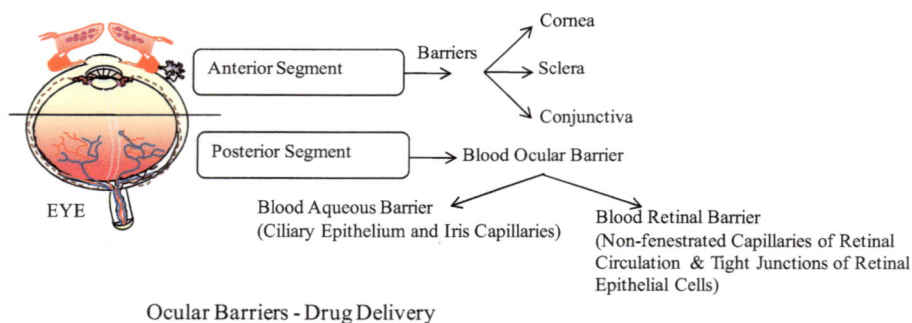

Ocular Barriers - Drug Delivery

Figure 2: Ocular barriers for drug delivery to anterior and posterior segments.

In addition, the presence of various efflux transporters further limits drug penetration after systemic administration [13,18,19]. Advancements in therapeutic approaches, surgical techniques, chemical technologies, formulation strategies and material sciences resulted in significant efforts to develop novel strategies for enhancing ocular bioavailability. Several novel drug delivery strategies such as the prodrug approach, ultrasound and microneedle are being widely studied. This chapter discusses a few promising novel ocular drug delivery strategies which may soon enter the clinic.

ULTRASOUND

As mentioned previously, impermeable nature of the cornea significantly limits drug entry [20-22]. The epithelium is the dominant barrier for penetration of hydrophilic drugs while the stroma is regarded the primary barrier for lipophilic drugs [8,9]. Various physical methods including iontophoresis and sonophoresis have been employed for changing barrier properties of the cornea. Sonophoresis involves the use of ultrasound for increasing the absorption of topically applied compounds. This technique was initially utilized for enhancing systemic bioavailability of transdermally applied drugs. Unlike the conventional passive diffusion process, the ultrasound application enhances drug transport by either thermal effects (due to absorption of sound waves) or non-thermal effects (cavitation, microstreaming and acoustic streaming) [23-27]. Cavitation is caused by formation of vapor bubbles in the region where liquid pressure falls below its vapor pressure [28]. The vapor bubbles collapse forming a high speed jet in a small region which is capable of causing pits on the surface of biological membranes [29-31]. This technique was used in transcorneal drug delivery for the treatment of corneal inflammation, wound and healing retinal dystrophy [25, 32-36]. The utility of sonophoresis in topically administered drugs has been widely reported. Recently, application of this technique in ocular gene delivery has been reported. Nuritdinov [37] achieved a 5-fold increase in corneal permeability of fluorescein after application of 880 kHz ultrasound. Tsok *et al*. [38] studied permeability of 99mTc-pertechnetate, ^{125}I and ^{45}CaCl$_2$ in the rabbit eye tissues including the aqueous and vitreous humor, cornea, iris, sclera, crystalline lens, choroid and retina following ultrasound application in varying frequencies (127, 295, 470, 660, 880, 1000, 2750 kHz). Frequency plays a key role in determining drug permeability across various ocular tissues. Sonophoresis at a frequency of 470, 660, 880 kHz and intensities of 0.2 to 0.3 W/cm^2 produced a 10 fold enhancement in corneal permeability.

Zderic *et al*. [39] studied the efficacy of 1-s bursts of 20-kHz ultrasound, at I(SAPA) of 14 W/cm^2 (I(SATA) of 2 W/cm^2) in raising *in vitro* corneal permeability of anti-glaucoma drugs of varying lipophilicity. The donor compartment was filled with phosphate buffer saline and the receiver compartment was filled with a commercial ophthalmic solution of atenolol, timolol, betaxolol and carteolol. Ultrasound was applied with a liquid processor containing a vibrating transducer tip operating for duration of 10, 30 and 60 min. In the control experiment, the cornea was exposed to drug solutions, but no ultrasound was applied. An increase in corneal permeability of atenolol, carteolol, timolol and betaxolol by 2.6, 2.8, 1.9 and 4.4 times respectively was observed. The same group further investigated the efficacy of ultrasound in enhancing corneal permeability of hydrophilic drug molecules. The researchers examined the mechanism involved in the enhancement of sodium fluorescein through rabbit cornea. *In vitro* permeability of sodium fluorescein improved by 2.1, 2.5and 4.2 times when ultrasound was applied at 0.19, 0.34and 0.56 W/cm^2, respectively for 5 min. The dye concentrations in aqueous humor were 2.4, 3.8 and 10.6 times relative to sham treatment at 0.19, 0.34 and 0.56 W/cm^2 respectively. The report suggested that the rise in permeability resulted from structural changes in the cornea [31].

Sonoda *et al.* [40] observed a significant improvement in the *in vitro* (rabbit corneal epithelial cells) and *in vivo* (rabbit cornea) gene transfer in the presence of microbubble mediated ultrasound. Zheng *et al.* [41] demonstrated that ultra sound targeted microbubbles destruction (UTMD) is capable of enhancing the transfection efficiency of the recombinant adeno-associated virus and plasmid in ARPE-19 cell line.

Ultrasound has the potential to raise ocular bioavailability and can be utilized as a minimally invasive method for ocular drug delivery. But its clinical application is of great concern as the technique may result in structural alteration of the epithelial layer. Feasibility of ultrasound in a clinical setting requires a more complete and detailed safety study.

MICRONEEDLE

Drug delivery to the inner compartments of the eye is very challenging. Posterior segment access *via* non-invasive or minimal invasive techniques would be more patient compliant and will offer significant advantages in treating diseases like age related macular degeneration, diabetic macular edema and proliferative vitreoretinopathy. Microneedle is a novel strategy to deliver drugs into inner compartments by topical administration. This drug delivery strategy confers various advantages by reducing pain, tissue damage and as a result more patient compliant. Moreover, due to the small needle size the device is predicted to avoid nerves innervating tissues and pain associated with damage by injection (Jiang J 2008, Ph.D. Dissertation - Ocular Drug Delivery Using Microneedles, Georgia Institute of Technology). Microneedle as a drug delivery technique has been successfully demonstrated to deliver vaccines, polymer encapsulated drugs and peptides (insulin) *via* transdermal route [42-44]. Studies by Jian *et al.*, 2007 successfully demonstrated that macromolecules can be delivered employing microneedles to the inner ocular compartments *via* intra-scleral and intra-corneal routes (Jiang *et al.* AICHE Annual Meeting, Abstract 96395). *In vitro* experiments demonstrated that hollow microneedles can successfully deliver drugs in humans *via* intrascleral route. These experiments for the first time demonstrated that microneedles can efficiently deliver higher drug concentrations to inner ocular compartments in a minimally invasive manner relative to traditional methods. *In vivo* studies using topical administration of drug loaded microneedles was also performed by Jiang *et al.* in rabbit model, which indicated a ~60 fold increase in fluorescein concentration in the anterior chamber compared to equivalent drug alone as control. Also, no cytotoxicity or tissue damage was observed in these studies.

This recent drug delivery strategy holds a significant promise for delivery to the posterior segment *via* topical administration. Various disease states that may be benefited in future by employing microneedles include, glaucoma, diabetic retinopathy and age related macular degeneration.

PRODRUG

Cornea forms the primary barrier for anterior segment ocular drug delivery and Conjuctiva/Sclera forms the barriers for drug administered topically to target the posterior segment eye diseases. While different techniques were explored to overcome these barriers, prodrug strategy has been a promising approach with demonstrated *in vitro* and *in vivo* therapeutic efficacies. Understanding the ability of corneal and other ocular tissues to metabolize the drug molecules is of prime importance for the prodrug strategy. In the design of prodrugs, a promoiety is linked to the active drug by chemical synthetic procedures [45]. This prodrug derivatization is widely utilized in the optimization of various physicochemical properties of a drug molecule including aqueous solubility, chemical and enzymatic stability and lipophilicity. Hydrolysis of the ester or amide linkage that binds the promoiety to the active drug by the peptidase and esterase enzymes will result in active drug release. Various factors such as affinity of the prodrug linkage to enzymatic hydrolysis, enzyme turnover rate capacity *etc.* affect the enzymatic hydrolysis. Enzymatic acivity of esterases was found to be at highest level in the ocular tissues in the following order: iris-ciliary body > cornea > aqueous humor. Butylcholinesterase (BuChE) is the major esterase enzyme present in the ocular tissues along with acetylcholinesterase (AChE). However, the esterase enzyme levels were found to vary in albino rabbit corneas, a major animal model in ocular drug research. Another prominent class of enzyme system responsible for the hydrolysis of "amide link" of the peptide prodrugs are peptidases/proteases. Endo-peptidases are known to cleave the internal peptide bonds and Exo-peptidases are known to cleave the external bonds. Enzymatic acivity of peptidases was found to be at highest level in the ocular tissues in the following order: corneal epithelium ≥ iris-ciliary body > conjunctiva > corneal stroma [45]. Efflux and influx transporters are expressed on the cell membrane. Promoieties are designed to mimic the nutrients, peptides and other molecules transported by the influx transporters on the cell membrane. Research indicated that prodrug approach significantly enhanced the absorption profiles of various drug molecules. The predicted mechanism for enhanced bioavailability at target site is due to prodrug being transported across the membrane barrier by the promoiety transporter.

Prodrug strategy has been successfully investigated to enhance the efficacy and ocular bioavailability of several topically applied compounds. Research indicated that peptidases (Amino, dipeptidyl and amino-dipeptidyl) are responsible for drug hydrolysis in rabbit ocular tissue homogenates of tear fluid, cornea, lens body, iris-ciliary system and conjunctiva [46].

Hussain *et al.* [47] introduced the concept of prodrugs in ophthalmic drug delivery in 1976. This article reported that dipivalyl ester prodrug of epinephrine (DPE) can overcome the problem of inefficient absorption of epinephrine through the lipoidal corneal epithelium. DPE absorption improved 8-10 times more than the parent drug because of higher lipophilicity and acceptable aqueous solubility [48]. Moreover, the drug loss *via* systemic circulation was reduced 100-400 times leading to lower systemic levels and reduced cardiovascular side effects [47]. Since then the concept of prodrug derivatization has been employed for improving ocular delivery of various antivirals, antiglaucoma agents and steroids.

SELECTED CASE STUDIES OF VARIOUS OPHTHALMIC PRODRUGS

Prostaglandin $F_{2\alpha}$

Prostaglandins (PGs) are effective in reducing intraocular pressure in mammals [49]. However, these compounds are fairly lipophilic and the therapy is associated with several ocular side effects such as conjunctival hyperemia, color changes in eye lashes, periocular skin pigmentation and darkening of the iris due to nonspecific binding [50]. Prodrug derivatization has been successfully utilized for enhancing the potency and safety of PGs (Fig. **3**).

Various 1-methyl and 1-benzyl ester prodrugs were synthesized by esterification of the 1-carboxylic acid group (Fig. **3**). The ester prodrugs were found to be 2-3 fold more lipophilic than $PGF_{2\alpha}$ and showed higher *in vitro* corneal permeability (25-40 fold). Although ester prodrugs exhibited improved ocular hypotensive effect by alleviating the concentration of $PGF_{2\alpha}$ in intraocular tissues (*e.g.*, aqueous humor, ciliary body, iris) the problem of ocular side effects still remained unresolved [51,52].

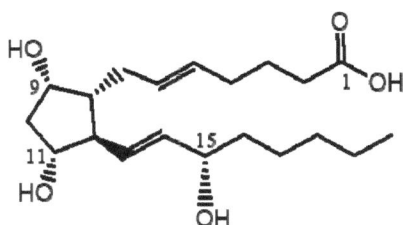

Figure 3: Prostaglandin F2α.

A series of $PGF_{2\alpha}$-mono and diesters with acyl group(s) at the 9, 11 and 15 have been synthesized as an alternative strategy to reduce or eliminate ocular surface side effects of $PGF_{2\alpha}$ [53,54]. Among them, $PGF_{2\alpha}$-11-acyl-, $PGF_{2\alpha}$-15-acyl- and

PGF$_{2\alpha}$-11,15-diacyl esters seemed to be promising, as they lowered intraocular pressure with mild ocular side effects. Esters of PGF$_{2\alpha}$ showed higher corneal permeability but slow bioconversion into PGF$_{2\alpha}$ leading to poor bioavailability [53-55].

Latanoprost was the first prostaglandin prodrug approved by FDA in 1996 for IOP reduction in patients with open angle glaucoma or ocular hypertension. The compound showed higher affinity to the prostaglandin F (FP) receptors and thus lower conjunctival hyperemia [56]. Currently, several prostaglandin prodrugs are on the market which includes bimatoprost (Lumigan®), travoprost (Travatan®) and unoprostone isopropyl (Rescula®) (Fig. **4**). Latanoprost, travoprost, unoprostone isopropyl are isopropyl esters of their parent acids. Bimatoprost is an N-ethyl amide of the parent acid, which has been reported to be a prostanoid FP receptor agonist [57]. Matsumura *et al.* synthesized tafluprost, an ester prodrug of the 15, 15-difluoro-prostaglandin F$_{2\alpha}$ which showed 10 times more affinity for FP receptor relative to latanoprost [58].

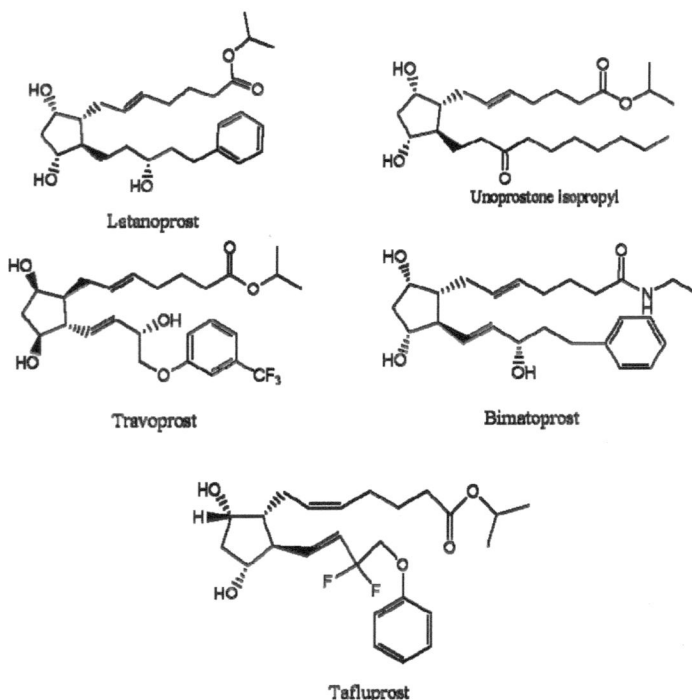

Figure 4: Various prostaglandin analogues.

SA9000

Ethacrynic acid is a commercially available diuretic which indicated for the treatment of elevated intraocular pressure [59,60]. Poor corneal permeability and lower tissue concentration require the application of higher concentrations (3-4%w/v) of ethacrynic acid which in turn results in severe ocular side effects such as conjunctival hyperemia [61]. Shimazaki *et al.* [62] synthesized SA9000 (ethacrynic acid analogue) which displays higher intrinsic corneal permeability than the parent drug (Fig. **5**).

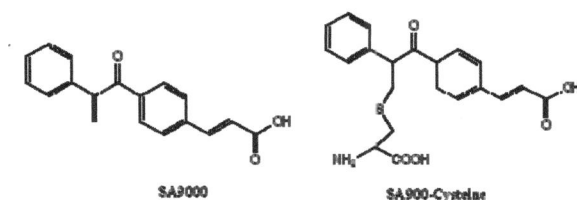

Figure 5: Structures of SA9000 and SA9000-cysteine.

In vivo studies with SA9000 demonstrated that a single dose of SA9000 (0.3%) could produce significant reduction in IOP lasting for 3 days. However, the inherent thiol reactivity resulted in corneal hyperemia and conjunctival chemosis. Arnold *et al.* [63] synthesized a cysteine adduct of SA9000 and studied the effect on the intraocular pressure in rabbits. This study concluded that SA9000-cystein adduct (0.3%) could significantly reduce IOP with no apparent ocular irritation. Moreover, corneal hyperemia was significantly lower following topical administration of 0.9% SA9000-cystein adducts relative to 0.3% SA9000.

Cyclosporine

Cyclosporine A (CsA) is a powerful immunosuppressive agent indicated in the treatment of dry eye syndrome, uveitis and prevention of corneal graft rejection [64, 65]. CsA is highly lipophilic in nature and hence its formulation into eye drops is not feasible [66]. It is currently marketed as topical oil-in-water emulsion under the trade name Restasis®, (Allergan Inc., Irvine, CA). However, this formulation is associated with side-effects such as burning, pain, stinging, redness, or itching resulting in poor ocular tolerance [67]. To overcome the undesirable side effects of cyclosporine A

(CsA), a water soluble prodrug of CsA called UNIL088 was synthesized. UNIL088 exhibits excellent ocular tolerability after single and chronic administrations. Lallemande *et al.* [68] demonstrated that ~20% of UNIL088 was converted to CsA in 30 min in the presence of rabbit tears, mainly by enzymatic hydrolysis. Topical administration of UNIL088 resulted in sustained therapeutic concentrations of CsA in tear fluids. UNIL088 seems to be a promising drug for the therapy of the dry eye syndrome and avoiding the corneal graft rejection [69]. Possible pathways of UNIL088 hydrolysis are given in (Fig. **6**).

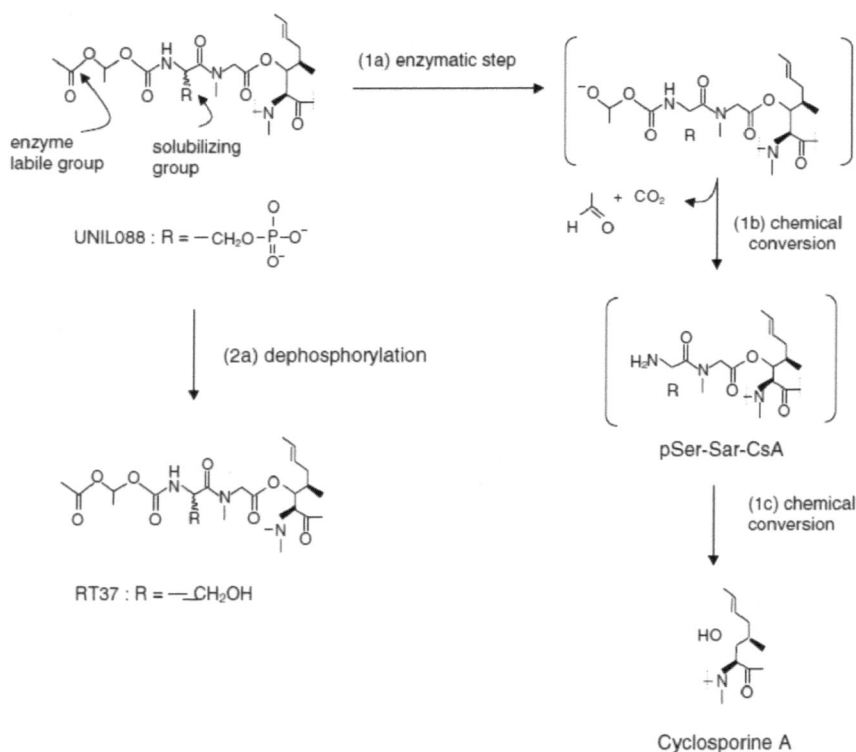

Figure 6: Possible pathway of UNIL088 hydrolysis. Figure is reproduced with permission from Lallemand *et al.* 2007 [69].

Nepafenac

Nepafenac is an amide prodrug of amfenac, a potent cyclooxygenase inhibitor which suppresses PGE2 synthesis (Fig. **7**). Nepafenac has a higher therapeutic index value compared to amfenac [70]. Recently, FDA has approved 0.1% nepafenac ophthalmic suspension for the treatment of pain and inflammation after cataract surgery [71]. Gamache *et al.* [72] showed that topically applied nepafenac (0.1%) can significantly inhibit the synthesis of PGs in the retina–choroid by about 55% for 4 hours, while diclofenac (0.1%), has only a minimal effect [73]. Moreover, nepafenac is also effective in the treatment of retinal neovascularization in a rat model following topical administration. Nepafenac can readily penetrate the cornea and get converted into amfenac, a potent cyclooxygenase (COX)-1 and COX-2 inhibitor [74].

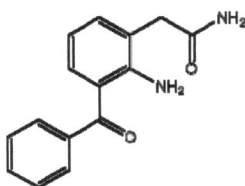

Figure 7: Structure of Nepafenac.

Takahashi *et al.* demonstrated that nepafenac; following topical application to the cornea can effectively inhibit retinal and choroidal neovascularization. These important findings clearly suggest the use of nepafenac in the treatment of anterior and posterior segment diseases because of its ability to readily permeate through the cornea and get converted into parent drug amfenac in the iris/ciliary body and retina/choroid [73].

TG100572

Doukas *et al.* [75] developed several benzotriazine inhibitors designed to target VEGFr2, Src for treatment of AMD. Among them, TG100572 was found to be most potent, dual inhibitor of both VEGFr2 and the Src family kinases. Major disadvantage associated with this compound is its short half life in ocular tissues. Its aqueous solubility is very low (maximum formulation concentration~0.7%), making it difficult to achieve sufficient concentration in posterior segment. Various ester prodrugs of TG100572 were developed to improve delivery to the back of the eye after topical administration. TG100801, an ester prodrug of TG100572 following topical administration, was readily converted to the parent compound in the eye. It demonstrated favourable ocular pharmacokinetics and negligible systemic level and indicated promise for the laser induced choroidal neovascularization model [76]. Table **1** summarizes ocular pharmacokinetic parameters.

Table 1: Exposure level of TG100572 in ocular tissue after single bilateral administration of TG100572 and TG100801 in mice. Table reproduced with permission from Palanki *et al.* 2008 [76]

Compound administered	Compound measured	Ocular tissue	T_{max} (hr)	$C_{max}(\mu M)$	AUC (h.ug/mL)
TG100572	TG100572	Retina	0.5	3.6	3.2
		Choroid/sclera	0.5	23	240
		Cornea	0.5	64	560
TG100801	TG100572	Retina	24	2.4	35
		Choroid/sclera	24	29	540
		Cornea	7	33	670

Prodrug derivatization is proven to be an effective method for both anterior and posterior segment drug delivery. Ocular bioavailability can be significantly improved by synthesizing prodrugs with optimal solubility, stability and partition coefficient. Several approved ocular prodrugs are on the market for the treatment of anterior segment disease. In future, topical application of prodrug can be a promising strategy for the treatment of posterior segment diseases which are otherwise difficult to treat by topical application.

TRANSPORTER TARGETED PRODRUG APPROACH

Various influx transporters are located on the corneal epithelium, conjunctiva and blood retinal barrier. These proteins play a role in the transport of vitral nutrients and other xenobiotics across the biological membranes in the vital organs [77]. Ocular bioavailability can be significantly enhanced by targeting influx transporters utilizing transporter targeted ligands. The prodrugs can act as substrates for the transporters and can be translocated across epithelial membrane. In addition transporter targeted prodrug approach, may also increase ocular bioavailability by evasion of various efflux pumps. Presence of efflux pumps on various ocular barriers has been recently identified from our laboratory. Karla *et al.* [78] demonstrated the presence of wide array of MRP class of efflux pumps on the human cornea which confer significant drug resistance [13,19,79]. These transporters decrease permeability of glaucoma treating agents (bimatoprost, latanoprost) and antiviral agents (acyclovir) across human corneal epithelium. Cornea is the major barrier for anterior segment drug delivery. A scheme demonstrating the localization of various efflux transporters on the cornea has been shown in Fig. **8**.

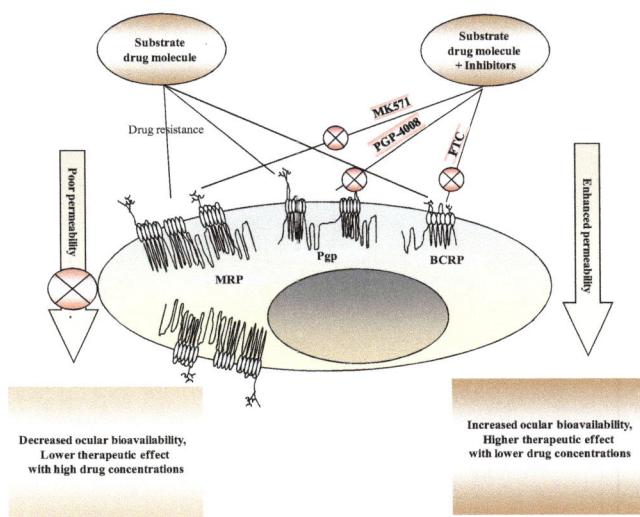

Figure 8: Schematic representation of possible localization of efflux transporters in human corneal epithelial cell. Pgp and BCRP are shown to be present on apical side. MRP has different homologues which are distributed on apical and basal side. Employing specific Pgp inhibitor (PGP-4008), MRP inhibitor (MK-571) and BCRP inhibitor (FTC) is shown to increase the permeability of drugs across corneal epithelium.

As the scheme depicts, Pgp, MRP and BCRP are localized on the apical side of cornea. A few homologues of MRP are known to be present on the basolateral side of cornea [13]. The scheme demonstrates that specific inhibitors can increase drug permeability across the cornea. Prodrug approach targeting various influx transporters can be highly advantageous, as prodrugs were shown to bypass efflux transporters on cornea [80]. Recent findings from our laboratory indicate that cornea expresses various influx transporters. The cornea expresses peptide and amino acid transporters [80,81]. Acyclovir (ACV), a nucleoside analogue commonly indicated in the treatment of ocular herpes keratitis exhibited poor permeability across the cornea. Topical administration of ACV was shown to be ineffective leading to treatment failure [82]. Peptide and amino acid prodrugs of ACV were shown to have increased corneal permeability and anti-viral efficacy [83,84]. Table **2** published from our laboratory represents increased permeability of ACV upon prodrug derivatization to peptide and amino acid prodrugs. Table **3** also published from our work demonstrated excellent anti-viral efficacy of both amino acid and peptide prodrugs of ACV.

Table 2: Increased permeability of (Valine-ACV) amino acid and (Valine-Valine-ACV) peptide prodrugs of ACV. Table reproduced with permission from Anand *et al.* 2003 [85] (*p<0.05)

Drug	Papp × 106 cm/sec (±S.D)
ACV	4.24 (± 1.41)
VACV	12.10 (± 0.44)
VVACV	9.91 (± 2.40)

Table 3: *In vitro* antiviral efficacy of amino acid and peptide prodrugs of ACV. Table reproduced with permission from Anand *et al.* 2003 [85]

Drug	HSV-1(μM)	HSV-2(μM)
ACV	EC50 = 7.1	EC50 = 6.6
VACV	EC50 = 9.1	EC50 = 7.77
VVACV	EC50 = 6.14	EC50 = 22.7

EC50 – Concentration for 50%viral cytopathogenicity inhibition.

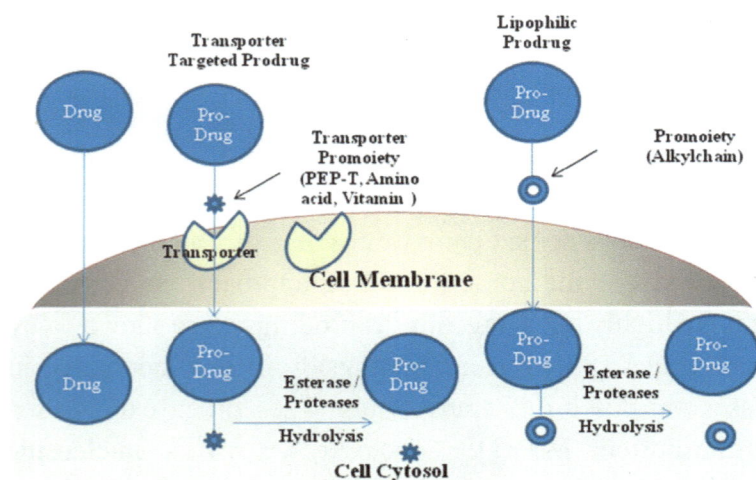

Figure 9: Targeted prodrug and lipophilic prodrug strategies. Structure, mode of permeation and release of active drug moiety at site of action.

Prodrugs are recognized as substrates by influx transporters on the BRB, cornea and conjunctiva. Thus, it can also increase drug penetration into ocular tissues. The inactive prodrug is converted to active drug moiety by various enzymes such as, peptidases and esterases [85]. A schematic representation of cellular entry and conversion is shown in Fig. **9**.

CONCLUSION

Drug delivery to various ocular compartments (anterior and posterior segment) is equally challenging. Advancements in the field of synthetic and medicinal chemistry facilitated the design, synthesis and development of novel therapeutic agents for the treatment of ocular diseases. Despite of the high developmental cost, most drug molecules fail in clinical trials because of their poor physicochemical properties. As a result extensive efforts have been devoted to the development of novel drug delivery strategies. Iontophoresis, sonophoresis, microneedles and transporter targeted prodrug approach are some of the technologies which can significantly enhance the ocular bioavailability. Several transporters/receptors have been identified and functionally characterized on various ocular barriers such as cornea, conjunctiva, BRB and retina. Transporter/receptor targeted prodrug approach has dual advantages: *i.e.*, modulations of P-gp/MRP mediated efflux of drugs; and enhance the drug uptake *via* influx pumps. Exploitation of these transporter/receptors may enhance ocular drug bioavailability following topical, systemic, intravitreal, or transscleral/subconjunctival administrations.

ACKNOWLEDGEMENTS

This publication was supported by the National Institutes of Health grants NIHKL2RR031974, R01 EY 09171-16, R01 EY 1065-14 and AACP 2012 New Investigator Grant. Sections of the article and figures are reproduced from the thesis published by the primary author (Copyright holder).

CONFLICT OF INTEREST

The author(s) confirm that this chapter content has no conflict of interest.

REFERENCES

[1]   Kaplan HJ. Anatomy and function of the eye. Chem Immunol Allergy 2007; 92: 4-10.

[2]   Gaudana R, Jwala J, Boddu SH, Mitra AK. Recent perspectives in ocular drug delivery. Pharm Res 2009; 26(5): 1197-216.

[3]   Lee VH, Robinson JR. Topical ocular drug delivery: recent developments and future challenges. J Ocul Pharmacol 1986; 2(1): 67-108.

[4]   Janoria KG, Gunda S, Boddu SH, Mitra AK. Novel approaches to retinal drug delivery. Expert Opin Drug Deliv 2007; 4(4): 371-88.

[5]   Kearns VR, Williams RL. Drug delivery systems for the eye. Expet Rev Med Dev 2009; 6(3): 277-90.

[6]   Lee VH, Robinson JR. Mechanistic and quantitative evaluation of precorneal pilocarpine disposition in albino rabbits. J Pharm Sci 1979; 68(6): 673-84.

[7]   Dingeldein SA, Klyce SD. Imaging of the cornea. Cornea 1988; 7(3): 170-82.

[8]   Prausnitz MR, Noonan JS. Permeability of cornea, sclera and conjunctiva: a literature analysis for drug delivery to the eye. J Pharm Sci 1998; 87(12): 1479-88.

[9]   Huang HS, Schoenwald RD, Lach JL. Corneal penetration behavior of beta-blocking agents II: Assessment of barrier contributions. J Pharm Sci 1983; 72(11): 1272-9.

[10]   Anumolu SS, Singh Y, Gao D, Stein S, Sinko PJ. Design and evaluation of novel fast forming pilocarpine-loaded ocular hydrogels for sustained pharmacological response. J Control Release 2009; 137(2): 152-9.

[11]   Kaur IP, Smitha R. Penetration enhancers and ocular bioadhesives: two new avenues for ophthalmic drug delivery. Drug Dev Ind Pharm 2002; 28(4): 353-69.

[12]   Saha P, Yang JJ, Lee VH. Existence of a p-glycoprotein drug efflux pump in cultured rabbit conjunctival epithelial cells. Investig Ophthalmol Vis Sci 1998; 39(7): 1221-6.

[13]   Karla PK, Quinn TL, Herndon BL, Thomas P, Pal D, Mitra A. Expression of multidrug resistance associated protein 5 (MRP5) on cornea and its role in drug efflux. J Ocul Pharmacol Ther 2009; 25(2): 121-32.

[14]   Lee SS, Robinson MR. Novel drug delivery systems for retinal diseases. A review. Ophthalmic Res 2009; 41(3): 124-35.

[15]   Baum J, Peyman GA, Barza M. Intravitreal administration of antibiotic in the treatment of bacterial endophthalmitis. III. Consensus. Survey of ophthalmology 1982; 26(4): 204-6.

[16]   Velez G, Whitcup SM. New developments in sustained release drug delivery for the treatment of intraocular disease. Br J Ophthalmol 1999; 83(11): 1225-9.

[17]   Cunha-Vaz JG. The blood-ocular barriers: past, presentand future. Documenta ophthalmologica 1997; 93(1-2): 149-57.

[18]   Dey S, Patel J, Anand BS, et al. Molecular evidence and functional expression of P-glycoprotein (MDR1) in human and rabbit cornea and corneal epithelial cell lines. Investig Ophthalmol Vis Sci 2003; 44(7): 2909-18.

[19]   Karla PK, Earla R, Boddu SH, Johnston TP, Pal D, Mitra A. Molecular expression and functional evidence of a drug efflux pump (BCRP) in human corneal epithelial cells. Curr Eye Res 2009; 34(1): 1-9.

[20]   Doane MG, Jensen AD, Dohlman CH. Penetration routes of topically applied eye medications. Am J Ophthalmol 1978; 85(3): 383-6.

[21]   Ke TL, Clark AF, Gracy RW. Age-related permeability changes in rabbit corneas. J Ocul Pharmacol Ther 1999; 15(6): 513-23.

[22]   Lee VH. New directions in the optimization of ocular drug delivery. J Ocul Pharmacol 1990; 6(2): 157-64.

[23]   Filippenko VI, Tret'iak VV. The treatment of eye diseases using the Gamma-G ultrasonic apparatus. Voen Med Zh 1989; (8): 30-1.

[24]   Cherkasov IS, Marmur RK, Radkovskaia A, Loskova LM. Phonophoresis of hypotensive agents in the treatment of simple glaucoma. Oftalmol Zh 1974; 29(2): 114-8.

[25]   Gvarishvili EP, Dushin NV. Effect of superphonoelectrophoresis on chorioretinal dystrophy. Vestn Oftalmol 1999; 115(4): 19-21.

[26]   Silverman RH. High-resolution ultrasound imaging of the eye - a review. Clin Experiment Ophthalmol 2009; 37(1): 54-67.

[27]   Fielding JA. Ocular ultrasound. Clin Radiol 1996; 51(8): 533-44.

[28]   Miller DL. A review of the ultrasonic bioeffects of microsonation, gas-body activationand related cavitation-like phenomena. Ultrasound Med Biol 1987; 13(8): 443-70.

[29]   Tachibana K, Tachibana S. The use of ultrasound for drug delivery. Echocardiography 2001; 18(4): 323-8.

[30]   Tang H, Mitragotri S, Blankschtein D, Langer R. Theoretical description of transdermal transport of hydrophilic permeants: application to low-frequency sonophoresis. J Pharm Sci 2001; 90(5): 545-68.

[31]   Zderic V, Clark JI, Vaezy S. Drug delivery into the eye with the use of ultrasound. J Ultrasound Med 2004; 23(10): 1349-59.

[32]   Egorov EA, Kriukova MB, Khabush T, Kriukov AI. Results of intraocular pharmaco-physical therapy in inflammatory diseases of the cornea. Vestn Oftalmol 1995; 111(1): 31-4.

[33]   Marmur RK, Moiseeva NN, Korkhov SS. Current state and perspectives of further development of phonophoresis of drugs in ophthalmology (review of the literature). Oftalmol Zh 1979; 34(2): 68-73.

[34]   Iakimenko SA, Chalanova RI. Phonophoresis of the proteolytic enzymes lekozim or kollalizin in the combined therapy of eye burns. Oftalmol Zh 1990; (6): 321-4.

[35]   Iakimenko SA, Chalanova RI, Artemov AV. The use of lekozim phonophoresis for the treatment of eye burns. Oftalmol Zh 1989; (8): 492-7.

[36]   Tsok RM. Phonophoresis in various diseases of the anterior segment of the eye. Oftalmol Zh 1979; 34(2): 73-6.

[37]   Nuritdinov VA. Phonophoresis and cavitation. Vestn Oftalmol 1981; (1): 56-8.

[38]   Tsok RM, Gereliuk IP, Tsok OB, Kaminskii Iu M. The effect of ultrasonic oscillations of different frequencies on radionuclide accumulation in the eye tissues. Oftalmol Zh 1990; (1): 46-9.

[39]   Zderic V, Vaezy S, Martin RW, Clark JI. Ocular drug delivery using 20-kHz ultrasound. Ultrasound Med Biol 2002; 28(6): 823-9.

[40]   Sonoda S, Tachibana K, Uchino E, *et al.* Gene transfer to corneal epithelium and keratocytes mediated by ultrasound with microbubbles. Investig Ophthalmol Vis Sci 2006; 47(2): 558-64.

[41]   Zheng XZ, Li HL, Du LF, Wang HP, Gu Q. Comparative analysis of gene transfer to human and rat retinal pigment epithelium cell line by a combinatorial use of recombinant adeno- associated virus and ultrasound or/and microbubbles. Bosn J Basic Med Sci 2009; 9(3): 174-81.

[42]   Wang PC, Wester BA, Rajaraman S, Paik SJ, Kim SH, Allen MG. Hollow polymer microneedle array fabricated by photolithography process combined with micromolding technique. Conf Proc IEEE Eng Med Biol Soc 2009; 1: 7026-9.

[43]   Prausnitz MR, Mikszta JA, Cormier Mandrianov AK. Microneedle-based vaccines. Current topics in microbiology and immunology 2009; 333: 369-93.

[44]   Gupta J, Felner EI, Prausnitz MR. Minimally invasive insulin delivery in subjects with type 1 diabetes using hollow microneedles. Diabetes Technol Ther 2009; 11(6): 329-37.

[45]   Talluri RS, Hariharan S, Karla PK, Mitra AK. Drug delivery to cornea and conjunctiva-esterase and protease directed prodrug design, in Ocular Periphery and Disorders. Darlene A. Dartt PB, Patricia D'Amore RD, Linda Mcloon & Jerry Niederkorn, editors: Elsevier, Academic Press; 2011.

[46]   Kashi SD, Lee VH. Hydrolysis of enkephalins in homogenates of anterior segment tissues of the albino rabbit eye. Invest Ophthalmol Vis Sci 1986; 27(8): 1300-3.

[47]   Hussain A, Truelove JE. Prodrug approaches to enhancement of physicochemical properties of drugs IV: novel epinephrine prodrug. J Pharm Sci 1976; 65(10): 1510-2.

[48]   Wei CPanderson JA, Leopold I. Ocular absorption and metabolism of topically applied epinephrine and a dipivalyl ester of epinephrine. Invest Ophthalmol Vis Sci 1978; 17(4): 315-21.

[49]   Bito LZ, Draga A, Blanco J, Camras CB. Long-term maintenance of reduced intraocular pressure by daily or twice daily topical application of prostaglandins to cat or rhesus monkey eyes. Invest Ophthalmol Vis Sci 1983; 24(3): 312-9.

[50]   Bito LZ. Prostaglandins. Old concepts and new perspectives. Arch Ophthalmol 1987; 105(8): 1036-9.

[51]   Villumsen J, Alm A, Soderstrom M. Prostaglandin F2 alpha-isopropylester eye drops: effect on intraocular pressure in open-angle glaucoma. Br J ophthalmol 1989; 73(12): 975-9.

[52]   Bito LZ, Baroody RA. The ocular pharmacokinetics of eicosanoids and their derivatives. 1. Comparison of ocular eicosanoid penetration and distribution following the topical application of PGF2 alpha, PGF2 alpha-1-methyl ester and PGF2 alpha-1-isopropyl ester. Exp Eye Res 1987; 44(2): 217-26.

[53]   Cheng-Bennett A, Chan MF, Chen G, et al. Studies on a novel series of acyl ester prodrugs of prostaglandin F2 alpha. Br J Ophthalmol 1994; 78(7): 560-7.

[54]   Woodward DF, Chan MF, Burke JA, et al. Studies on the ocular hypotensive effects of prostaglandin F2 alpha ester prodrugs and receptor selective prostaglandin analogs. J Ocul Pharmacol 1994; 10(1): 177-93.

[55]   Chien DS, Tang-Liu DD, Woodward DF. Ocular penetration and bioconversion of prostaglandin F2 alpha prodrugs in rabbit cornea and conjunctiva. J Pharm Sci 1997; 86(10): 1180-6.

[56]   Alm A, Grierson I, Shields MB. Side effects associated with prostaglandin analog therapy. Surv Ophthalmol 2008; 53(Suppl1): S93-105.

[57]   Sharif NA, Kelly CR, Crider JY, Williams GW, Xu SX. Ocular hypotensive FP prostaglandin (PG) analogs: PG receptor subtype binding affinities and selectivities and agonist potencies at FP and other PG receptors in cultured cells. J Ocul Pharmacol Ther 2003; 19(6): 501-15.

[58]   Takagi Y, Nakajima T, Shimazaki A, et al. Pharmacological characteristics of AFP-168 (tafluprost), a new prostanoid FP receptor agonist, as an ocular hypotensive drug. Exp Eye Res 2004; 78(4): 767-76.

[59]   Tingey DP, Ozment RR, Schroeder A, Epstein DL. The effect of intracameral ethacrynic acid on the intraocular pressure of living monkeys. Am J Ophthalmol 1992; 113(6): 706-11.

[60]   Wang RF, Podos SM, Serle JB, Lee PY, Neufeld AH, Deschenes R. Effects of topical ethacrynic acid ointment *vs.* timolol on intraocular pressure in glaucomatous monkey eyes. Arch Ophthalmol 1994; 112(3): 390-4.

[61]   Tingey DP, Schroeder A, Epstein MP, Epstein DL. Effects of topical ethacrynic acid adducts on intraocular pressure in rabbits and monkeys. Arch Ophthalmol 1992; 110(5): 699-702.

[62]   Shimazaki A, Suhara H, Ichikawa M, *et al.* New ethacrynic acid derivatives as potent cytoskeletal modulators in trabecular meshwork cells. Biol Pharma Bull 2004; 27(6): 846-50.

[63]   Arnold JJ, Choksi Y, Chen X, *et al.* Eyedrops containing SA9000 prodrugs result in sustained reductions in intraocular pressure in rabbits. J Ocul Pharmacol Ther 2009; 25(3): 179-86.

[64]   Foets B, Missotten L, Vanderveeren P, Goossens W. Prolonged survival of allogeneic corneal grafts in rabbits treated with topically applied cyclosporin A: systemic absorption and local immunosuppressive effect. Br J Ophthalmol 1985; 69(8): 600-3.

[65]   Perry HD, Solomon R, Donnenfeld ED, *et al.* Evaluation of topical cyclosporine for the treatment of dry eye disease. Arch Ophthalmol 2008; 126(8): 1046-50.

[66]   Lallemand F, Felt-Baeyens O, Besseghir K, Behar-Cohen F, Gurny R. Cyclosporine A delivery to the eye: a pharmaceutical challenge. Eur J Pharm Biopharm 2003; 56(3): 307-18..

[67]   Sall K, Stevenson OD, Mundorf TK, Reis BL. Two multicenter, randomized studies of the efficacy and safety of cyclosporine ophthalmic emulsion in moderate to severe dry eye disease. CsA Phase 3 Study Group. Ophthalmology 2000; 107(4): 631-9.

[68]   Lallemand F, Felt-Baeyens O, Rudaz S, *et al.* Conversion of cyclosporine A prodrugs in human tears *vs.* rabbits tears. Eur J Pharm Biopharm 2005; 59(1): 51-6.

[69]   Lallemand F, Varesio E, Felt-Baeyens O, Bossy L, Hopfgartner G, Gurny R. Biological conversion of a water-soluble prodrug of cyclosporine A. Eur J Pharm Biopharm 2007; 67(2): 555-61.

[70]   Walsh DA, Moran HW, Shamblee DA, *et al.* Antiinflammatory agents. 4. Syntheses and biological evaluation of potential prodrugs of 2-amino-3-benzoylbenzeneacetic acid and 2-amino-3-(4-chlorobenzoyl)benzeneacetic acid. J Med Chem 1990; 33(8): 2296-304.

[71]   Gaynes B., Onyekwuluje A. Topical ophthalmic NSAIDs: a discussion with focus on nepafenac ophthalmic suspension. Clin Ophthalmol. 2008; 2(2): 355-68.

[72]   Gamache DA, Graff G, Brady MT, Spellman JM, Yanni JM. Nepafenac, a unique nonsteroidal prodrug with potential utility in the treatment of trauma-induced ocular inflammation: I. Assessment of anti-inflammatory efficacy. Inflammation 2000; 24(4): 357-70.

[73]   Ke TL, Graff G, Spellman JM, Yanni JM. Nepafenac, a unique nonsteroidal prodrug with potential utility in the treatment of trauma-induced ocular inflammation: II. *In vitro* bioactivation and permeation of external ocular barriers. Inflammation 2000; 24(4): 371-84.

[74]   Takahashi K, Saishin Y, Saishin Y, *et al.* Topical nepafenac inhibits ocular neovascularization. Invest Ophthalmol Vis Sci 2003; 44(1): 409-15.

[75]   Doukas J, Mahesh S, Umeda N, *et al.* Topical administration of a multi-targeted kinase inhibitor suppresses choroidal neovascularization and retinal edema. J cell physiol 2008; 216(1): 29-37.

[76] Palanki MS, Akiyama H, Campochiaro P, *et al.* Development of prodrug 4-chloro-3-(5-methyl-3-{[4-(2-pyrrolidin-1-ylethoxy)phenyl]amino}-1,2,4-be nzotriazin-7-yl)phenyl benzoate (TG100801): a topically administered therapeutic candidate in clinical trials for the treatment of age-related macular degeneration. J Med Chem 2008; 51(6): 1546-59.

[77] Mannermaa E, Vellonen KS, Urtti A. Drug transport in corneal epithelium and blood-retina barrier: emerging role of transporters in ocular pharmacokinetics. Adv Drug Deliv Rev 2006; 58(11): 1136-63.

[78] Karla PK, Pal D, Mitra AK. Molecular evidence and functional expression of multidrug resistance associated protein (MRP) in rabbit corneal epithelial cells. Exp Eye Res 2007; 84(1): 53-60.

[79] Karla PK, Pal D, Quinn T, Mitra AK. Molecular evidence and functional expression of a novel drug efflux pump (ABCC2) in human corneal epithelium and rabbit cornea and its role in ocular drug efflux. Int J Pharm 2007; 336(1): 12-21.

[80] Anand BS, Katragadda S, Mitra AK. Pharmacokinetics of novel dipeptide ester prodrugs of acyclovir after oral administration: intestinal absorption and liver metabolism. J Pharmacol Exp Ther 2004; 311(2): 659-67.

[81] Jain-Vakkalagadda B, Dey S, Pal D, Mitra AK. Identification and functional characterization of a Na+-independent large neutral amino acid transporter, LAT1, in human and rabbit cornea. Invest Ophthalmol Vis Sci 2003; 44(7): 2919-27.

[82] Trousdale MD, Dunkel EC, Nesburn AB. Effect of acyclovir on acute and latent herpes simplex virus infections in the rabbit. Invest Ophthalmol Vis Sci 1980; 19(11): 1336-41.

[83] Anand BS, Mitra AK. Mechanism of corneal permeation of L-valyl ester of acyclovir: targeting the oligopeptide transporter on the rabbit cornea. Pharm Res 2002; 19(8): 1194-202.

[84] Anand BS, Hill JM, Dey S, Maruyama K, *et al. In vivo* antiviral efficacy of a dipeptide acyclovir prodrug, val-val-acyclovir, against HSV-1 epithelial and stromal keratitis in the rabbit eye model. Invest Ophthalmol Vis Sci 2003; 44(6): 2529-34.

[85] Anand B, Nashed Y, Mitra A. Novel dipeptide prodrugs of acyclovir for ocular herpes infections: Bioreversion, antiviral activity and transport across rabbit cornea. Curr Eye Res 2003; 26(3-4): 151-63.

Send Orders of Reprints at reprints@benthamscience.net

CHAPTER 8

Microdialysis - Utility in Establishing PK/PD Relationships in Ophthalmology

Kay D. Rittenhouse[1,*], Harisha Atluri[2], Sai HS. Boddu[3] and Ashim K. Mitra[4]

[1]Translational Medicine Ophthalmology, Specialty Care Business Unit, Pfizer Inc., USA; [2]Xeno Port Inc. Santa Clara, California, USA; [3]Department of Pharmacy Practice, College of Pharmacy and Pharmaceutical Sciences, The University of Toledo, Ohio, OH 43614, USA and [4]Division of Pharmaceutical Sciences, School of Pharmacy, University of Missouri-Kansas City, Kansas City, Missouri-64108, USA

Abstract: Ocular pharmacokinetics is a core component in the development of therapeutics for eye diseases. In this chapter, we provide a description of the following concepts and strategies that undergird when and where microdialysis may be a significant advance in the armamentarium of approaches for establishing PK/PD relationships in ophthalmology. We cover the following topics:

- Understanding the current limitations in PK/PD with conventional sampling approaches

- Progress report on advances in the use of microdialysis in ophthalmology

- Preclinical *vs.* clinical ocular PK cases studies

- Roadblocks to microdialysis in ophthalmology

  - Probe design and probe recovery

  - Bioanalytical limitations

  - Invasiveness of probe implantation

  - Analyte properties and perfusion flow rate

- Strategies for design of an ideal microdialysis experiment

- Next advances in microdialysis

Keywords: Microdialysis, eye, pharmacokinetics, drug delivery, posterior segment, anterior segment, microdialysis probes.

*Address correspondence to Kay D. Rittenhouse: Translational Medicine Ophthalmology, Clinical Development and Medical Affairs, Specialty Care Business Unit, Pfizer Inc., 10777 Science Center Drive CB4, San Diego, CA 92121 Tel: 858-638-3710; E-mail:kay.rittenhouse@pfizer.com

LIMITATIONS IN PK/PD WITH CONVENTIONAL APPROACHES

The eye is a small but complex organ of the body. Current knowledge of physiological processes within the eye has led to greater appreciation for approaches used to understand various endogenous *versus* xenobiotic modulation of the processes and factors that influence the intraocular drug disposition. Vitreous, a jelly like substance of ~99% water containing a number of important glycosaminoglycans, collagens and hyaluronates, has been characterized as an unstirred compartment. Unlike aqueous humor, vitreous is not regenerated after removal [1]. Recent studies have shown that vitreous has predictable clearance pathways for molecules, based on specific characteristics of candidates under study [2]. Retina, a specialized portion of the eye containing various types of neuronal cells, is a metabolically active organ. At the vitreo-retinal interface, endogenous substances have been measured using a variety of techniques, including vitreous sampling with microdialysis [3, 4]. Recently, the scientific community has focused on posterior segment delivery as well as characteristics of drug disposition following posterior segment administration [5]. Because of this heightened interest, there has been an exponential increase in papers examining the posterior segment ocular pharmacokinetics of candidate drugs, both small molecule and biologicals like monoclonal antibodies, pegylated aptamers and siRNA's. Routine employment of intravitreous routes of administration is a relatively recent event. Previously, intermittent procedures involving intravitreal injections were used such as treating endophalmitis with potent antibiotics and triamcinolone acetonide used off label for treating ocular inflammatory diseases such as uveitis and diabetic macular edema [5]. Implants such as Vitrasert®, a ganciclovir non-erodible device placed in the vitreous of immunocompromised HIV positive subjects, were developed in the 1990's for cytomegaloviral (CMV) retinitis [6]. Vitravene® was the first aptamer approved for intravitreal injection for CMV retinitis [7]. Retisert®, a fluocinolone acetonide non-erodible implant, was approved for the treatment of posterior uveitis and involves surgical placement of the implant at the pars plana region of the eye in the vitreous [8]. Macugen®, a pegylated aptamer that inhibits VEGF165 mediated choroidal neovascularization in wet AMD, paved the way for more common employment of intravitreous drug administration with an approved dosing frequency of every 6 weeks [9]. Lucentis® was approved shortly after Macugen and is currently considered as a standard of care for treating CNV in wet AMD [10]. Avastin®, the full length monoclonal antibody against VEGF-A, which is approved for renal carcinoma, has been used off label for wet AMD. Both Lucentis and Avastin employ intravitreal dosing at a frequency of every 4 weeks [11, 12].

Topical ocular drug delivery has an established history in the treatment of ocular inflammations, seasonal allergic conjunctivitis and hypertension in glaucoma. Thus, a large body of studies examining intraocular drug disposition following topical administration is available in a number of animal species. Although the topical route of drug administration has been exploited for treating anterior segment diseases like conjunctivitis and ocular hypertension, a few reports have also examined topical routes for delivery of drugs to posterior segment targets at sufficiently potent concentrations to treat posterior segment diseases [13].

POTENTIAL ARTIFACTS IN PK OR PD DATA DEVELOPED USING STANDARD TECHNIQUE

Conventional ocular pharmacokinetic studies in animal models involve sampling of various ocular tissues and fluids by dissecting the eye. Techniques used to extrapolate from animals to humans for estimation of intraocular exposures to drugs involve interspecies scaling with ocular compartment size. For example, in Table **1**, information concerning interspecies scaling of various relevant organelles in several animal species is presented. Scaling based on anatomic size is a useful approach for understanding human exposure and is routinely used to extrapolate nonclinical toxicology data and animal exposure, as an alternative to human exposure.

Table 1: Inter-species Scaling: Translating Intraocular Dose From Animals To Humans – reported in milliliters unless otherwise indicated [14-18]

	Horse [18]	Cow [18]	Human [18]	Dog [18]	Cat [18]	Rabbit [18]	Rat [14, 15]	Mouse [16, 17]
Anterior Chamber	2.4	1.7	0.3	0.4	0.6	0.3		
Posterior chamber	1.6	1.5	0.06	0.2	0.3	0.06		
Lens	3.1	2.2	0.2	0.5	0.3	0.2	0.02 - 0.03	0.6 (μL)
Vitreous volume	28.8	20.9	3.9	3.2	2.8	1.5	0.05	0.005

Recent papers have highlighted potential artifacts in the use of conventional approaches for obtaining ocular pharmacokinetic data. During the course of developing a conscious animal model for estimating anterior segment disposition of topically administered drugs [19, 20], Rittenhouse *et al.* [21] examined inter-species differences in aqueous humor exposure to topically administered propranolol. They also noted that aqueous humor sampling of propranolol in conscious *versus* anesthetized rabbits resulted in significant differences in the estimation of intraocular exposure. This data, reanalyzed and presented in a graphical form, highlights appreciable overestimation of exposure that was obtained using anesthetized animals (Fig. **1**). As a result of these studies, the question arises whether pharmacokinetic data obtained from conventional approaches (euthanized animals) provide accurate estimates or prediction of human exposure. Recent approaches to minimize such artifacts include the incorporation of flash freezing of tissue samples so that potential postmortem changes in disposition due to cessation of blood flow are minimized.

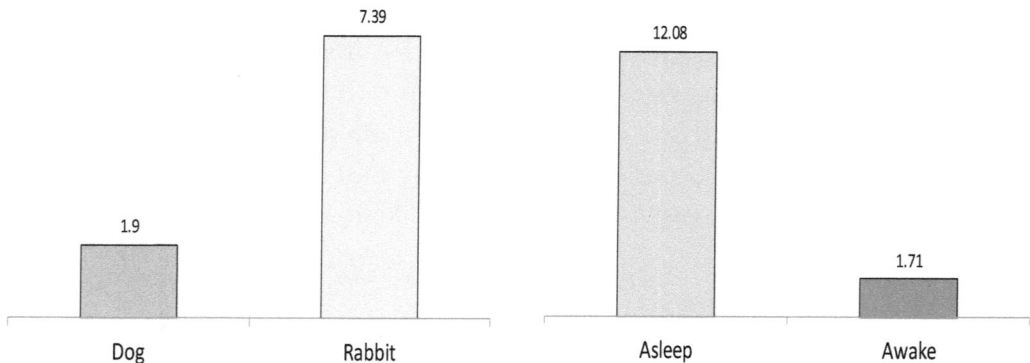

Figure 1: Impact of species and anesthesia on aqueous humor exposure to topically administered drug. R - dog *vs.*rabbit and L - asleep *vs.* awake rabbits (reported as dose normalized C_{max} ($\mu g/mL/\mu g$)).

PROGRESS REPORT ON ADVANCES IN MICRODIALYSIS IN OPHTHALMOLOGY

The eye is an isolated organ with unique physiological and anatomical characteristics. Complex fluid dynamics and protective blood ocular barriers contribute to regional pharmacokinetics (PK) and pharmacodynamics (PD) of drug molecules. There are multiple routes through which drugs can be administered to the eye including topical, transscleral, intravitreal, periocular (subconjunctival, retrobulbar, peribulbar and posterior sub-Tenon injections) and systemic administration. Each route of delivery renders the drug molecules susceptible to unique and intricate mechanisms of transport, distribution and elimination from the eye. Various barriers to ocular drug delivery are illustrated in Fig. **2**.

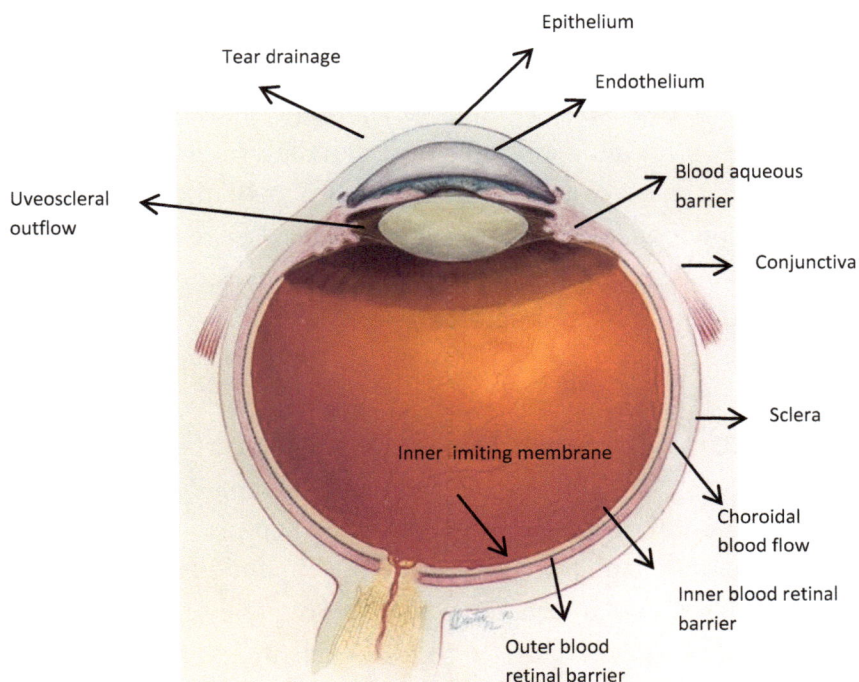

Figure 2: Different barriers to ocular drug delivery including cornea, tear drainage, episcleral blood flow, blood aqueous barriers, convection flow of aqueous humor and blood retinal barriers. Adapted from National Institutes of Health Ref#: NEA01. Used by permission.

Microdialysis can be a valuable tool to examine drug concentrations in inaccessible ocular fluid compartments and to study ocular PK/PD of drug molecules. Traditionally, it was assumed that the drug concentration in plasma is reflective of the drug concentration at the target site; this is generally true for systemically administered drugs with highly perfused target organs [22]. However, the plasma concentration time profile may be inadequate for characterizing the time course of the pharmacological effect. This condition is even true of target organs or compartments that are secluded from the systemic circulation through physiological and anatomical barriers such as the brain and the eye [23]. Since the early accounts of using dialysis sacs to study tissue biochemistry in the 1960s [24], there have been significant advancements in the microdialysis probe development, surgical procedures and sampling and analytical techniques. Application of microdialysis in clinical research is emerging mainly in the area of neurointensive care and other physiological and pathological conditions [25].

Previously, Rittenhouse *et al*. [26] and Duvvuri *et al*. [27] have provided excellent comprehensive reviews on the application of microdialysis in the assessment of drug delivery to the eye. We hereby provide a recap of the earlier work and advances in ocular microdialysis since the time of the last reviews published by these authors. Microdialysis literature is presented as two sections: anterior (Table **2**) and posterior segment (Table **3**) microdialysis.

Anterior Segment Microdialysis

Typically drug concentrations in the aqueous humor are determined by repeated paracentesis; therefore, many animals are required to reliably determine ocular pharmacokinetics. Some of the earlier reports on the application of microdialysis to sample aqueous humor came from Fukuda *et al*. [28] and Sato *et al*. [29] where the investigators studied ocular penetration of fluoroquinolones in anesthetized rabbits. In a subsequent study, Ohtori *et al*. [30] evaluated the kinetics of topical beta-adrenergic antagonists carteolol and timolol in pigmented rabbit aqueous humor. They successfully utilized microdialysis technique to continuously monitor aqueous levels of beta-blockers and to analyze pharmacokinetic parameters while requiring much fewer animals than conventional sampling with paracentesis. The authors used a microdialysis probe made of regenerated cellulose with molecular weight cutoff (MWCO) of 50,000 Da and *in vitro* probe recovery ranging from 18 to 22 %. Rittenhouse *et al*. [19] studied the pharmacokinetics of propranolol in aqueous humor of anesthetized dogs and rabbits after intracameral and topical administration. They employed a linear probe with a polycarbonate membrane. The authors demonstrated interspecies differences in propranolol disposition in rabbit and dog anterior segment. Rittenhouse and colleagues were the first to develop a conscious rabbit model of anterior segment sampling, which allowed complete recovery of the animal from anesthesia and local physiological perturbations due to probe placement. Implantation of the probe in anterior chamber can pose unique challenges such as initial leakage of aqueous humor, increase in protein concentrations, intraocular inflammation, decrease in intraocular pressure, or compromised blood aqueous barrier function that can alter the aqueous kinetics of drugs. In a study using microdialysis for anterior segment sampling, ascorbate was utilized as an aqueous humor turnover marker and a pharmacodynamic surrogate to study alteration in aqueous secretion. In this elegant study, Rittenhouse *et al.* characterized the transport kinetics of ascorbate in aqueous humor and plasma of conscious rabbits by placing a probe in the anterior chamber of one eye and the posterior chamber of the contralateral eye. They employed a complex pharmacokinetic model to assess the rate of secretion of exogenously administered ascorbate from blood to the posterior chamber and its transport into and clearance from the anterior chamber. There has been an increased number of reports published on ocular microdialysis since the year 2000. Refinement to the existing methodology was made and novel ocular microdialysis techniques were developed for gaining insights into mechanisms of ocular pharmacokinetics and pharmacodynamics. Recently there have been a number of publications reporting the application of microdialysis to study the ocular bioavailability of drugs from different ophthalmic delivery systems and formulations [31-34]. In these reports, aqueous humor concentrations were determined following topical administration. To mention a few examples, increased bioavailability from timolol thermosetting gel compared to a conventional solution formulation was reported by Wei *et al.* [35]. Aggarwal *et al.* [34] reported increased and sustained levels of acetazolamide in aqueous humor from niosomal formulation compared to control suspension.

Several pharmacokinetic models of varying complexity have been proposed for estimating ocular absorption, distribution and elimination of topically administered drugs. However, precise estimates of corneal absorption could not be obtained due to precorneal loss and flip flop kinetics of drugs in the anterior chamber. Absorption across the cornea is often a slower process than elimination from the eye and an erroneous assignment of slopes is possible. Topical infusion model has been described previously by which accurate estimates of the ocular absorption rate constant can be obtained with a more straight forward pharmacokinetic method. With constant input of drug through the cornea, absorption, distribution and elimination can be determined independently of the number of peripheral compartments that are operative. Constant concentration was maintained through the use of a plastic cylindrical well containing the drug solution. Researchers from Dr. Mitra's laboratory have conceptualized the use of a combination of the topical well infusion model and aqueous humor microdialysis sampling for precise prediction of ocular absorption (Fig. **3**).

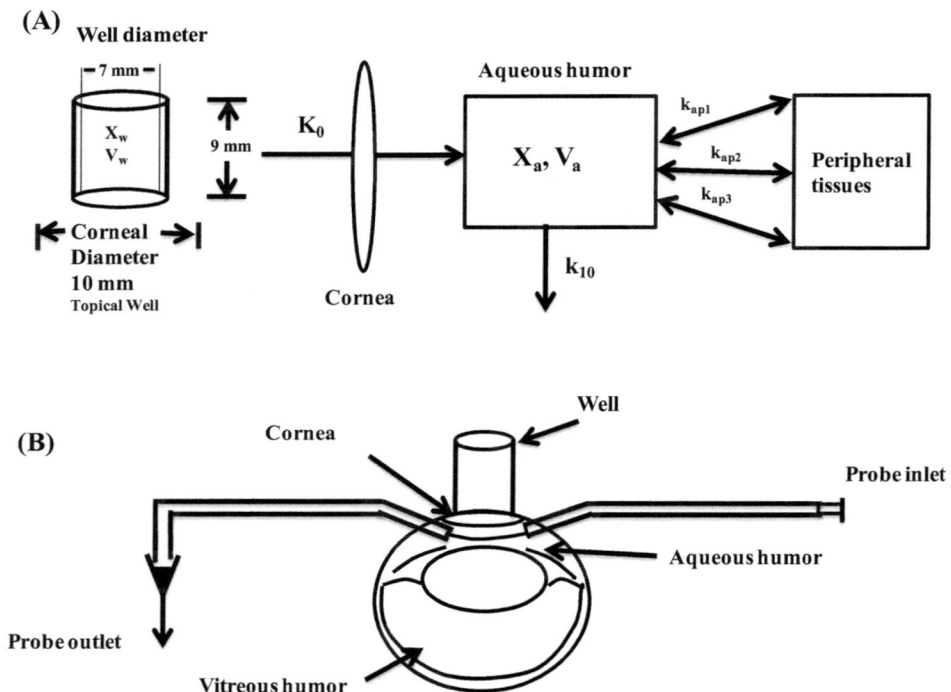

Figure 3: Schematic representation of mathematical model (A) and topical infusion (B) to the rabbit eye [2].

Using this method Dey *et al.* [36] have shown that P-glycoprotein (P-gp) restricts topical erythromycin absorption across the cornea, which can be inhibited by known P-gp inhibitors. Anand *et al.* [37] and Katragadda *et al.* [38] have investigated ocular pharmacokinetics of acyclovir dipeptide and amino acid ester prodrugs following continuous topical infusion. Recently, Karla *et al.* [39] investigated the functional role of multidrug resistance associated protein 5 (MRP5) expressed on the cornea using the topical infusion model.

Table 2: Ocular studies using anterior segment microdialysis from 1995 to present

Author	Probe description	Animal used	Anesthetized/Conscious	Problem examined
Fukuda *et al.* [28]	Probes were inserted into the temporal cornea *via* the anterior chamber and exteriorized out of the nasal cornea	Rabbit	Unconscious	Application of microdialysis for studying the intraocular disposition of fluoroquinolones in aqueous humor
Sato *et al.* [29]	Same as above [28]	Rabbit	Unconscious	Studied the pharmacokinetics of norfloxacin and lomefloxacin in domestic rabbit aqueous humor
Ohtori *et al.* [30]	Probe with a microdialysis membrane (diameter, 0.2 mm and length, 5 mm) was implanted and perfused with Ringer's solution.	Rabbit	Conscious	Studied the ocular pharmacokinetics of timolol and carteolol after recovery from anesthesia.
Rittenhouse *et al.* [21]	CMA/20 microdialysis probes with a 10 mm, polycarbonate membrane (MWCO: 20 kDa) was used	Dog and Rabbit	Unconscious	Examined the pharmacokinetics and inter-species differences of propranolol in aqueous humor in dogs and New Zealand white rabbits.
Rittenhouse *et al.* [19]	Same as above [21]	Rabbit	Conscious	Examined the effects of anesthesia and aqueous humor protein concentrations on ocular disposition of propranolol.
Rittenhouse *et al.* [20, 40]	Same as above [21]	Rabbit	Conscious	Examined the endogenous ascorbate concentration in aqueous humor
Rittenhouse *et al.* [40]	Same as above [21]	Rabbit	Conscious	Examined the pharmacodynamics of beta-blocker modulation of aqueous humor production
Macha and Mitra [41]	CMA/20 microdialysis probes with 0.5 x 10 mm, polycarbonate membrane and 14 mm shaft was used for vitreous sampling. Linear probes (MD-2000, 0.32 x 10 mm, polyacrylo nitrile membrane and 0.22 mm tubing) was used for aqueous sampling	Rabbit	Unconscious	Developed and validated a dual probe microdialysis technique.
Macha and Mitra [42]	Same as above [41]	Rabbits	Unconscious	Investigated the presence of peptide transporters in rabbit retina and delineated the ocular disposition of cephalosporins (cephalexin, cefazolin) in aqueous and vitreous humor.
Macha and Mitra [43]	Same as above [41]	Rabbits	Unconscious	Studied the ocular disposition of ganciclovir and its acyl monoester prodrugs (acetate, propionate, butyrateand valerate) following intravitreal administration using dual probe microdialysis technique.

Table 2: contd….

Author	Probe description	Animal used	Anesthetized/Conscious	Problem examined
Atluri and Mitra [44]	Same as above [41]	Rabbits	Unconscious	Studied the ocular disposition of short chain aliphatic alcohols (14C-methanol, 14C-1-propanol, 14C-1-pentanoland 14C-1-heptanol) using dual probe microdialysis technique.
Dias *et al.* [45]	Same as above [41]	Rabbits	Unconscious	Studied the ocular penetration of acyclovir and its peptide prodrugs (valacyclovir and val-valacyclovir) in aqueous and vitreous humor following systemic administration.
Wei *et al.* [126]	KH-1 microsyringe pump model (Chemistry Institute of Academy Sinica, Beijing, China) with a 1.0 mL glass syringe and a LM-10 linear microdialysis probe (10 mm dialysis membrane (Bioanalytical systems Inc., USA) was used for the studies.	Rabbits	Conscious	Studied the ocular pharmacokinetics of timolol from a thermosetting gel-based formulation in rabbit aqueous humor following topical administration.
Dey *et al.* [36]	A CMA/100 microdialysis pump obtained from CMA/Microdialysis (Acton, MA) and linear probes (MD-2000, 0.32 × 10 mm, polyacronitrile membrane, 0.22-mm tubing) obtained from BAS Bioanalytical Systems (West Lafayette, IN) was used for aqueous humor sampling	Rabbits	Unconscious	Investigated the pharmacokinetics of erythromycin in rabbit corneas after single-dose infusion. Also studied the role of P-gp as a barrier to *in vivo* ocular drug absorption.
Gunda *et al.* [46]	Same as above [41]	Rabbits	Unconscious	Investigated the corneal absorption and anterior chamber pharmacokinetics of dipeptide monoester prodrugs of ganciclovir (valine-, glycine-valine-, valine-valine-, tyrosine-valine) a topical well model.
Anand *et al.* [37]	Same as above [41]	Rabbits	Unconscious	Studied the corneal absorption of the dipeptide prodrugs of acyclovir (ACV) L-valine-ACV, glycine-valine-ACV, valine-valine-ACVand valine-tyrosine-ACV using a corneal well model with linear probes implanted in aqueous humor.
Agarwal *et al.* [34]	Same as above [41]	Rabbits	Unconscious	Studied the aqueous humor disposition of acetazolamide from bioadhesive coated niosomal formulation (ACZREVbio) and aqueous suspension containing 1% (w/v) Tween 80.

Author	Probe description	Animal used	Anesthetized/Conscious	Problem examined
Cao *et al.* [130]	LM-10 Linear Microdialysis Probes, BASi, USA.	Rabbits	Conscious	Evaluated the ocular disposition of timolol maleate in poly(N-isopropylacrylamide)-chitosan (thermosensitive *in situ* gel-forming polymer) following topical administration.
Liu *et al.* [32]	LM-10 microdialysis probe (Bioanalytical System)	Rabbits	Conscious	Evaluated the relative ocular bioavailability of gatifloxacin from an ion-activated *in situ* ophthalmic gel by microdialysis.
Katragadda *et al.* [38]	Same as above [41]	Rabbits	Unconscious	Evaluated the corneal absorption of the amino acid prodrugs of acyclovir (L-alanine-acyclovir, L-serine- acyclovir, L-isoleucine- acyclovir, gamma-glutamate-acyclovir and L-valine- acyclovir) using a topical well model and microdialysis.
Fu *et al.* [31]	A linear probe (MD-2005, Bioanalytical Systems, USA) and CMA/100 microinjection pump (Acton, MA, USA) was implanted into the aqueous humor	Rabbits	Unconscious	Studied the ocular disposition of S(-)-satropane from an *in situ* gelling polymer.
Li *et al.* [47]	LM-10 microdialysis probe (Bioanalytical System, USA)	Rabbits	Conscious	Developed and evaluated the ocular disposition of ibuprofen from a liposomal formulation in conscious rabbit aqueous humor following topical administration
Karla *et al.* [39]	Same as above [41]	Rabbits	Unconscious	Demonstrated the presence of nucleoside/nucleotide efflux transporter in cornea and its relevance in modulating antiviral and glaucoma drug absorption.
Liu *et al.* [48]				Evaluated the effects of labrasol on rabbit corneal permeability of baicalin
Hariharan *et al.* [49]	Same as above [41]	Rabbits	Unconscious	Evaluated the *in vivo* functional activity of multi-drug resistant protein-2 (MRP2) on rabbit corneal epithelium and further studied the modulation of P-gp and MRP2 mediated efflux of erythromycin when co-administered with corticosteroids using a topical well model and microdialysis.

Posterior Segment Microdialysis

Application of microdialysis for ocular drug sampling was first attempted by Gunnarson *et al.* [50]. The authors sampled rabbit vitreous humor using a specially devised probe made of cuprofan membrane matrix with 3 kDa MCWO. They studied the penetration of radiolabelled water and mannitol into the vitreous humor following intracarotid injections in albino rabbits. They also examined the concentrations of endogenous compounds glutamine, phosphoethanolamine and gamma-aminobutyric acid (GABA). Subsequently, Ben-Nun and colleagues employed the microdialysis technique to obtain a complete pharmacokinetic profile in the cat eye. The pharmacokinetics of aminoglycoside gentamicin in cat vitreous was characterized using a specially designed semi permeable probe made of regenerated cellulose with 35 kDa MCWO [51]. The intraocular fluid dynamics were not altered and no inflammatory reaction was observed with the probe implantation for up to 11 h. In another study, Ben-Nun *et al.* utilized microdialysis to demonstrate the differences in pharmacokinetics of gentamicin in normal and bacterial endophthalmitis induced eyes [52]. The authors also examined the feasibility of controlled and sustained delivery of gentamicin through a specially designed device made of hollow haemodialysis fibers. They observed sustained gentamicin vitreous levels using dialysis membrane as opposed to localized peak levels caused by direct intravitreal administration.

The scope of application of microdialysis in ocular pharmacokinetics and ocular drug delivery systems was remarkably enhanced by development of a conscious animal model to sample ocular fluids for prolonged periods of time. This chronic model also eliminates the local and systemic physiological effects of anesthesia on ocular disposition of drugs. In 1991, Waga and colleagues were the first to develop a viable conscious animal model to sample vitreous humor in chronic experiments [53]. This is a significant advancement in posterior segment microdialysis, where probes could be placed in vitreous humor for up to 161 days as opposed to acute microdialysis experiments reported thus far. Waga *et al.* [3] also characterized the pharmacokinetics of ceftazidime in rabbit vitreous following chronic implantation of probes in normal and inflammation induced eyes. The results were also compared with that obtained from traditional pharmacokinetic sampling methods. In later experiments, concentric probes were employed and delivery of different drugs to the vitreous body with probes made of polycarbonate and polyamide membranes were examined [4,54,55]. The authors were also successful in administration of ^{125}I labeled nerve growth factor to the rabbit vitreous *via* a polyether sulphone (PES) membrane probe with a 100 kDa MCWO [56]. Further application and development of chronic microdialysis technique was progressed by Zhang *et al.* [57] and Dais *et al.* [58] for long term sampling of vitreous humor. Hughes and colleagues [59] established an acute surgical procedure in the anesthetized rabbit vitreous using a concentric probe design (CMA-12, CMA/AB Microdialysis, Stockholm, Sweden) and with minimal invasiveness to the eye. The effect of pigmentation on disposition of acycloguanosines, acyclovir (ACV) and ganciclovir (GCV) was studied in New Zealand albino rabbits and Dutch Belt pigmented rabbits. Melanin binding of acyclovir and ganciclovir resulted in lowering of the rate of vitreous elimination by 2 to 3 fold in pigmented rabbits compared to albino rabbits ($t_{1/2}$ = 5.59 *vs.* 2.62 hr for GCV and 8.63 *vs.* 2.98 hr for ACV).

Posterior Segment Microdialysis After Year 2000

Anand *et al.* [60] carried out validation of a conscious animal model with permanently implanted vitreous probes in rabbits. The model was validated by fluorescein disposition studies and modulation of vitreous protein levels was monitored. A dual probe microdialysis technique was developed to simultaneously sample aqueous and vitreous humors by adapting the approach reported by Hughes *et al.* [41]. A concentric probe from CMA (CMA/20, CMA microdialysis, Acton MA) was implanted in vitreous humor and a linear probe (MD 2000, Bioanalytical systems, West Lafayette, IN) was inserted into the anterior chamber. Intraocular pressure and protein concentrations in aqueous and vitreous humor were measured for up to 12 h post probe implantation. The permeability index for fluorescein following systemic administration was determined in order to assess blood-aqueous and blood-retinal barrier integrity. The authors observed initial drop in IOP, which was attributed to eye proptosis and loss of aqueous humor with probe placement. The IOP reverted back to normal within 2 h after the implantation of the probes. The aqueous protein increased significantly compared to basal levels (within 5 fold) but the vitreous protein concentration was not significantly different from the baseline. The permeability index values were found to be 9.48 +/- 4.25% and 1.99 +/- 0.66% for the anterior and vitreous chambers, respectively, consistent with earlier reports. Dual probe microdialysis model is a valuable technique to obtain a thorough characterization of ocular kinetics of drugs by simultaneously studying anterior and posterior compartments along with plasma kinetics.

This technique was employed to explore the possibility of improving the intravitreal pharmacokinetic profile of ganciclovir (GCV) *via* prodrug derivatization [43, 62, 63]. Majumdar *et al.* [63] studied intravitreal kinetics of series of dipeptide monoester GCV prodrugs, designed to target the peptide transporter expressed on the retina following intravitreal administration in rabbits. Vitreal pharmacokinetic profiles and retinal concentrations of four GCV dipeptide esters: L-Valine, L-Valine-L-Valine, L-Tyrosine-L-Valine and L-Glycine-L-Valine were studied and compared to the parent drug GCV. They observed that L-Glycine-L-Valine ester has sustained GCV levels compared to other esters in the vitreous humor and retina (Fig. **4**). The authors noted from the retinal uptake studies that L-Glycine-L-Valine-GCV is not a substrate of the retinal peptide transporter. However, greater stability in the vitreous humor and the ability to generate both hydrophilic GCV and lipophilic Valine-GCV, at the same time, allowed L-Glycine-L-Valine-GCV to maintain higher retinal and vitreal GCV concentrations. This study shows that a combination of factors such as physicochemical properties, enzymatic stability in ocular tissue and transporter mediated uptake dictate the kinetics of intravitreally administered drugs.

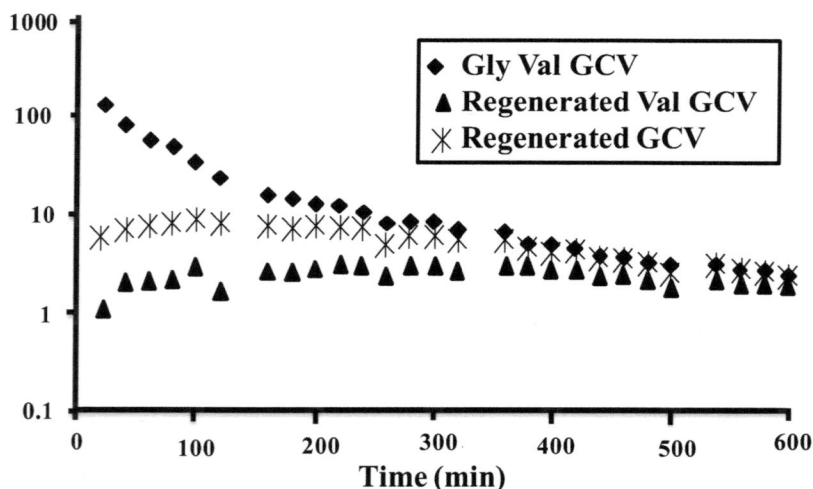

Figure 4: Vitreous concentration-time profiles of Gly-Val-GCV and regenerated ganciclovir (GCV) and Val-GCV [3].

There are a number of reports that employed dual probe microdialysis to delineate mechanisms of elimination from and penetration into the anterior and posterior segments of the eye [42, 44, 45, 64-67]. The role of peptide transporters expressed on retina and blood retinal barrier on vitreal drug elimination was investigated by Macha *et al.* [42]. Ocular clearance of peptide transporter substrates such as cephalosporins was investigated in the presence and absence of specific inhibitors. Dias *et al.* [45] examined the transport of a model dipeptide glycylsarcosine across blood ocular barriers following systemic administration. They concluded that the oligopeptide transport system was involved in ocular uptake of glycylsarcosine from systemic circulation. Investigations into the expression and orientation of drug efflux proteins on the retina were carried out by Duvvuri *et al.* [64] using dual probe ocular microdialysis model. Ocular pharmacokinetics of quinidine, a model P-glycoprotein/multi-drug resistance protein (MRP) substrate, was investigated following intravitreal and systemic administration in the presence and absence of verapamil, a known inhibitor. Atluri *et al.* [65] elucidated the functional activity of a large neutral amino acid transporter (LAT) in the rabbit retina by studying intravitreal pharmacokinetics of L-phenylalanine, a known substrate for LAT. This study concluded that lipophilicity can be considered as one of the primary physicochemical properties that determine ocular drug disposition [27]. The same group also investigated the effect of lipophilicity, diffusivity and aqueous solubility on ocular drug disposition by studying the vitreous pharmacokinetics of short-chain aliphatic alcohols. Microdialysis probes were implanted in both anterior and vitreous chamber of the rabbit eye to sample aqueous and vitreous humors simultaneously. Interestingly, the elimination rate constants of alcohols from the vitreous decreased with ascending chain length and lipophilicity (methanol to 1-heptanol) [44].

A number of other investigators used microdialysis to study the role of transporters in ocular drug disposition [66-69]. Investigators from the University of Toyama employed a rat microdialysis model to study efflux transport of organic anions across the rat blood retinal barrier (BRB) [66, 69]. This is the first report of using rat as an animal model for ocular microdialysis. The rational for using rat model for these studies is that the retinas in humans and rats are well vascularized and have an inner BRB as opposed to relatively avascular retina in the rabbit. A custom designed microdialysis probe (TEP-50) was constructed by Eicom (Kyoto, Japan). The length of the probe membrane (cellulose membrane) was 2.0mm with 50 kDa MWCO.

Katayama *et al.* [66] studied the vitreal elimination of estradiol 17-beta glucuronide (E17βG) and D-mannitol, which are model compounds for amphipathic organic anions and bulk flow markers, respectively. The efflux transport of E17βG was significantly inhibited by organic anions, such as probenecid, sulfobromophthalein, digoxin and dehydroepiandrosterone sulfate. However, no inhibition was observed with para-aminohippuric acid. This study demonstrated the role of organic anion transporting polypeptide 1a4 in mediating the efflux of E17βG across the rat BRB [66]. Hosoya *et al.* [69] characterized the role of rat organic anion transporter (Oat3) in efflux transport at the inner BRB. The contribution of rat Oat3 to the efflux of its substrates [para-aminohippuric acid (PAH), benzylpenicillin (PCG) and mercaptopurine (6-MP)], from the vitreous humor/retina to the circulating blood across the inner BRB was evaluated using the microdialysis method. The elimination rate of these substrates was reduced in the presence of Oat3 inhibitors such as probenecid and PCG, whereas it was not inhibited by digoxin. The expression of Oat3 in the retina was further confirmed by RT-PCR and Western blot analysis. These results support the expression of Oat3 at the inner BRB and reveal its involvement in the vitreous humor/retina-to-blood transport of PAH, PCG and 6-MP.

Table 3: Ocular studies using posterior segment microdialysis from 1987 to present

Author	Probe description	Animal used	Anesthetized/Conscious	Problem examined
Macha *et al.* [41]	CMA/20 (0.5 × 10 mm) Polycarbonate membrane and 14 mm shaft MD 2000, 0.32 × 10 mm, polyacrylonitrile membrane and 0.22 mm tubing.	Male New Zealand Albino rabbits (2–4 kg). CMA probe inserted 3–4 mm below scleral limbus and MD-2000 probe inserted into the cornea by a 25-gauge needle	Anesthetized	Model development and validation by studying IOP variations, protein levels and ocular fluorescein kinetics following systemic and intravitreous administrations following probe implantation
Macha *et al.* [42]	Same as Ref. [41]	Same as Ref. [41]	Anesthetized	Delineated the effect of peptide transporter on ocular disposition of vitreously administered cephalosporins

Author	Probe description	Animal used	Anesthetized/Conscious	Problem examined
Macha *et al.* [43]	Same as Ref. [41]	Same as Ref. [41]	Anesthetized	Screened a series of mono-ester prodrugs of GCV for their efficacy as lead compounds in treatment of cytomegalovirus retinitis
Atluri *et al.* [44]	Same as Ref. [41]	Same as Ref. [41]	Anesthetized	Investigated the effect of lipophilicity on ocular clearance of intravitreously administered molecules
Duvvuri *et al.* [64]	Same as Ref. [41]	Same as Ref. [41]	Anesthetized	Examined the effect of efflux proteins on ocular kinetics of a model substrate following both intravitreous and systemic administrations
Macha *et al.* [62]	Same as Ref. [41]	Same as Ref. [41]	Anesthetized	Screened a series of diester prodrugs of GCV for their efficacy as lead compounds in treatment of cytomegalovirus retinitis
Zhang *et al.* [57]	7 mm cellulose membrane linear microdialysis probes; outer and inner diameter of 0.24 and 0.22 mm respectively, 50 kDa MWCO. 60 degree bend 8 mm tube for mounting inlet and outlet tubing. 1 μl/min perfusion rate; ringer's solution.	Albino rabbits 3.3–4 kg; 20-gauge needle 4–6 mm from limbus temporal to superior rectus muscle. Tubes inserted under eyelids, exteriorized between ears of rabbit	Not clearly stated, but likely conscious	Vitreous ascorbate concentrations perturbed by intense visible light exposure in the presence of intravenously administered fluorescein as photosensitizer
Dias *et al.* [58]	Same as Ref. [41]	Same as Ref. [41]	Conscious	Delineation of intravitreal disposition of GCV following intravitreous administration. Differences in disposition due to anesthesia investigated

Table 3: contd….

Author	Probe description	Animal used	Anesthetized/Conscious	Problem examined
Anand *et al.* [60]	MD 2000, 0.32 × 10 mm, polyacrylonitrile membrane and 0.22 mm tubing	Male New Zealand Albino rabbits (2–4 kg). MD-2000 probe inserted 3–4 mm below scleral limbus *via* 1 25-gauge needle and secured by conjunctival sutures	Conscious	Model development and validation by studying ocular fluorescein kinetics and protein concentrations
Duvvuri *et al.* [70]	Linear microdialysis probes (MD 2000) were procured from BAS microdialysis, (Lafayette, IN).	Male New Zealand albino rabbits (2–2.5 kg)	Conscious	Studied the controlled delivery of ganciclovir to the retina using drug-loaded poly(D,L-lactide-co-glycolide) (PLGA) microspheres dispersed in PLGA-PEG-PLGA gel
Okuno *et al.* [71]	Concentric microdialysis probe (regenerated cellulose, 30 mm length; A-I-30-015; Eicom, Kyoto, Japan)	Albino rabbits (2.7–3.2 kg)	Unconscious	Glutamate level in optic nerve head is increased by artificial elevation of intraocular pressure in rabbits
Majumdar *et al.* [63]	Concentric probes (CMA/20, 0.5 x 10 mm polycarbonate membrane and 14 mm shaft) employed for sampling the vitreous chamber were obtained from CMA/Microdialysis (Acton, MA).	Adult male New Zealand White (NZW) rabbits, weighing 2–2.5 kg. Probe was inserted approximately 3 mm below the corneal-scleral limbus.	Unconscious	Carried out vitreal pharmacokinetics of dipeptide monoester prodrugs of ganciclovir
Senthilkumari *et al.* [68]	Concentric probes (CMA/20, 0.5× 10-mm polycarbonate membrane having a 14-mm shaft)	Male New Zealand albino rabbits weighing 2.0–2.5kg	Unconscious	Evaluated the modulation of P-glycoprotein (P-gp) on the intraocular diposition of its substrates in rabbits

Author	Probe description	Animal used	Anesthetized/Conscious	Problem examined
Janoria *et al.* [67]	Concentric probes (CMA/20, 0.5 × 10 mm polycarbonate membrane and 14-mm shaft) and microinjection pump (CMA/100)	Male New Zealand Albino rabbits (2–4 kg). Probe implantation in the vitreous was carried out at 3 mm below the corneal-scleral limbus through the pars plana	Unconscious	Vitreal pharmacokinetics of biotinylated ganciclovir: Role of sodium-dependent multivitamin transporter expressed on retina

PRECLINICAL *VS.* CLINICAL OCULAR PHARMACOKINETICS

Systematic knowledge on ocular disposition in human eye is scarce due to inaccessibility of ocular fluids for continuous sampling. Studies in humans are usually performed as single dose studies on patients undergoing cataract extraction and without other ocular diseases. Samples from different subjects are typically pooled together to construct a pharmacokinetic profile leading to imprecise estimates and large variability in kinetic parameters. Nevertheless, study of ocular disposition of molecular probes such as fluorescein and sodium pertechnetate using non invasive imaging techniques has shed light on some of the mechanisms of disposition in the human eye [61, 72]. Rabbit has been routinely employed as an animal model to study ocular pharmacokinetics and pharmacodynamics. Although, anatomical and physiological differences limit direct extrapolation of data from preclinical species to humans, general understanding about mechanism of ocular penetration and disposition can be obtained. Earlier reports by Mishima *et al.* [23] have shown that kinetics of intraocular drug penetration for topically applied drugs follow a similar pattern in rabbit and human eyes. Also, time course of different response parameters was used to estimate intraocular pharmacokinetics based on the assumption that pharmacodynamics of the drug is a function of biophase drug concentration at a given time. Case studies have been presented below where data in humans and preclinical species is available. Since the kinetics of drugs follow different mechanisms in anterior and posterior segment, the ocular pharmacokinetics in preclinical species and humans are discussed in two separate sections: 1) anterior segment pharmacokinetics and 2) posterior segment pharmacokinetics. Moreover, suitability of different animal models to predict human ocular PK and their interspecies differences is discussed below.

Selection of Relevant Animal Model

Rabbit is the most commonly employed animal model to study ocular pharmacokinetics and pharmacodynamics. Rabbit eye is large enough to perform accurate ocular injections or delivery by special devices or implants in contrast to rat eye, which is too small to perform such studies. The monkey eye most closely resembles the human eye with regard to anatomy and physiology, including the presence of macula and is the preferred model to study biologics because of higher sequence homology to humans compared to other species [73]. Also, anatomical differences exist between monkey and rabbit eyes. Although globe size is similar between the two species, the anterior chamber and the lens of rabbit eye were 2.3-fold and 3.9-fold larger, respectively than similar areas of the monkey eye [73]. Rabbit vitreous volume is similar to some strains of monkey vitreous. However, pharmacokinetic studies in monkey are not as prevalent as in rabbits. Also, rabbit and human eye exhibit differences in blood retinal barrier properties. The retinal vessels are limited to a stripe of myelinated tissue that radiates horizontally from the optic nerve head, while the remainder of the retina is avascular and drug transport between the retina and blood is mainly *via* the outer BRB, the retinal pigment epithelium. The retinas in humans and rats are well vascularized and have an inner BRB as well as an outer BRB.

Case Studies

Anterior Segment Pharmacokinetics

The ocular bioavailability and disposition of topically applied drugs are predominantly determined by three distinct processes in the eye: 1) precorneal kinetics 2) permeability across the cornea and 3) elimination from the aqueous humor. The concentration of the drug in the precorneal tear film dictates the drug penetration into the anterior chamber. Saturation of the tear film and subsequent transport across the cornea depend on a variety of factors such as volume of the instilled fluid in the conjunctival sac, blinking rate, viscosity of the vehicle administered, and the rate of drug loss in the tears. Cornea is a multilayered structure with both hydrophobic and hydrophilic barrier characteristics. A good correlation was observed between the permeability of compounds across rabbit and human corneas [74]. Drug molecules that enter the anterior chamber through the cornea are mixed with the aqueous humor by convection movements. Drug mixed with the aqueous is eliminated with the drainage of aqueous humor or it binds to surrounding iris and ciliary body. Certain drugs may bind to the melanin pigment present in these tissues leading to slow release of the drug. A very small percentage of the drug reaches the posterior vitreous, retina and choroid from the anterior chamber.

Latanoprost

Latanoprost (Xalatan®) is a prostanoid selective FP receptor agonist that reduces the intraocular pressure (IOP) by increasing the flow of aqueous humor through the ciliary muscle bundles of the uveoscleral pathway [75]. It is found to be effective in long-term treatment of primary open angle glaucoma and ocular hypertension [75]. Latanoprost is a lipophilic isopropyl ester prodrug in which the carboxylic acid moiety in the α-chain has been esterified to increase the bioavailability of the drug in the eye. It is rapidly and completely hydrolyzed by esterases in the cornea to the biologically active acid [76]. Pharmacokinetic studies in humans have indicated that maximum aqueous concentrations of 15-30 ng/mL are reached in 1-2 h after topical administration of a 1.5 microgram clinical dose [77]. The half-life of latanoprost acid in the aqueous was 2-3 h. Similar time to peak concentrations (1 h) and half life (2.3 h) was observed following topical administration of latanoprost (1.06 micrograms) to rabbits [78]. However, much lower peak aqueous concentration was observed in rabbits (0.067 ng eq/mg) compared to humans (15-30 ng/mL). During the entire 24-hour period, the cornea showed substantially higher levels of latanoprost than the aqueous humor, iris and the ciliary body. Thus, there is a possibility that cornea could function as a slow release depot of the drug into the anterior parts of the eye. It was reported that reduction in IOP starts approximately 3 to 4 hours after administration and the maximum effect is reached after 8 to 12 hours (Xalatan Package Insert). This could be explained by slow release of drug from the cornea and aqueous kinetics do not appear to parallel the time course of pharmacodynamic effect. Ocular kinetic studies in monkey revealed that maximum concentration in the eye was reached after 1 h with an elimination half-life of 3-4 h [79]. Similar ocular distribution and elimination profiles were observed in monkeys and rabbits.

Betaxolol

Betaxolol, a beta-1 selective beta adrenergic receptor blocker, was developed for treating ocular hypertension or primary open angle glaucoma (Betoptic-S package insert). Human *vs.* cynomolgus monkey ocular pharmacokinetics were comprehensively evaluated following repeated dosing. Eyes (n=7) from glaucoma patients were enucleated following self-administration of 0.25% betaxolol twice daily for 28 days or longer and assayed for intraocular betaxolol concentrations. Similar data was collected in cynomolgus monkeys (n=3) after receiving 0.25% topical betaxolol twice daily for 30 days. Drug levels in specific intraocular tissues were determined. Betaxolol intraocular tissue concentrations and plasma were measured by HPLC and tandem mass spectrometry. With interspecies scaling factors using predicted vitreous volume assumed differences (~1.5 ml in monkey *vs.* ~4 ml in man), the human retina and optic nerve head exposures are higher in primates than humans, as would be expected. However, the increased optic nerve head exposure (~8-fold higher than humans) was disproportionately higher in primates than humans in comparison to retinal tissue exposures (~2-fold higher than humans), highlighting the complexities in the prediction of translatable ocular PK (Fig. **5**) [80].

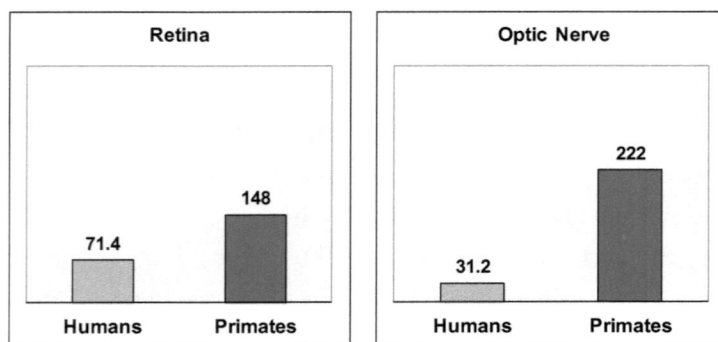

Figure 5: Human *vs.* Primate Ocular PK following topically administered Betaxolol - reported as μg/g exposure.

Posterior Segment Pharmacokinetics

Intravitreal injections provide more efficient drug delivery to the back of the eye compared to topical, systemic and periocular routes of administration [81]. Following intravitreal administration, small drug molecules diffuse within the vitreous body and into the anterior chamber at the same rate as they diffuse in free solution. After initial distribution in the vitreous body, molecules exit through two pathways: (a) through the anterior hyaloid membrane into the posterior chamber and out of the eye with the aqueous drainage and, (b) directly across the retinal surface. Typically hydrophilic and large molecules that cannot traverse the blood retinal barrier are eliminated through anterior route. Whereas, small, lipophilic and molecules that are substrates to the transporters present on blood retinal barrier are exited through retinal route.

Fluocinolone Acetonide

Glucocorticoids as a class are important therapeutic options in the treatment of various inflammatory components of ocular diseases. Due to their potency and systemic safety profile, local delivery to the eye *via* topical drops or *via* more advanced drug delivery platforms has been developed. Retisert, an intravitreal implant that delivers fluocinolone acetonide over 3 years, was developed with the aforementioned rationale. Retisert® was approved for treatment of posterior uveitis and incorporates a drug delivery platform based on the first intravitreal drug delivery device for ganciclovir administration in CMV retinitis, Vitrasert®. An important aspect of a sustained delivery approach is the confirmation of sustained and dose-related drug delivery at efficacious concentrations in relevant target tissues. Long term ocular pharmacokinetic studies were conducted in rabbit species to verify these concepts in an ocular scalable manner to the human eye [82]. Rabbit retina and vitreous concentrations were sustained over the 1 year period; aqueous levels were generally low and plasma levels below the limit of quantitation [82]. Early clinical studies showcased the evolution of the implant technology in posterior uveitis patients. The device was comprised of 1.5 mm tablet pellets of pure fluocinolone acetonide coated with polyvinyl alcohol (PVA) and silicone laminate and was affixed to a PVA suture. Sterilization involved a 5 hour heat treatment followed by gamma irradiation. The implant was sutured to the pars plana region for diffusion into vitreous. The surgical implantation procedure included local anesthesia followed by trimming the suture to a 2 mm suture strut-in device. A 0.5 mm hole was prepared and placed so that a suture could be used (nylon). Eyes had to be quiet, free of inflammation, prior to device surgical implantation. A limbal based conjunctival peritomy was prepared *via* 3-4 mm pars plana sclerotomy and the device placed in the infero-temporal quadrant. The device was then anchored using 8-0 or 10-0 nylon to the pars plana. In this study, four out of seven eyes had 3 line improvements in visual acuity, all subjects could eliminate periocular injections of steroids and there was a reduction in systemic steroid use of ~80%. These results confirm the advantages inherent in the local and sustained delivery of potent drugs like fluocinolone acetonide for treating chronic ocular diseases [83]. Two phase III clinical trials were conducted demonstrating reduction in the primary efficacy outcome: recurrence rate in the eye up to 34 weeks after implantation (see Table **4**) for the indication of non-infectious posterior uveitis; n=517 [71].

Table 4: Efficacy Results for Retisert in posterior uveitis [8]

Primary efficacy outcome	Recurrence rate in the eye at baseline before implantation	Recurrence rate up to 34 weeks after implantation
Implanted Eyes	51.4%	6.1%
Fellow Eyes (non-implanted)	20.3%	42.0%
Percentage of eyes requiring systemic steroids	52.9%	12.1%
Percentage of eyes requiring Topical steroids	35.7%,	16.5%

Although a local delivery approach reduces the relative systemic exposure to steroids, there were still a number of important dose related adverse events such as elevated IOP requiring pharmacological and/or surgical intervention and cataracts.

Ranibizumab (Lucentis ^{TM}) and Bevacizumab (Avastin^{TM})

Ranibizumab (rhuF$_{ab}$ V2; Lucentis) is a humanized monoclonal antibody fragment designed to bind to the receptor binding sites of active forms of VEGF-A, thereby blocking vessel permeability and angiogenesis in neovascular age-related macular degeneration (wet AMD). Lucentis 0.5 mg (0.05 mL) is recommended to be administered by intravitreal injection once a month [84]. The half life of ranibizumab in monkey vitreous following intravitreal administration was found to be approximately 3 days [85]. Ranibizumab cleared in parallel from the anterior chamber and retina with a similar half-life observed in vitreous. Peak concentrations in aqueous humor and retina were reached within 6 to 24 hr after administration of 500 and 2000 μg doses. This shows that the distribution and elimination of ranibizumab are mainly governed by diffusion within the vitreous and into the anterior chamber. Ranibizumab exposure in aqueous humor and the retina is 2 to 3.3 fold lower than in the vitreous. Moreover, ranibizumab concentrations were approximately two fold greater in neural retina than in the retinal pigment epithelium/Bruch's membrane/choriocapillaris. This demonstrates the ability of ranibizumab to penetrate into the retina in monkeys but it appears that ranibizumab could be freely diffused through the neural retina when compared to its limited uptake by tighter retinal pigment epithelium barrier. Mordenti *et al.* [86] has shown that full-length HER2 antibody (148 kDa) did not penetrate the inner limiting membrane of the retina at any of the time points examined; whereas, Fab antibody of vascular endothelial growth factor (48.3 kDa) diffused through the neural retina to the retinal pigment epithelial layer. Also, in line with the molecular weights of these compounds, the half-life in vitreous was 5.6 days for the full-length antibody and 3.2 days for the Fab antibody. Ranibizumab half-life in rabbit ocular compartments was also found to be around 3 days [87]. In humans, longer half-life can be expected since species with bigger eyes and longer diffusion paths would have slower vitreous clearance. The human eye is larger with vitreous volume of 4.5 mL *versus* 1.5 mL in rabbits and monkey. The vitreous elimination half life in humans was estimated to be ~9 days. This estimate was based on population pharmacokinetic analysis of disappearance rate of ranibizumab from serum following intravitreal administration.

Bevacizumab is a completely humanized murine monoclonal antibody against all isoforms of VEGFA. Bevacizumab was approved by the FDA for metastatic colon cancer. There are numerous studies investigating the efficacy of bevacizumab in patients with age related macular degeneration. Vitreous half-life of bevacizumab in Dutch-Belted rabbit eyes was found to be 4.32 days [88]. The aqueous levels peaked on the first day after intravitreal injection. Bevacizumab ocular kinetics was studied in patients diagnosed with cataract and concurrent macular edema. Aqueous humor samples were obtained during elective cataract surgery. The aqueous half-life of 1.5 mg intravitreally injected bevacizumab was found be 9.82 days. Since parallel decline in ranibizumab levels was observed in aqueous and vitreous humor, we can assume intravitreal half- life to be approximately 9 days. It will be difficult to predict the half-life in humans based on animal data; however longer half-life can be expected based on volume of the vitreous. With growing knowledge of ocular kinetics in preclinical species and humans, there could be increased understanding of inter species differences in pharmacokinetics and improvement in the predictive ability of preclinical data.

ROADBLOCKS TO MICRODIALYSIS IN OPHTHALMOLOGY

Ocular microdialysis was performed for the first time in late 1980's [26]. The unique physiology and anatomy of the eye presents numerous challenges to the successful development and delivery of drugs. The clinical outcomes of a therapeutic strategy designed to treat ocular diseases can be determined by monitoring the drug concentrations in ocular fluids. Microdialysis has gained a lot of importance in recent years for its ability to monitor drug substances in the extracellular space. This technique was employed for the first time in 1966, by Bito *et al.* [89] to estimate the concentrations of free amino acids in the microenvironment of brain. Ocular microdialysis has gained popularity for its ability to continuously monitor drug concentrations and substantially reduce the number of animals being used. However, requirements like sight preservation make this technique relatively difficult, requiring surgically related artifact [26]. In this section, various important parameters which need to be considered in ocular microdialysis experimentation are described.

Probe Design

A variety of probes have been employed in the study of anterior and posterior segment pharmacokinetics. The selection of a probe depends mainly on the analyte under investigation and implantation site (anterior chamber or posterior segment). Ben-Nun *et al.* [51] reported the use of a catheter for vitreous sampling in cat eyes. Later on, Waga *et al.* [53] developed special surgical procedure for the long-term implantation of the probes in rabbit vitreous using a newly designed probe. The dialysis membrane was made up of polycarbonate-polyether copolymer with inner and outer diameters of 400 and 520 mm respectively. The eye is a very sensitive organ and probe implantation results in immuno-protective cascades [53]. Both anterior and posterior segments provide unique challenges in the probe design for ocular microdialysis. The aqueous humor is relatively dynamic and prevents the formation of microenvironments surrounding the dialysis membrane. However, the long term probe implantation in aqueous humor results in the formation of a fibrin coat which in turn affects the analyte recovery [19]. Vitreous humor is relatively static with gelatinous consistency. Stemples *et al.* [90] reported the formation of transient flare following implantation of probes in rabbit vitreous. Moreover, implantation of improperly sterilized probes may result in formation of endophthalmitis. Waga *et al.* [3] demonstrated that the probes were well tolerated in the rabbit vitreous over duration of 30 days. Cataract formation was observed in a few cases when the improperly placed probes touched the lens. Currently, ocular microdialysis is usually carried out using linear and concentric probes. Linear probe consists of a hollow fiber dialysis membrane connected to small bore tubings on two ends making this useful for implantation in peripheral tissues (*e.g.* anterior segment). Concentric probe consists of cylindrical shaped dialysis membrane sealed at one end and attached to a solid metal cannula consisting of inner and outer tubing at the other end [91]. This probe is generally used in the posterior segment microdialysis.

Probe Membrane Properties

Several polymers such as regenerated celluloses, polyethersulfone, polyamides, polyacrylonitriles, cuprophan and polycarbonate-ethers with MWCO values ranging between 5 and 100 kDa have been employed in the preparation of semipermeable dialysis membrane [92]. Torto *et al.* [93] evaluated the performance and characteristics (extraction fraction, permeability factors, temperature stability and protein interaction) of membranes with MWCO between 3 and 100 kDa. Higher extraction fraction and non-specific membrane interaction were observed for polysulfone membranes in comparison to polyamide and polyethersulfone membranes. Moreover, no significant change in the extraction fraction and membrane texture was observed with increasing concentrations of analyte (even for a 250-fold change) and higher temperature (90 $^{\circ}$C) respectively.

Low MWCO membranes (5-30kDa) results in protein free samples with relatively higher recovery compared to higher MWCO membranes (≥ 100 kDa). This might be attributed to the ultrafiltration in which hydrostatic pressure forces the liquid against a semipermeable membrane. However, for sampling of larger protein and peptide molecules, custom made polyethylene polymer tubular membrane with MWCO-3000kDa has been reported [94]. Log % *in vitro* recovery of neuropeptides with MWCO ranging from 400-4500 Da exhibited a linear relationship using CMA/10 microdialysis probe [95]. Waga and Ehinger [4] investigated the passage of drugs through dialysis membranes based on the lipophilicity (corticosteroids: dexamethasone and triamcinolone, antibiotics: cefuroxim and benzylpenicillinand cytostatics: daunomycin and 5-fluorouracil) and molecular weight (formic acid: MW 70 Da, glucose: MW 189 Da, and inulin: MW. 5200 Da) following perfusion into microdialysis probes implanted in rabbit eyes. They concluded that lipophilic drugs stick to polycarbonate membrane and not to polyamide membranes. They could not observe any significant difference in the transport properties of drug molecules with change in dimensions and probe geometry of polycarbonate and polyamide membrane. Further, all drug molecules except inulin (high molecular weight) were found to diffuse through the polyamide membrane with a recovery of 10-20%. Irrespective of the above mentioned constraints, ocular microdialysis experimentation widely involves the use of concentric probes (CMA/20 with 0.5x 10 mm, polycarbonate membrane and 14 mm shaft) for vitreous humor sampling and linear probes (MD-2000, 0.32 x 10 mm, polyacrylo nitrile membrane and 0.22 mm tubing) for aqueous humor sampling [41].

Probe Recovery

Microdialysis sampling is typically performed under non-equilibrium conditions. Analyte concentration in the dialysate represents only a fraction of actual concentration present in the surrounding biological fluid or tissue matrix [96]. One of the major concerns associated with microdialysis is the effect of membrane permeability on the percentage recovery of substance. The dialysate sample collected during microdialysis does not represent the actual drug concentration present in the extracellular environment. Only a fraction of the drug passes through the dialysis membrane from extracellular fluid into the perfusate that is collected at regular time intervals. This fraction is known as recovery and it is defined as the ratio C_{out}/C_{in}, where in C_{out} is the concentration (μM) of the drug in the dialysate fluid and C_{in} is the concentration of the drug in the solution outside the membrane (Eq. 1). This is also known as relative recovery. For any drug substance the recovery is directly proportional to the length and diameter of the membrane, while inversely proportional to molecular weight, flow rate, temperatureand non-specific binding to the tubing and membrane [97, 98].

$$\text{Recovery}_{in\ vitro} = C_{out}/C_{in} \tag{1}$$

After determining the *in vitro* recovery of a drug dialysate, concentrations can be transformed into the actual anterior and vitreous chamber concentrations using Eq. 2 [99].

$$\hat{C}_{in} = \hat{C}_{out}/\text{Recovery}_{in\ vitro} \tag{2}$$

$\hat{C}_{out}$ is the concentration of drug in the sample collected and $\hat{C}_{in}$ is the concentration of drug in aqueous or vitreous humor. In ocular microdialysis experiments the probe is continuously perfused at a constant flow rate of 2 μL/min. The recovery of drugs generally varies from 15-18% in linear probes and 20-25% in concentric probes. In absolute recovery (Eq. 3) the actual amount or the mass of the analyte is calculated in a defined time period. It is the product of perfusion flow rate (F), relative recovery (R) and analyst concentration (C) in the external solution [100].

$$A = C * F * R \tag{3}$$

Recovery of drug molecules from the dialysis membrane is highly variable and governed mainly on the length and diameter of the membrane, flow rate or perfusion rate, temperature, molecular weight of analyte, molecular shape of analyte, molecular charge, binding of the substance to the dialysis membrane or outlet tubing and stability of the substance at the temperature and pH of the perfusion medium. These factors should be taken into consideration for increasing the analyte concentration in dialysis sample [101]. Optimal recovery of drugs following ocular microdialysis was obtained with the help of the commercially available CMA probe with a membrane length of 10 mm, shaft 14 mm and a cutoff value of 20 kDa [41]. The recovery of the analytes from surgically implanted probes is performed using retrodialysis (also known as reverse microdialysis). It requires the use of an internal standard with similar diffusion characteristics as analyte and should not interfere with the ocular disposition of analyte [38]. Dias and Mitra [58] investigated the ocular disposition of ^{3}[H]-ganciclovir in a conscious animal model using ^{14}C-mannitol as an internal standard. Initially the probe was placed in isotonic phosphate buffer saline (IPBS) and continuously perfused with the mixture of analyte and internal standard at 2 μL/min. At regular time intervals the samples were collected, analyzed and the recovery of analyte and internal standard were calculated individually using the below equation.

$$Recovery = (C_{in}-C_{out})/C_{in}$$

where, C_{out} is the concentration of analyte or internal standard leaving the probe and C_{in} is the concentration of analyte or internal standard entering the probe. Recovery of the two compounds is compared using an equation given below.

$$Recovery\ ratio = Recovery_{internal\ standard}/Recovery_{analyte}$$

After the probes are surgically implanted, the *in vivo* recovery of internal standard will be assessed to make sure the functionality and integrity of the probe. Similarly the disposition kinetics of analytes will be calculated using the predetermined recovery ratio of analyte.

Bio-Analytical Limitations

Analysis of biological samples plays a critical role in any pharmacokinetic study [102]. Unlike the conventional method in which ocular pharmacokinetic parameters are determined by pooling the data generated from various subjects, microdialysis experimentation results in small sample volumes with low concentration of analytes [103, 104]. This entails the use of highly sensitive and specific analytical method for the quantitative estimation of analytes in microdialysis samples. Generally ocular microdialysis involves the perfusion of isotonic phosphate buffer saline at 2 μL/min flow rate. Based on the duration of time interval, the sample volumes vary from 40–60 μL [60]. Typically the analyte concentrations vary from 1 pM to 1 µM. The major advantage associated with microdialysis over traditional blood or tissue sampling is the freedom to vary the temporal time depending on the sensitivity of the analytical method. Temporal resolution time is the duration over which microdialysis samples are collected. Unlike traditional blood sampling, microdialysis does not result in loss of body fluids and moreover the data can be collected in a continuous manner [105]. Microdialysis results in essentially protein free samples and hence do not need an extraction of analytes. Depending on analyte, various analytical methods such as liquid chromatography [43], mass spectrophotometry [45] and liquid scintillation counter [49] have been reported in literature. Liquid scintillation counter is relatively simple and less tedious without the requirement of analyte extraction. Further, using this technique it is possible to analyze two isotopes at the same time. Isotopes such as ^{14}C, ^{3}H and ^{125}I [49, 56] have been widely employed in ocular microdialysis studies. Although this technique offers high sensitivity, it is relatively expensive and requires disposal of radioactive substances. HPLC analysis using UV and fluorescent detectors is relatively cost effective. However, based on the sensitivity of the detection method, temporal resolution should be adjusted to obtain a sufficient volume of dialysate. Microdialysis samples can be directly injected into the chromatographic columns attached to a guard column without any further purification. Liquid chromatography attached to mass spectrometric detection (LCMS/MS) is utilized for the analysis of microdialysis samples due to its high sensitivity, selectivity and the ability to quantify small sample volumes with low analyte concentrations. However, the microdialysis samples cannot be directly injected because of the presence of high buffer concentrations. So the analytes should be extracted before injecting into the LCMS/MS system.

Invasiveness of Probe Implantation

Microdialysis is relatively less invasive in nature. However, following probe implantation an acute inflammatory response is produced due to the invasion by neutrophils and macrophages [19, 106]. The anatomical size of the eye presents numerous obstacles for appropriate normal and pathological examination. The sensitivity of eye further complicates the situation due to a series of immunoprotective cascade pathways [19]. The nature of the ocular microdialysis experimentation permits these studies only in animal models [53, 107]. Microdialysis technique is relatively complex and success of an experiment depends mainly on the surgical experience of the personnel. The sight of the animal needs to be preserved throughout the experimental duration while performing microdialysis in a conscious animal model [108]. This model involves the implantation for duration of 30 days depending on the nature of the experiment. So it is necessary to apply anti-inflammatory agents such as 0.1% dexamethasone phosphate to counter any inflammation or redness of sclera/conjunctiva. Moreover, the probes should be flushed with IPBS containing antibiotics (penicillin and streptomycin) to prevent any bacterial growth around the probe membrane. The anatomical dimensions of eye offer many difficulties during probe implantation and examination of pathological conditions [53]. This requires expertise and development of alternative ways to overcome surgically related artifacts. For small organs such as the eye it is very important to maintain fluid balance for obtaining the precise pharmacokinetic values. Studies by Rittenhouse *et al.* [19] concluded that alterations in aqueous humor protein concentrations may considerably vary ocular pharmacokinetic parameters. An appropriate recovery period must be allowed to recover the physiological fluid loss occurred during the implantation of probes. The recovery period of animals varies depending on the model (unconscious or conscious animal model) and region (anterior or posterior segment) of probe implantation. In an unconscious animal model, the IOP and protein content of the eyes retain their normal values in approximately 2 h following probe implantation [41]. However, in a conscious animal model the IOP and protein content for anterior chamber and posterior segment microdialysis retain their normal values in approximately 5 and 2 days respectively [19, 60].

Analyte Properties and Perfusion Flow Rate

Physicochemical properties of drug molecules such as molecular weight and log P significantly affect the probe recovery. Kendrick [95] observed the effect of molecular weight on *in vitro* probe recovery of 40 analytes using CMA/10 microdialysis probe at 2 µL/min flow rate. Kendrick concluded that the log % *in vitro* recovery of neuropeptides with MWCO ranging from 400-4500 Da exhibited an inverse linear relationship. Moreover, the relative recovery was highest for amino acids (33-40%) followed by monoamines (22-30%) and neuropeptides (1.5-24%) [109]. Hydrophobic drug molecules like neurotensin, neuropeptides Y and estradiols tend to have lower recovery values due to their sticky nature. Such molecules require longer equilibration times for attaining a steady level in recovery [110]. Waga and Ehinger [4] reported that lipophilic molecules tend to stick to polycarbonate and not to polyamides and moreover the high molecular weight drug molecules such as inulin (MW. 5200 Da) have relatively low recovery compared to low molecular weight substances. Apart from the lipophilicity and the molecular weight of the analyte, the recovery of the analyte depends on the flow rate of perfusion fluid. At lower flow rates (<0.1 µL/min) the relative recovery of analyte equals to 1 [111, 112]. However, low perfusion rates may require higher temporal resolution depending on the sensitivity of analytical methods. Absolute recovery of an analyte is inversely proportionally to perfusate flow rate up to 2µL/min [99]. Generally ocular microdialysis is carried out at a flow rate of 2 or 3 µL/min with IPBS and the dialysate is collected every 20-30 min [38, 60].

STRATEGIES FOR DESIGN OF AN IDEAL MICRODIALYSIS EXPERIMENT

Based on the preliminary information about ocular microdialysis variables, an ideal experimentation procedure should involve the proper selection of probe, perfusion rate depending on the nature of the drug molecules (hydrophilic or lipophilic) and sensitivity of bioanalytical method. Generally a CMA/100 microinjection pump is used for the perfusion of IPBS through the dialysis probes. Design of probe depends mainly on the microdialysis model and the sampling site. Sampling of aqueous humor utilizing an unconscious animal model involves the use of linear probes (MD-2000, 0.32 x 10 mm, polyacrylo nitrile membrane and 0.22 mm tubing), while for a conscious animal model both concentric (custom made CMA/20 custom, 4 mm polycarbonate membrane, 20 kD MCWO) and linear probes (LM-10 Linear Microdialysis Probes, 10 mm membrane window) have been utilized [19, 41, 47]. Sampling of vitreous humor in an unconscious animal model involves the use of a concentric probe (CMA/20 with 0.5 x10 mm, polycarbonate membrane and 14 mm shaft), while in a conscious animal model linear microdialysis probes (polyacrylonitrile membrane with 10 mm length) are employed [41, 58]. Information regarding the physicochemical characteristics of the analyte (lipophilicity and molecular weight) and analytical sensitivity plays a critical role in the design of microdialysis experiments. Generally the recovery of hydrophilic molecules is higher compared to lipophilic molecules. Very few studies correlating the effect of lipophilicity and membrane properties were carried out using ocular microdialysis [4]. Further use of probes made of polyamide membranes increases the recovery of lipophilic drug molecules [4]. However, such correlations can be exploited from the microdialysis carried out in other organs. Recovery of sticky drug molecules can be increased by perfusion with bovine serum albumin, cyclodextrins, chelating agents, solid supports, colloids or antibodies [109, 113-115]. Mackie *et al.* [116] observed a maximum probe recovery of 66% at a flow of 1 μl/min, using Ringer solution consisting of BSA (70 mg/mL) as perfusion medium. Khramov *et al.* [117] studied the effects of β-cyclodextrin or 2-hydroxypropyl-β-cyclodextrin on the relative recovery of hydrophobic tricyclic drugs such as imipramine, desipramine, amitriptyline, carbamazepine and promethazine. Addition of β-cyclodextrin (≤2% w/v) or 2-hydroxypropyl-β-cyclodextrin (≤5% w/v) increased the relative recovery of carbamazepine, imipramine, desipramine, amitriptyline and promethazine by 136, 268, 298, 634 and 987% respectively. Ao and Steken [118] studied the relative recovery of amitryptiline, carbamazepine, hydroquinone, ibuprofenand 4-nitrophenol using different water-soluble, epichlorohydrin-based cyclodextrin polymers (CD-EPS). They observed a higher recovery of analytes in the presence of CD-EPS when compared to native alpha, beta and gamma cyclodextrins in polycarbonate membrane with 20 kDa MWCO. Pich *et al.* [119] observed a 2-fold increase in the recovery of corticotropin-releasing factor following addition of antibodies into the perfusion fluid. Fletcher and Stenken [120] studied the effect of cyclodextrins (β-cyclodextrin, 2-hydroxypropyl-β-cyclodextrinand γ-cyclodextrin) and antibodies as affinity agents in increasing the probe recovery of two neuropeptides, methionine-enkephalin and leucine-enkephalin. The recovery of neuropeptides was increased by 2 and 2.5 folds using cyclodextrin and antibodies respectively.

FUTURE ADVANCES IN MICRODIALYSIS

The utility of microdialysis in characterizing ocular disposition of small molecules has been studied over 3 decades. There has also been some greater awareness of technical hurdles such as handling lipophilic/sticky substrates, efficiency of probe recovery and the ability of bioanalytical techniques to quantify substrates. Nevertheless, significant and impactful factors supporting the continued use of microdialysis include understanding the artifacts possible with conventional terminal animal ocular PK studies. Conventional approaches may result in over-estimation of intraocular drug exposure and less precision in animal to human predictions. A number of biologicals have been recently introduced providing viable therapeutic options for treating important ocular diseases. Microdialysis technologies must adapt to sampling macromolecules in intraocular regions in order to remain a relevant tool for these types of substrates. In the small molecule space, strategies to improve probe recovery for sticky molecules become a key analytical challenge to be met. The interplay of drug properties and biological barriers within the eye has been studied extensively in recent years. Coupling this expanded knowledge with technical advances in microdialysis will maintain a window of opportunity for its continued importance for characterizing ocular pharmacokinetics and enhancing animal to human predictions of exposure.

ACKNOWLEDGEMENTS

This work was partly supported by the National Institutes of Health grants R01 EY 09171-16 and R01 EY 10659-12.

CONFLICT OF INTEREST

The author(s) confirm that this chapter content has no conflict of interest.

REFERENCES

[1]   Brubaker RF. Flow of aqueous humor in humans [The Friedenwald Lecture]. Invest Ophthalmol Visual Sci 1991; 32(13): 3145-66.
[2]   Mitra AK (ed). Ophthalmic drug delivery systems. New York: Dekker; 1993. xii, 502 p. p.
[3]   Waga J, Nilsson-Ehle I, Ljungberg B, Skarin A, Stahle L, Ehinger B. Microdialysis for pharmacokinetic studies of ceftazidime in rabbit vitreous. J Ocul Pharmacol Ther 1999; 15(5): 455-63.
[4]   Waga J, Ehinger B. Passage of drugs through different intraocular microdialysis membranes. Graefes Arch Clin Exp Ophthalmol 1995; 233(1): 31-7.

[5]   Boddu SH, Jwala J, Vaishya R, *et al*. Novel nanoparticulate gel formulations of steroids for the treatment of macular edema. J Ocul Pharmacol Ther; 2010; 26(1): 37-48.

[6]   Bourges JL, Bloquel C, Thomas A, *et al*. Intraocular implants for extended drug delivery: therapeutic applications. Adv Drug Deliv Rev 2006; 58(11): 1182-202.

[7]   Fattal E, Bochot A. Antisense oligonucleotides, aptamers and SiRNA: promises for the treatment of ocular diseases. Arch Soc Esp Oftalmol. 2006; 81(1): 3-6.

[8]   Jaffe GJ, Martin D, Callanan D, Pearson PA, Levy B, Comstock T. Fluocinolone acetonide implant (Retisert) for noninfectious posterior uveitis: thirty-four-week results of a multicenter randomized clinical study. Ophthalmology 2006; 113(6): 1020-7.

[9]   Lee JH, Canny MD, De Erkenez A, *et al*. A therapeutic aptamer inhibits angiogenesis by specifically targeting the heparin binding domain of VEGF165. Proc Natl Acad Sci U S A 2005; 102(52): 18902-7.

[10] Waisbourd M, Loewenstein A, Goldstein M, Leibovitch I. Targeting vascular endothelial growth factor: a promising strategy for treating age-related macular degeneration. Drugs Aging 2007; 24(8): 643-62.

[11] Los M, Roodhart JM, Voest EE. Target practice: lessons from phase III trials with bevacizumab and vatalanib in the treatment of advanced colorectal cancer. The Oncologist 2007; 12(4): 443-50.

[12] Steinbrook R. The price of sight--ranibizumab, bevacizumab and the treatment of macular degeneration. N Engl J Med 2006; 355(14): 1409-12.

[13] Kern TS, Miller CM, Du Y, *et al*. Topical administration of nepafenac inhibits diabetes-induced retinal microvascular disease and underlying abnormalities of retinal metabolism and physiology. Diabetes 2007; 56(2): 373-9.

[14] Yu DY, Cringle SJ, Alder VA, Su EN. Intraretinal oxygen distribution in rats as a function of systemic blood pressure. Am J Physiol 1994; 267(6 Pt 2):H2498-507.

[15] Patterson JW. The effect of ouabain on volume regulation in the rat lens. Invest Ophthalmol Visual Sci 1981; 20(1): 40-6.

[16] Remtulla S, Hallett PE. A schematic eye for the mouse and comparisons with the rat. Vision Res 1985; 25(1): 21-31.

[17] Augusteyn RC. The effect of light deprivation on the mouse lens. Exp Eye Res 1998; 66(5): 669-74.

[18] Gum G. Physiology of the eye. In: Gelatt K, editor. Essentials of veterinary ophthalmology Baltimore: Lippincott Williams & Wilkins; 1999. p. 169

[19] Rittenhouse KD, Peiffer RL, Jr., Pollack GM. Microdialysis evaluation of the ocular pharmacokinetics of propranolol in the conscious rabbit. Pharma Res 1999; 16(5): 736-42.

[20] Rittenhouse KD, Peiffer RL, Jr., Pollack GM. Assessment of ascorbate ocular disposition in the conscious rabbit: an approach using the microdialysis technique. Curr Eye Res 2000; 20(5): 351-60.

[21] Rittenhouse KD, Peiffer RL, Jr., Pollack GM. Evaluation of microdialysis sampling of aqueous humor for *in vivo* models of ocular absorption and disposition. J Pharm Biomed Anal 1998; 16(6): 951-9.

[22] Boddu SH, Gunda S, Earla R, Mitra AK. Ocular microdialysis: a continuous sampling technique to study pharmacokinetics and pharmacodynamics in the eye. Bioanalysis 2010; 2(3): 487-507.

[23] Mishima S. Clinical pharmacokinetics of the eye. Proctor lecture. Invest Ophthalmol Vis Sci 1981; 21(4): 504-41.

[24] Ungerstedt U. Microdialysis--principles and applications for studies in animals and man. J Intern Med 1991; 230(4): 365-73.

[25] Muller M. Science, medicineand the future: Microdialysis. BMJ 2002;324(7337):588-91.

[26] Rittenhouse KD, Pollack GM. Microdialysis and drug delivery to the eye. Adv Drug Deliv Rev 2000; 45(2-3): 229-41.

[27] Duvvuri S, Rittenhouse KD, Mitra AK. Microdialysis assessment of drug delivery systems for vitreoretinal targets. Adv Drug Deliv Rev 2005; 57(14): 2080-91.

[28] Fukuda M, Mikitani M, Ueda T, Inatomi M, Koide Y, Kurata T. Application of microdialysis on analysis of pharmacokinetics in domestic rabbits aqueous humor. J Jpn Ophthalmol Soc 1995; 99: 400–5.

[29] Sato H, Fukuda S, Inatomi M, *et al*. Pharmacokinetics of norfloxacin and lomefloxacin in domestic rabbit aqueous humor analyzed by microdialysis. J Jpn Ophthalmol Soc 1996; 100: 513–9.

[30] Ohtori R, Sato H, Fukuda S, *et al*. Pharmacokinetics of topical beta-adrenergic antagonists in rabbit aqueous humor evaluated with the microdialysis method. Exp Eye Res 1998; 66(4): 487-94.

[31] Fu J, Feng X, Yuan H, *et al*. Study of ocular pharmacokinetics of *in situ* gel system for S(-)-satropane evaluated by microdialysis. J Pharm Biomed Anal. 2008; 48(3): 840-3.

[32] Liu Z, Yang XG, Li X, Pan W, Li J. Study on the ocular pharmacokinetics of ion-activated *in situ* gelling ophthalmic delivery system for gatifloxacin by microdialysis. Drug Dev Ind Pharm 2007; 33(12): 1327-31.

[33] Liu Z, Pan W, Nie S, Zhang L, Yang X, Li J. Preparation and evaluation of sustained ophthalmic gel of enoxacin. Drug Dev Ind Pharm 2005; 31(10): 969-75.

[34] Aggarwal D, Pal D, Mitra AK, Kaur IP. Study of the extent of ocular absorption of acetazolamide from a developed niosomal formulation, by microdialysis sampling of aqueous humor. Int J Pharm 2007; 338(1-2): 21-6.

[35] Wei G, Ding PT, Zheng JM, Lu WY. Pharmacokinetics of timolol in aqueous humor sampled by microdialysis after topical administration of thermosetting gels. Biomed Chromatogr 2006; 20(1): 67-71.

[36] Dey S, Gunda S, Mitra AK. Pharmacokinetics of erythromycin in rabbit corneas after single-dose infusion: role of P-glycoprotein as a barrier to *in vivo* ocular drug absorption. J Pharmacol Exp Ther 2004; 311(1): 246-55.

[37] Anand BS, Katragadda S, Gunda S, Mitra AK. *In vivo* ocular pharmacokinetics of acyclovir dipeptide ester prodrugs by microdialysis in rabbits. Mol Pharm 2006; 3(4): 431-40.

[38] Katragadda S, Gunda S, Hariharan S, Mitra AK. Ocular pharmacokinetics of acyclovir amino acid ester prodrugs in the anterior chamber: evaluation of their utility in treating ocular HSV infections. Int J Pharm 2008; 359(1-2): 15-24.

[39] Karla PK, Quinn TL, Herndon BL, Thomas P, Pal D, Mitra A. Expression of multidrug resistance associated protein 5 (MRP5) on cornea and its role in drug efflux. J Ocul Pharmacol Ther 2009; 25(2): 121-32.

[40] Rittenhouse KD, Pollack GM. Pharmacodynamics of beta-blocker modulation of aqueous humor production. Exp Eye Res 2000; 70(4): 429-39.

[41] Macha S, Mitra AK. Ocular pharmacokinetics in rabbits using a novel dual probe microdialysis technique. Exp Eye Res 2001; 72(3): 289-99.

[42] Macha S, Mitra AK. Ocular pharmacokinetics of cephalosporins using microdialysis. J Ocul Pharmacol Ther 2001; 17(5): 485-98.

[43] Macha S, Mitra AK. Ocular disposition of ganciclovir and its monoester prodrugs following intravitreal administration using microdialysis. Drug Metab Dispos 2002; 30(6): 670-5.

[44] Atluri H, Mitra AK. Disposition of short-chain aliphatic alcohols in rabbit vitreous by ocular microdialysis. Exp Eye Res 2003; 76(3): 315-20.

[45] Dias C, Nashed Y, Atluri H, Mitra A. Ocular penetration of acyclovir and its peptide prodrugs valacyclovir and val-valacyclovir following systemic administration in rabbits: An evaluation using ocular microdialysis and LC-MS. Curr Eye Res 2002; 25(4): 243-52.

[46] Gunda S, Hariharan S, Mitra AK. Corneal absorption and anterior chamber pharmacokinetics of dipeptide monoester prodrugs of ganciclovir (GCV): *in vivo* comparative evaluation of these prodrugs with Val-GCV and GCV in rabbits. J Ocul Pharmacol Ther 2006; 22(6): 465-76.

[47] Li X, Nie SF, Kong J, Li N, Ju CY, Pan WS. A controlled-release ocular delivery system for ibuprofen based on nanostructured lipid carriers. Int J Pharm 2008; 363(1-2): 177-82.

[48] Liu Z, Zhang X, Li J, Liu R, Shu L, Jin J. Effects of labrasol on the corneal drug delivery of baicalin. Drug Deliv 2009; 16(7): 399-404.

[49] Hariharan S, Gunda S, Mishra GP, Pal D, Mitra AK. Enhanced corneal absorption of erythromycin by modulating P-glycoprotein and MRP mediated efflux with corticosteroids. Pharm Res 2009; 26(5): 1270-82.

[50] Gunnarson G, Jakobsson AK, Hamberger A, Sjostrand J. Free amino acids in the pre-retinal vitreous space. Effect of high potassium and nipecotic acid. Exp Eye Res 1987; 44(2): 235-44.

[51] Ben-Nun J, Cooper RL, Cringle SJ, Constable IJ. Ocular dialysis. A new technique for *in vivo* intraocular pharmacokinetic measurements. Arch Ophthalmol 1988; 106(2): 254-9.

[52] Ben-Nun J, Joyce DA, Cooper RL, Cringle SJ, Constable IJ. Pharmacokinetics of intravitreal injection. Assessment of a gentamicin model by ocular dialysis. Invest Ophthalmol Visual Sci 1989; 30(6): 1055-61.

[53] Waga J, Ohta A, Ehinger B. Intraocular microdialysis with permanently implanted probes in rabbit. Acta Ophthalmologica 1991; 69(5): 618-24.

[54] Waga J, Ehinger B. Intravitreal concentrations of some drugs administered with microdialysis. Acta Ophthalmol Scand 1997; 75(1): 36-40.

[55] Waga J. Ganciclovir delivery through an intravitreal microdialysis probe in rabbit. Acta Ophthalmol Scand 2000; 78(3): 369-71.

[56] Waga J, Ehinger B. NGF administered by microdialysis into rabbit vitreous. Acta Ophthalmol Scand 2000; 78(2): 154-5.

[57] Zhang XM, Ohishi K, Hiramitsu T. Microdialysis measurement of ascorbic acid in rabbit vitreous after photodynamic reaction. Exp Eye Res 2001; 73(3): 303-9.

[58] Dias CS, Mitra AK. Posterior segment ocular pharmacokinetics using microdialysis in a conscious rabbit model. Invest Ophthalmol Visual Sci 2003; 44(1): 300-5.

[59] Hughes PM, Krishnamoorthy R, Mitra AK. Vitreous disposition of two acycloguanosine antivirals in the albino and pigmented rabbit models: a novel ocular microdialysis technique. J Ocul Pharmacol Ther 1996; 12(2): 209-24.

[60] Anand BS, Atluri H, Mitra AK. Validation of an ocular microdialysis technique in rabbits with permanently implanted vitreous probes: systemic and intravitreal pharmacokinetics of fluorescein. Int J Pharm 2004; 281(1-2): 79-88.

[61]   Knudsen LL, Nielsen-Kudsk F. Anterior chamber and vitreous fluorescein kinetics in normal and diabetic subjects. Acta Ophthalmol Scand 1998; 76(4): 396-400.
[62]   Macha S, Duvvuri S, Mitra AK. Ocular disposition of novel lipophilic diester prodrugs of ganciclovir following intravitreal administration using microdialysis. Curr Eye Res 2004; 28(2): 77-84.
[63]   Majumdar S, Kansara V, Mitra AK. Vitreal pharmacokinetics of dipeptide monoester prodrugs of ganciclovir. J Ocul Pharmacol Ther 2006; 22(4): 231-41.
[64]   Duvvuri S, Gandhi MD, Mitra AK. Effect of P-glycoprotein on the ocular disposition of a model substrate, quinidine. Curr Eye Res 2003; 27(6): 345-53.
[65]   Atluri H, Talluri RS, Mitra AK. Functional activity of a large neutral amino acid transporter (LAT) in rabbit retina: a study involving the *in vivo* retinal uptake and vitreal pharmacokinetics of L-phenyl alanine. Int J Pharm 2008; 347(1-2): 23-30.
[66]   Katayama K, Ohshima Y, Tomi M, Hosoya K. Application of microdialysis to evaluate the efflux transport of estradiol 17-beta glucuronide across the rat blood-retinal barrier. J Neurosci Methods 2006; 156(1-2): 249-56.
[67]   Janoria KG, Boddu SH, Wang Z, *et al.* Vitreal pharmacokinetics of biotinylated ganciclovir: role of sodium-dependent multivitamin transporter expressed on retina. J Ocul Pharmacol Ther 2009; 25(1): 39-49.
[68]   Senthilkumari S, Velpandian T, Biswas NR, Saxena R, Ghose S. Evaluation of the modulation of P-glycoprotein (P-gp) on the intraocular disposition of its substrate in rabbits. Curr Eye Res 2008; 33(4): 333-43.
[69]   Hosoya K, Makihara A, Tsujikawa Y, *et al.* Roles of inner blood-retinal barrier organic anion transporter 3 in the vitreous/retina-to-blood efflux transport of p-aminohippuric acid, benzylpenicillinand 6-mercaptopurine. J Pharmacol Exp Ther 2009; 329(1): 87-93.
[70]   Duvvuri S, Janoria KG, Pal D, Mitra AK. Controlled delivery of ganciclovir to the retina with drug-loaded Poly(d,L-lactide-co-glycolide) (PLGA) microspheres dispersed in PLGA-PEG-PLGA Gel: a novel intravitreal delivery system for the treatment of cytomegalovirus retinitis. J Ocul Pharmacol Ther 2007; 23(3): 264-74.
[71]   Okuno T, Oku H, Sugiyama T, Ikeda T. Glutamate level in optic nerve head is increased by artificial elevation of intraocular pressure in rabbits. Exp Eye Res 2006; 82(3): 465-70.
[72]   Murai Y. [Study of tear flow using radioactive isotope (author's transl)]. Nippon Ganka Gakkai Zasshi 1975; 79(10): 1405-13.
[73]   Short BG. Safety evaluation of ocular drug delivery formulations: techniques and practical considerations. Toxicol Pathol 2008; 36(1): 49-62.
[74]   Van Der Bijl P, Engelbrecht AH, Van Eyk AD, Meyer D. Comparative permeability of human and rabbit corneas to cyclosporin and tritiated water. J Ocul Pharmacol Ther 2002; 18(5): 419-27.
[75]   Ravinet E, Mermoud A, Brignoli R. Four years later: a clinical update on latanoprost. Eur J Ophthalmol 2003; 13(2): 162-75.
[76]   Basu S, Sjoquist B, Stjernschantz J, Resul B. Corneal permeability to and ocular metabolism of phenyl substituted prostaglandin esters *in vitro*. Prostaglandins Leukot Essent Fatty Acids 1994; 50(4): 161-8.
[77]   Sjoquist B, Stjernschantz J. Ocular and systemic pharmacokinetics of latanoprost in humans. Surv Ophthalmol 2002; 47(Suppl 1): S6-12.
[78]   Sjoquist B, Basu S, Byding P, Bergh K, Stjernschantz J. The pharmacokinetics of a new antiglaucoma drug, latanoprost, in the rabbit. Drug Metab Dispos 1998; 26(8): 745-54.

[79]   Sjoquist B, Johansson A, Stjernschantz J. Pharmacokinetics of latanoprost in the cynomolgus monkey. 3rd communication: tissue distribution after topical administration on the eye studied by whole body autoradiography. Arzneimittelforschung 1999; 49(3): 240-9.

[80]   Hollo G, Whitson JT, Faulkner R, *et al.* Concentrations of betaxolol in ocular tissues of patients with glaucoma and normal monkeys after 1 month of topical ocular administration. Invest Ophthalmol Visual Sci 2006; 47(1): 235-40.

[81]   Geroski DH, Edelhauser HF. Drug delivery for posterior segment eye disease. Invest Ophthalmol Visual Sci 2000; 41(5): 961-4.

[82]   Driot JY, Novack GD, Rittenhouse KD, Milazzo C, Pearson PA. Ocular pharmacokinetics of fluocinolone acetonide after Retisert intravitreal implantation in rabbits over a 1-year period. J Ocul Pharmacol Ther 2004; 20(3): 269-75.

[83]   Jaffe GJ, Ben-Nun J, Guo H, Dunn JP, Ashton P. Fluocinolone acetonide sustained drug delivery device to treat severe uveitis. Ophthalmology 2000; 107(11): 2024-33.

[84]   Sharei V, Hohn F, Kohler T, Hattenbach LO, Mirshahi A. Course of intraocular pressure after intravitreal injection of 0.05 mL ranibizumab (Lucentis). Eur J Ophthalmol 2010; 20(1): 174-9.

[85]   Gaudreault J, Fei D, Rusit J, Suboc P, Shiu V. Preclinical pharmacokinetics of Ranibizumab (rhuFabV2) after a single intravitreal administration. Invest Ophthalmol Visual Sci 2005; 46(2): 726-33.

[86]   Mordenti J, Cuthbertson RA, Ferrara N, *et al.* Comparisons of the intraocular tissue distribution, pharmacokineticsand safety of 125I-labeled full-length and Fab antibodies in rhesus monkeys following intravitreal administration. Toxicol Pathol 1999; 27(5): 536-44.

[87]   Gaudreault J, Fei D, Beyer JC, *et al.* Pharmacokinetics and retinal distribution of ranibizumab, a humanized antibody fragment directed against VEGF-A, following intravitreal administration in rabbits. Retina 2007; 27(9): 1260-6.

[88]   Bakri SJ, Snyder MR, Reid JM, Pulido JS, Ezzat MK, Singh RJ. Pharmacokinetics of intravitreal ranibizumab (Lucentis). Ophthalmology 2007; 114(12): 2179-82.

[89]   Bito L, Davson H, Levin E, Murray M, Snider N. The concentrations of free amino acids and other electrolytes in cerebrospinal fluid, *in vivo* dialysate of brainand blood plasma of the dog. J Neurochem 1966; 13(11): 1057-67.

[90]   Stempels N, Tassignon MJ, Sarre S. A removable ocular microdialysis system for measuring vitreous biogenic amines. Graefes Arch Clin Exp Ophthalmol. 1993; 231(11): 651-5.

[91]   Hernandez L, Stanley BG, Hoebel BG. A small, removable microdialysis probe. Life Sci 1986; 39(26): 2629-37.

[92]   Wang X, Stenken JA. Microdialysis sampling membrane performance during *in vitro* macromolecule collection. Anal Chem 2006; 78(17): 6026-34.

[93]   Torto N, Bang J, Richardson S, *et al.* Optimal membrane choice for microdialysis sampling of oligosaccharides. J Chromatogr A. 1998; 806(2): 265-78.

[94]   Winter CD, Iannotti F, Pringle AK, Trikkas C, Clough GF, Church MK. A microdialysis method for the recovery of IL-1beta, IL-6 and nerve growth factor from human brain *in vivo*. J Neurosci Methods 2002; 119(1): 45-50.

[95]   Kendrick KM. Microdialysis measurement of *in vivo* neuropeptide release. J Neurosci Methods 1990; 34(1-3): 35-46.

[96]   Hansen DK, Davies MI, Lunte SM, Lunte CE. Pharmacokinetic and metabolism studies using microdialysis sampling. J Pharm Sci 1999; 88(1): 14-27.

[97] Menacherry S, Hubert W, Justice JB, Jr. *In vivo* calibration of microdialysis probes for exogenous compounds. Anal Chem 1992; 64(6): 577-83.

[98] Zetterstrom T, Sharp T, Collin AK, Ungerstedt U. *In vivo* measurement of extracellular dopamine and DOPAC in rat striatum after various dopamine-releasing drugs; implications for the origin of extracellular DOPAC. Eur J Pharmacol 1988; 148(3): 327-34.

[99] Benveniste H, Huttemeier PC. Microdialysis--theory and application. Prog Neurobiol 1990; 35(3): 195-215.

[100] Wages SA, Church WH, Justice JB, Jr. Sampling considerations for on-line microbore liquid chromatography of brain dialysate. Anal Chem 1986; 58(8): 1649-56.

[101] Plock N, Kloft C. Microdialysis--theoretical background and recent implementation in applied life-sciences. Eur J Pharm Sci 2005; 25(1): 1-24.

[102] Peng GW, Chiou WL. Analysis of drugs and other toxic substances in biological samples for pharmacokinetic studies. J Chromatogr 1990; 531: 3-50.

[103] Sheiner LB, Rosenberg B, Marathe VV. Estimation of population characteristics of pharmacokinetic parameters from routine clinical data. J Pharmacokinet Biopharm. 1977; 5(5): 445-79.

[104] Drusano GL, Liu W, Perkins R, *et al.* Determination of robust ocular pharmacokinetic parameters in serum and vitreous humor of albino rabbits following systemic administration of ciprofloxacin from sparse data sets by using IT2S, a population pharmacokinetic modeling program. Antimicrob Agents Chemother 1995; 39(8): 1683-7.

[105] Riley C, Ault J, Lunte C. On-line microdialysis sampling. In: Riley CM, Lough WJ, Wainer IW, editors. Pharmaceutical and biomedical applications of liquid chromatography. 1st ed. [New York]: Pergamon; 1994. p. 193-239.

[106] Davies MI, Lunte CE. Microdialysis sampling for hepatic metabolism studies. Impact of microdialysis probe design and implantation technique on liver tissue. Drug Metab Dispos. 1995; 23(10): 1072-9.

[107] Schoenwald RD. Ocular Pharmacokinetics and Pharmacodynamics. In: Mitra AK, editor. Ophthalmic drug delivery systems. New York: Dekker; 1993. p. 83–110.

[108] Riordan-Evan P, Tabbara KF. Anatomy and embryology of the eye. In: Vaughan D, Asbury T, Riordan-Eva P, editors. General ophthalmology. 13th ed. Norwalk, Conn.: Appleton & Lange; 1992. p. 1–23.

[109] Kendrick KM. Use of microdialysis in neuroendocrinology. Methods Enzymol 1989; 168: 182-205.

[110] Thompson AC, Justice JB, Jr., McDonald JK. Quantitative microdialysis of neuropeptide Y. J Neurosci Methods 1995; 60(1-2): 189-98.

[111] Van Wylen DG, Park TS, Rubio R, Berne RM. Increases in cerebral interstitial fluid adenosine concentration during hypoxia, local potassium infusionand ischemia. J Cereb Blood Flow Metab 1986; 6(5): 522-8.

[112] Delgado JM, Lerma J, Martin del Rio R, Solis JM. Dialytrode technology and local profiles of amino acids in the awake cat brain. J Neurochem 1984; 42(5): 1218-28.

[113] Lambert PD, Wilding JP, Turton MD, Ghatei MA, Bloom SR. Effect of food deprivation and streptozotocin-induced diabetes on hypothalamic neuropeptide Y release as measured by a radioimmunoassay-linked microdialysis procedure. Brain Research 1994; 656(1): 135-40.

[114] Pettersson A, Amirkhani A, Arvidsson B, Markides K, Bergquist J. A feasibility study of solid supported enhanced microdialysis. Anal Chem 2004; 76(6): 1678-82.

[115] Hamrin K, Rosdahl H, Ungerstedt U, Henriksson J. Microdialysis in human skeletal muscle: effects of adding a colloid to the perfusate. J Appl Physiol 2002; 92(1): 385-93.

[116] Mackie CE, English HE, Lelievre E, Gordon BH, Genissel P, Robinson BV. Radioimmunoassay for the measurement of S9788 in serum and microdialysis samples. J Pharm Biomed Anal 1997; 15(7): 917-28.

[117] Khramov AN, Stenken JA. Enhanced microdialysis recovery of some tricyclic antidepressants and structurally related drugs by cyclodextrin-mediated transport. The Analyst 1999; 124(7): 1027-33.

[118] Ao X, Stenken JA. Water-soluble cyclodextrin polymers for enhanced relative recovery of hydrophobic analytes during microdialysis sampling. The Analyst 2003; 128(9): 1143-9.

[119] Pich EM, Koob GF, Heilig M, Menzaghi F, Vale W, Weiss F. Corticotropin-releasing factor release from the mediobasal hypothalamus of the rat as measured by microdialysis. Neuroscience 1993; 55(3): 695-707.

[120] Fletcher HJ, Stenken JA. An *in vitro* comparison of microdialysis relative recovery of Met- and Leu-enkephalin using cyclodextrins and antibodies as affinity agents. Analytica Chimica Acta 2008; 620(1-2): 170-5.

CHAPTER 9

Recent Patents and Regulatory Aspects on Ophthalmic Drug Delivery Systems

Soumyajit Majumdar[1,2,*], Ketan Hippalgaonkar[1], Tushar Hingorani[1] and Walter G. Chambliss[1,2]

[1]*Department of Pharmaceutics, University of Mississippi, University, MS 38677, USA and* [2]*Research Institute of Pharmaceutical Sciences, University of Mississippi, University, MS 38677, USA*

Abstract: The eye is protected from the external environment by various physiological and anatomical barriers. These barriers, through their protective actions, drastically diminish the ocular bioavailability of drugs. In the last decade, a number of innovations attempting to improve the ocular bioavailability of therapeutic agents have been reported. In the present chapter, some of the US patents and patent applications related to ocular drug delivery, published in the last decade, have been discussed. Additionally, an overview of US regulatory requirements and guidelines concerning transformation of innovations into commercial ophthalmic products have been presented.

Keywords: Ophthalmic, ocular, eye, patent, patent application, regulatory, investigational new drug, NDA, CMC, orphan drug, non-clinical, clinical trials, implants, ocular drug delivery, intravitreal, polymers, peptides, cGMP, GCP.

INTRODUCTION

The human eye is a very well protected organ. Designing ophthalmic formulations that do not compromise the protective barriers of the eye, yet deliver therapeutic drug concentrations into the anterior and posterior ocular segments are a challenging task. Topical application is the preferred route for ocular drug delivery. However, several factors severely limit the effectiveness of this route. It is thought that almost 90% of the topically administered agent undergoes precorneal drug loss. Moreover, a better understanding of the disease process and targets and the use of computational and high throughput screening techniques in drug discovery is yielding highly potent drug candidates with less favorable

---

*Address correspondence to Soumyajit Majumdar: 111 Faser Hall, Department of Pharmaceutics, School of Pharmacy, The University of Mississippi, University, MS 38677, USA; Tel: (662)-915 3793; Fax: (662)-915-1177; E-mail: majumso@olemiss.edu

Ashim K. Mitra (Ed)

physicochemical properties and aqueous solubility from a drug delivery point of view. As a result, researchers have actively been seeking to develop noninvasive or minimally invasive strategies to deliver drugs into the deep seated ocular tissues, as evident from a rapid rise in the number of patents filed in this field over the last decade. A major thrust has been on the treatment of posterior segment diseases which are difficult to treat using traditional methods [1]. In this chapter some of the recent US patents (published after 2003) and patent applications concerning ocular drug delivery will be discussed. Additionally, an overview of the US regulatory guidelines and requirements that concern ophthalmic products will be introduced.

U.S. PATENT

A patent for an invention is the grant of property rights to the inventor, issued by the United States Patent and Trademark Office. For an inventor it means that he/she has exclusive rights to the invention.

Patent is a form of intellectual property. For an invention to be patentable it should be a novel idea. The inventor should prove the condition of novelty and non-obviousness. The invention should not have been described in any published literature and should not be obvious from the prior art. If the inventor discloses the invention publicly, it has to be patented within one year or he loses the rights to patenting.

Types of U.S. Patents

There are three basic types of patents: utility patents, design patents and plant patents. For areas concerning patents in ocular drug delivery, the two most important types of patents are utility patents and design patents.

Utility Patents: It is issued for a new invention such as a new drug molecule or a new drug delivery vehicle (eg. solid lipid nanoparticles). It may also be granted for a new method for manufacturing (e.g a novel technique to manufacture liposomes). They are usually granted for a period of twenty years.

Design Patents: It is issued for a new, original design for an article. For example a design patent may be granted for an improved electrode for ocular iontophoresis that reduces irritation during drug delivery. Design patents are usually granted for a period of fourteen years.

Sections in a U.S. Patent Application

A typical non-provisional patent application consists of a written document and an oath or declaration.

- A Title

- An Abstract

- Drawings

- Field of Invention

- Prior Art

- Summary of the Invention

- Detailed Description

- Particular Examples

- Claims

Types of Patent Applications

There are two types of patent applications, provisional patent applications and non-provisional patent applications. Provisional patent applications are fairly new and have been offered since June 1995 by the United States Patent and Trademark Office (USPTO). An inventor can apply either for a provisional/non-provisional patent application depending on his/her needs. Provisional patents are cheaper to apply and are valid for twelve months. After 12 months the protection provided by provisional patent application would expire and the inventor has to apply for a non-provisional application. An inventor who is sure of his idea and has sufficient funds can directly apply for a non-provisional patent application.

Provisional patent applications are similar to non-provisional patents but claims, oath and declaration are not required. Advantages for filing a provisional patent are:

1. Commercialization potential of the invention can be tested in one year before non-provisional patent application.

2. It gives the inventor sufficient time if he does not himself wish to commercialize the invention to find a sponsor who would be interested in buying/licensing the said application and would be ready to bear the higher cost of non-provisional patent application.

3. Another advantage of filing a provisional patent application is that when a subsequent non-provisional patent application is filed it still receives the same twenty year protection. But if the inventor decides to convert his provisional patent application to non- provisional patent application rather than applying for a new non-provisional application the term of the patent will be considered from the original date of filing of the provisional patent application.

4. Inventor can file multiple provisional patent applications as he completes his work which could then be combined into single non-provisional patent application to reduce costs.

5. Provisional patents are not published thus maintains confidentiality of invention compared to a non-provisional patent application which are mostly published after eighteen months from the date of application.

After one year, provisional application protection would expire and an inventor has to apply for a non-provisional patent to receive patent protection.

Steps in Acquiring a U.S. Patent

When an inventor is faced with the prospect of patenting his invention the important steps are as follows:

1. Patent Full-Text and Image database has to be searched to confirm whether the idea has already been patented.

2. An electronic application has to be made and fees have to be paid.

3. After the USPTO grants a patent, the inventor has to keep paying maintenance fees to keep the invention under protection.

In the following paragraphs some examples of novel ideas to enhance ocular drug delivery has been presented.

RECENT PATENTS AND PATENT APPLICATIONS IN THE FIELD OF OCULAR DRUG DELIVERY

Solutions and Smart Gels

A 2006 patent describes stable and long acting aqueous formulations of azalide antibiotics [2]. Azithromycin, an azalide, is a broad spectrum antibiotic supplied as a tablet/suspension for oral use or as a powder for reconstitution to be used parenterally. Azithromycin is unstable in aqueous solution. The patentees observed that azithromycin formulated using DuraSite® technology was stable for 24 months at 5°C or for 12 months at 25°C. Durasite® technology uses a crosslinked polyacrylic acid synthetic polymer which is reported to stabilize the drug in solution. Additionally, the crosslinked polyacrylic polymer is bioadhesive and increases viscosity leading to greater retention of azithromycin on the ocular surface and thus to reduced dosing frequency. Azithromycin for ophthalmic use (using the Durasite® technology) is currently marketed as AzaSite® by InsiteVision Inc. It is available as a 1% ophthalmic solution to be applied twice a day for two days and once daily for the next five days.

An ocular solution for treating inflammation secondary to other eye diseases or autoimmune disorders has been described in a patent application [3]. The formulation consists of the sodium salt of mycophenolic acid (MPA) as the primary active ingredient. MPA specifically inhibits ionosine monophosphate dehydrogenase which is involved in triggering inflammatory processes. MPA is currently marketed as a sodium salt (Myfortic®, Novartis) or as an ester prodrug mycophenolate mofetil (CellCept®, Roche), to be given orally to prevent solid organ transplant rejection. Cellcept® is also approved for intravenous use (hydrochloride salt of mycophenolate mofetil). On topical administration, the sodium salt of MPA formulated at physiological pH value penetrates into the anterior and posterior chambers of the eye. Mycophenolic acid has a pKa of 4.5 and would be negatively charged in the tear fluid. The penetration into the eye occurs even though the sodium salt of MPA is less lipophilic than its ester prodrug mycophenolate mofetil (MFA). An example describes preparation of 1.4

% ophthalmic solution. Water (80% of the final volume) was heated to 80° C. Mycophenolic acid (4% w/v) and glycerin (0.8% w/v) were then added. Heating was stopped and 10% sodium hydroxide was added and mixed until MPA went into solution and volume was made up after final pH was adjusted. Animal studies described in the patent suggest that the topical formulation is well tolerated and may be effective in significantly reducing inflammation.

Mixed micelle ophthalmic solutions consisting of calcineurin inhibitors or mTOR inhibitors have been described in another patent application [4]. The formulation consists of calcineurin inhibitor/mTOR inhibitor and two surfactants. One surfactant has an HLB greater than 10 and another has an HLB greater than 13. The difference between the two surfactants has to be greater than about three. In an example described in the patent application, voclosporin (0.2 % w/v) and vitamin E TPGS (2 % w/v) and octoxynol 40 (2% w/v) were dissolved in 10 mL 95% ethanol. Ethanol was evaporated in rotatory vacuum evaporator for 12 hours to get a thin dry film. To this 50 mL of water was added and sonicated for 20 mins to form mixed micelles. In another 40 mL of deionized water PVP-K-90 (1.2% w/v), buffering agents and other osmotic excipients (sodium chloride) were added. This buffered polymer solution was added to the mixed micelle solution and pH was adjusted to 6.8. The final volume was then made up. The formulations were found to be biocompatible.

Corneal wounds from injury or refractive surgery could lead to a fibrotic response. A patent application claims that ethyl pyruvate or other esters/amides of alpha-ketoalkonoic acid could be useful in preventing the fibrotic response during wound healing [5], without major tissue damage. In a mouse model of corneal wound healing ethyl pyruvate treated group (10µL, 5% w/v every 90 mins) showed significantly reduced stromal light scattering and edema. The mechanism of action for ethyl pyruvate or its derivatives is still to be elucidated.

A pH and temperature sensitive *in situ* gelling formulation containing a combination of Carbopol® and Pluronic® is described in a 2003 patent [6]. Recommended concentrations of Carbopol® are 0.3-0.4% (w/v), more preferably 0.3% (w/v) and the concentration of Pluronic® is 14% (w/v). At pH 4 and 25°C this combination of polymers produces a free flowing liquid but on contact with the tear film at pH 7.4 and 37°C it forms a gel.

Another reversible gelling system is described in a patent issued to Xia [7]. In this case, a block polymer of propylene oxide and ethylene oxide is used in combination with hydroxypropyl methylcellulose. The viscosity of the block co-polymer is dependent on temperature. On contact with the ocular surface the viscosity of the block co-polymer increases. Hydroxypropyl methylcellulose is used to further improve the durability of the gel formed. An antihistaminic drug incorporated in this formulation was able to exert a therapeutic effect for 6-8 hours, compared to 1 hour for the control formulation.

A patent by Singh *et al.* describes novel gum compositions as viscosity enhancers for ophthalmic formulations [8]. The novel gum compositions comprise of at least two polymers selected from konjac, scleroglucan, hydroxypropyl guar, propyleneglycol alginate, sodium alginate, carbopol 971, pectin and agrose. Using more than one gum in a formulation provides a means to produce gels with more specific viscosity and gelling behavior. Most gels made from natural gelling agents lose viscosity when they come in contact with tear fluid. By using combinations of natural gums, formulations may be developed which can show an increase or a decrease in viscosity on contact with tear fluid.

Matrix controlled drug delivery systems made of cationic siloxanyl macromonomers have been described in a patent application. The matrix system is primarily intended for back of the eye delivery. Drug release rate can be controlled/modified by varying the HLB of the silicon containing monomers [9]. Matrix diffusion controlled systems in a variety of shapes can be formulated.

Contact Lenses

An alternative to bioadhesive polymers and viscosity imparting agents, to increase the residence time of the drug in the tear film, is medicated contact lenses. An ocular drug delivery system that consists of nanoparticles, less than 200 nm in size, in a contact lens has been described by Chauhan *et al* [10]. The drug is encapsulated in a vehicle, such as microemulsion/ liposome and then dispersed in the contact lens matrix such as poly 2-hydroxyethyl methacrylate to produce soft contact lenses. A sufficiently transparent drug loaded contact lens is obtained when the size of the encapsulated nanoparticles used is between 50 to 200 nm and the loading of the nanoparticles in the contact lens matrix is kept sufficiently low.

Advancing the field of drug loaded contact lenses, Bryne *et al* have described contact lenses made of drug loaded biomimetic recognitive polymeric hydrogels [11]. An advantage of using this ocular delivery system is that the drug is released when the contact lens touches a biological membrane. The recognitive polymeric hydrogel is formed using cross linking monomers and functionalized monomers. The biotemplate is bound to the functionalized monomer preferably through weak interactions. The cross linking monomer is co-polymerized with the functional monomer to form a contact lens. After formation of the contact lens the biotemplate can be partially washed off and the open sites on the functional polymer can be used to bind the drug. The biotemplate may be an amino acid, an oligopeptide or a tissue target or pseudo-tissue target for drug molecules. The biotemplate enhances the loading capacity of drug molecules to the hydrogel matrix through weak bonds and provides a controlled release of the drug over a period of time as the weak bonds break. Additionally, the biotemplate can be completely washed off and the uncomplexed sites can then be used to bind the drug to the recognitive polymeric hydrogel.

In another patent application, Abdulrazik describes targeting the central nervous system (CNS) through the ocular route [12]. Drugs having poor corneal permeability could permeate through the conjunctiva/sclera into the choroid followed by passive diffusion across the choroid to reach the retina. The exact pathway through which the drug permeates has not yet been elucidated. The authors suggest that drugs given topically in the eye could reach the brain due to sharing of sensory neurons by both organs. As an example, delivery of topically applied brimonidine to target the CNS has been described. Permeation of brimonidine across the conjunctiva was found to be higher than that across the cornea. High concentration of brimonidine was found in brain tissues following application of a single 50 µL drop in the *cul de sac*. Extremely low concentration of brimonidine was detected in the blood, indicating that the drug did not use the ocular-blood-brain pathway. Alternative routes, such as absorption through the olfactory mucosa after nasolacrimal drainage, were ruled out due to the low concentrations of brominidine detected in the olfactory bulbs.

Iontophoresis

Iontophoresis is a non-invasive drug delivery system used to deliver ionized drug molecules across, or into a membrane, with the help of a small electric current.

Iontophoresis works on the principle that electrodes will repel ionized drug molecules of the same charge leading to higher transcorneal/transcleral fluxes. In an ocular iontophoretic system, the electrode, with a charge similar to that of the ionized drug molecule, is placed in the eye and the other electrode is placed elsewhere on the body to complete the circuit. The drug is placed in the eye either in a cup that is continuously infused with drug solution or incorporated in a gel.

Topical glucocorticoid therapy is not effective in delivering drugs to the back of the eye. Either high dose corticosteroids need to be given systemically or periocular/intravitreal injections are required. Even if the drug is administered by periocular/intravitreal injection, due to the relatively short half-lives (few hours), multiple injections have to be administered. Delivery of triamcinolone acetonide/triamcinolone acetonide phosphate to the posterior segment of the eye using iontophoresis has been described by Hugichi *et al* [13]. A constant dielectric system of two milliampere was applied for 15 mins. A depot forming agent was used to sustain the release of triamcinolone acetonide phosphate in the rabbit eyes. After ten minutes about 700 µg and at the end of 24 hours about 20 µg of triamcinolone acetonide/triamcinolone acetonide phosphate was still present in the conjunctiva, sclera and vitreous humor.

Particulates and Other Disperse Systems

Particulate drug delivery systems consists of small drug loaded polymer particulates that are suspended in a liquid carrier. Biodegradable/non-biodegradable polymers or ion exchange resins are used in particulate formulations. In most cases, particulates are used topically or injected intravitreally or periocularly. When used topically, particulates are not rapidly drained away from the eye and therefore provide prolonged drug release. Microparticles/nanoparticles are also injected intravitreally for intraocular use.

In a 2006 patent application, a particulate system, that can be administered either sub-conjuctivally or intravitreally, to deliver and maintain drug concentration in the posterior segment of the eye has been described. Sub-conjunctival injection is preferred over intravitreal injection since it is easy to administer and is associated with less complications. The application describes a delivery system that has drug suspended in the matrix (such as a gel or a solution that gels in the physiological environment) that forms a depot when administered into the subconjunctival space [14]. The drug being insoluble in the vehicle is slowly released *in vivo*. This system can be used to effectively deliver drugs for posterior segment diseases over a prolonged period of time.

A 2009 patent discloses polymeric microparticles/microspheres for the delivery of a alpha-2 receptor agonist. The microparticles/microspheres are administered subconjuctivally and provide controlled release of the drug for the treatment of ocular diseases such as glaucoma [15].

Another 2009 patent discloses a method of producing nanoparticles/microparticles by altering the ternary agent concentration and process temperature [16]. An example in the patent describes a system consisting of a non-solvent (water), solvent (Tetrahydrofuran-THF), ternary agent (NaCl), surfactant (Pluronic F127), a monomer and polymerization initiator for the monomer. It was discovered that in a 1M sodium chloride solution in water at 10°C THF was completely soluble while at 45 °C solubility of THF reduced to 10 percent. To manufacture the drug containing nanoparticles/microparticles, 30% THF solution containing the drug, the monomer and the polymerization initiator was added to 1M sodium chloride in an aqueous surfactant solution. The mixture was cooled to 10°C. At this temperature THF is completely soluble in the surfactant-salt solution and forms a homogenous solution. When this homogenous mixture was transferred to a flask at 45°C and stirred, the insoluble THF was emulsified by the surfactant in the salt solution. Exposure to UV light initiated polymerization of the monomers in the emulsified THF droplets leading to the formation of nanoparticles/microparticles depending on the conditions used. THF was removed by vacuum and the resulting particles were collected by filtration. The greater the amount of THF used, the lower the concentration of the monomer in THF and the smaller the particles. The concentration of salt used also influenced the solubility of THF at a particular temperature and affected the particle size.

Hofland *et al.* in a patent application described ophthalmic liposomal formulations [17]. The lipid phase consists of a combination of a neutral lipid, a cationic lipid and a mucoadhesive compound. The drug is entrapped within the liposome. Since the mucosal layer covering the cornea is negatively charged, incorporation of cationic lipid gives the liposome a net positive charge allowing it to coat the negatively charged mucus. Increased ophthalmic residence is thus achieved. The mucoadhesive agent in the liposome also helps it to adhere to the ocular surface and may lead to even longer residence times. Liposomes adhering to the mucosal surface form a depot from which the drug is slowly released. An example in the application describes a formulation that led to an improved delivery of diclofenac to the anterior chamber of the eye.

In another patent application, Karaoka *et al.* described formulation of polymeric micelles containing a photosensitive drug [18]. In photodynamic therapy, a photosensitive drug is administered and subsequently activated by light of a specific wavelength. Photo-activation leads to release of highly reactive singlet oxygen by the photosensitive drug. Targeting is achieved by higher accumulation of the photosensitive drug in the diseased tissue compared to healthy tissue. The micelles are formed of polymers having a hydrophilic end and a hydrophobic end. The core of the micelle is formed by the hydrophobic polymer chain while the shell is made from the hydrophilic end. This provides a hydrophobic core in which poorly water soluble drugs can be incorporated. The size of the polymeric nanoparticles is between 10-100 nm. The photosensitive drug incorporated polymer micelles are injected intravenously. The micelles can effectively deliver the drug to the posterior segment of the eye as well as improve solubility and stability of the agent used for photodynamic therapy.

Implants

Implants are classified as biodegradable or non-biodegradable and provide controlled release of a drug for extended periods of time. Non-biodegradable implants have the advantage of more accurately controlling drug release over longer periods of time but have to be surgically removed once their load gets depleted. An implant is able to by-pass most of the barriers encountered in topical/systemic drug delivery approaches. Minor surgery is usually required to place the implant at the site of action [19]. A patent by Robinson *et al.* describes ocular implant devices for delivering therapeutic agents to the eye [20]. Sub-conjunctival and intravitreal implants are described. Drug is continuously delivered to the eye by dual mode release kinetics of the insert. A dual mode insert consists of both a loading dose and maintenance dose in the same implant and therefore provides a smooth transition from a high release rate to a slow release rate. A matrix layer consists of drug (1-50%), drug permeable polymer (superhydrolyzed polyvinyl acetate, 5-50%) and a water soluble polymer (hydroxypropylmethyl cellulose (HPMC), methyl cellulose, hydroxypropyl cellulose or methyl cellulose, 0.05-90%). This layer carries the loading dose of the drug. The super hydrolyzed PVA releases the drug by slow bioerosion and diffusion through the matrix. As the preloaded drug from the matrix is exhausted the inner core releases additional drug at a controlled rate which provides the maintenance dose. The super hydrolyzed PVA is most preferablly 99.3 % w or more hydrolyzed. The molecular weight of the water soluble polymer, HPMC is most preferably 85,000.

A patent application by Asgharian *et al.* describes an implantable, drug containing, styrene elastomer matrix [21]. It is claimed that the styrene elastomer matrix is superior since it provides controlled drug release over prolonged periods of time and is safer than bio-erodible polymers as they do not generate erosion by-products such as acids or alcohols. The styrene elastomers are copolymers consisting of styrene with mid-blocks of butadiene/propylene/butylene to provide an elastomeric matrix. Styrene elastomers can be molded into a variety of shapes for implantation in the eye.

A 2008 patent application by Wong describes a delivery system for an immunosuppressive agent to reduce or prevent neovascularization in the eye [22]. The implant consists of a bioerodible polymer and an immunosuppressive agent. The authors suggest that after ocular transplantation procedures a systemic immunosuppressive therapy may not provide adequate drug concentrations in the ocular tissues and thereby lead to transplant rejections. Since the ocular globe is very well protected, large doses of systemic immunosuppressive therapy may be required leading to generalized side effects. Local drug administration using bioerodible implants may provide better dug delivery while lowering chances of transplant rejection and systemic side effects. These delivery systems may be placed in the anterior chamber for corneal transplants or in the posterior chamber for back of the eye transplant procedures. In a rat model of penetrating keratoplasty model, all of the donor corneas were rejected in the control group (second week) and 80% of the corneas were rejected in the comparative treatment group (0.5% topical dexamethasone solution) by the end of 8th week. None of the corneas were rejected in the group treated with the dexamethasone loaded implant. Additional patent applications have been filed for delivery systems made of bioerodible polymer containing immunosuppressive agent and auxiallary agents [23].

Another patent application describes ocular implants made by a double extrusion process [24]. A mixture of PLGA and esterified PLGA is used to control drug release. The un-esterified PLGA takes up water at a faster rate and is thus hydrolyzed before the esterified PLGA. A 3:1 ratio of PLGA: PLGA ester is most preferable. For double extrusion, a 3:1 ratio of PLGA to esterified PLGA was taken and intimately mixed with the drug. This mixture was then extruded as filaments. Filaments were pelletized and extruded again. A conventional compressed implant exhibits an initial burst release of the medication. In comparison, ocular implants made by the extrusion process did not show an initial burst release of the medication. Also, the extruded implants were observed to completely release the drug *in vivo* compared to the compressed implants which showed that some drug was retained in the implant.

A patent application by Burkstrand *et al.* describes biodegradable implants made from polysaccharides for ocular drug delivery [25]. Using a polymerizable group, natural polysaccharides are crosslinked to form a biodegradable matrix. Low molecular weight polysaccharides, having little or no branching, are preferred such as amylase, maltodextrin and polyadlitol. Enzymatic cleavage of the cross linked polysaccharide releases the drug at the site in the eye. The polysaccharides formed in the process are common physiological components and are thus non-toxic. Impants that last from 1 to 3 months may be fabricated.

A biocompatible intraocular implant consisting of a biodegradable polymer and a prostamide is described in a patent application [26]. The biodegradable intraocular implant was shown to be useful in controlling the release of bimatoprost for extended periods in the eye. The drug is mixed with a biodegradable polymer/polymer mixture and is either compressed or extruded to form an implant. The implant is then placed in the vitreous fluid. Implants composed of bimatoprost/PLA were found to be effective in reducing intraocular pressure in humans for about six months. Bimatoprost in a combination of PLA and PLGA were useful in controlling elevated intraocular pressure for about 2 years.

A 2009 patent application describes the synthesis of biocompatible and biodegradable polymers which can provide pseudo zero order release of water insoluble drug compounds under physiologic conditions. The water insoluble drug is blended with a diphenolic polymer such as polycarbonate or polyacrylate [27].

A patent application by Meng *et al.* describes implantable drug delivery devices which can be refilled [28]. The device consists of a needle entry port, a refillable drug reservoir and a cannula. A check valve is present between the needle entry port and the drug reservoir. The needle entry port is used to deliver the refill to the drug reservoir. The cannula acts to direct the drug to the target site. The injection of a liquid medication into the injection port forces the liquid through the check valve into the drug reservoir. The drug is then slowly released from the cannula towards the targeted site. A visualization ring may be added on the opening point for easier placement of the needle into the injection port. The device can be placed over the conjunctiva and the cannula releases medication into the posterior segment of the eye.

A 2005 patent by Santini Jr. *et al* describes microchip device arrays as ocular implants for drug delivery [29]. The device consists of an array of small microchip devices which can be mounted on a flexible support. Due to its flexible nature it can be implanted over a curved surface such as the sclera. The device contains drug reservoirs that can hold multiple drugs. The device may also contain sensors so that accurate amount of certain drugs may be released in response to changes in surrounding environment.

Delivery of Peptides

A 2006 patent describes non-invasive delivery of genes into ocular cells [30]. Genes are delivered in pegylated liposomes combined with ocular receptor targeting. Gene delivery is usually done by viral vectors or non-viral vectors. Viral vectors carrying the therapeutic gene have to be administered by intravitreal or sub-retinal injection in the eye since they cannot reach the retina after intravenous injection. Another problem is development of antibodies to viral vectors even after single injection. If in subsequent administrations same vector is used it would cause inflammation in the eye. Even after such invasive delivery mechanisms, the virus transduces an area of only about 100 μm from the site of injection. Liposomes with diameters less than 200 nm, preferably those in the size range of 50 to 150 nm, especially with an external diameter of 80 nm are preferred. Transportable peptides such as insulin are conjugated on the surface of the liposome to help it cross the BBB. PEG, sphingomyelin or other organic polymers could be used as conjugating agents to attach transportable peptides to the surface of the liposome. The liposome encapsulated gene showed improved delivery to the retina.

Nanoparticles, comprised of a biodegradable polymer and co-polymer, encapsulating therapeutic siRNA are described in a patent application by Lyons *et al* [31]. The siRNA may be complexed with a cationic polymer, such as protamine, before encapsulation in nanoparticles. Nanoparticles in the range of 100-200 nm are most preferred. In an example provided in the patent application, the siRNA is dissolved in water and emulsified in a chloroform solution containing the matrix polymer PLGA. This emulsion is added to protein binding buffer (PBB) containing PVA and homogenized leading to the formation of nanoparticles. The nanoparticles are collected using utracentrifugation and resuspended in solution or may be incorporated into hydrogels.

REGULATORY CONSIDERATIONS

Conceptualization of a novel idea or a discovery of a novel molecule for ocular drug delivery has to be followed by a methodical approach to ensure successful translation into a marketable product.

The regulatory agencies expectations for ophthalmic products have always been among the most demanding of all pharmaceutical products. In addition to cGMP requirements, Federal laws in the United States require ophthalmic products to meet additional requirements. 21 CFR 211.167 addresses control of foreign particles and harsh or abrasive substances in ophthalmic ointments [32]. 21 CFR

200.50 requires ophthalmic drug and medical device products to be sterile and pyrogen free. It also requires the primary packaging components to be sterile and tamper proof [33].

Sterilization of ophthalmic products is generally achieved by either terminal sterilization or aseptic processing techniques. In terminal sterilization the ophthalmic product is manufactured and packaged in a clean environment and then sterilized using heat or radiation. In aseptic processing each component is individually sterilized, or several components are combined and sterilized and the final package assembled in a sterile environment. The FDA has provided guidance for sterile drug products manufactured by aseptic processing [34]. Terminal sterilization generally provides greater assurance of sterility of the final product [35]. However, when heat labile plastic containers or ingredients are used, aspect processing is the preferred method of sterilization. The use of aseptic processing requires additional process validation data and justification during regulatory submissions [35]. Sterilization can lead to changes in implant material or release of toxic residual products which can induce intraocular inflammation. Therefore, effect of sterilization procedures on drug delivery systems should also be tested before its use in humans.

Ophthalmic products are also expected to be isotonic and compatible with the ocular tissues. Ideally, every topical ophthalmic solution would be buffered at 7.4, the pH of the lachrymal fluid. However, many drugs have lower stability and solubility at this pH. Hence the formulator sometimes must compromise between drug stability and patient's comfort. If buffers are required, their capacity is kept as low as possible, to enable rapid neutralization by the tear fluid. The effect of buffers on tonicity must also be taken into account and is another reason for minimally buffered ophthalmic formulations [36].

21 CFR 200.50 also requires that all multi-dose ophthalmic formulations should contain one or more preservatives, or should be packed and labeled in a manner that it offers adequate protection and minimizes the risk of injury/infection [33].

Non-Clinical Safety Studies

Prior to initiation of human clinical trials, FDA requires adequate non-clinical toxicity and safety information of an Investigational New Drug. However, sufficient FDA guidance on the regulatory requirements for the assessment of non-clinical safety of ocular drugs are currently not available [37]. The International Committee on Harmonization (ICH) guidelines on non-clinical safety studies for the conduct of human clinical trials for all pharmaceuticals, including ocular drugs, requires systematic evaluation of non-clinical toxicology, tolerance, pharmacokinetic, genotoxicity, carcinogenicity and reproduction toxicity studies of a drug [38,39]. Additionally, FDA regulations require that all the non-clinical safety studies for IND, NDA or any other regulatory submission should be conducted in compliance with good laboratories practices (GLP) (21 CFR 58) [40].

Single and Repeat Dose Toxicity: For compounds that are to be administered as a single dose, two weeks acute toxicity has to be evaluated in two mammalian species prior to human exposure. For repeated dose toxicity studies the recommended duration of toxicity study is based on the duration of testing, therapeutic indication and scale of the proposed clinical trial. These studies are usually performed in two species (one non-rodent). For example, 2-week, 1-, 3- or 6- month's toxicity data would support any of the clinical development phases for up to 2-weeks, 1-, 3- or 6- months, respectively. If any of the clinical trials last beyond these periods, 6 month rodent and chronic non-rodent studies are required [38]. However, these requirements may vary with the ocular drug or delivery system. For example, non clinical development of Retisert involved a 1-year intravitreal implant toxicity study in Dutch-Belted rabbits, a 4-week and a 1-year intravitreal implant toxicity in dogs [41].

Local Tolerance Studies: Assessment of ocular tolerance of ophthalmic products in non-clinical studies is extremely important prior to human exposure [41]. The type and extent of testing are usually determined based on the duration and frequency of exposure of the eye to the ophthalmic product. European regulatory agencies recommend single and repeat dose ocular tolerance test, in rabbits, for medicinal products indented for administration in the eye. In these studies ocular tissues, exposed or not exposed to the product, are evaluated for tolerance [42].

Pharmacokinetic Studies: Following ocular administration, a drug can potentially enter into the systemic circulation (through the conjunctival vasculature and lacrimal drainage system) and exert systemic side effects. For example systemic absorption of topical timolol may endanger patients with congestive heart failure and asthma [43]. Therefore, to determine the systemic exposure of topical agents, pharmacokinetic studies of drug candidates are usually conduced in nonclinical settings prior to human exposure. Usually one species is sufficient [41]. Another important factor that has to be considered in establishing the pharmacokinetic properties of the agent is the degree of binding to melanin. Binding to melanin in the ocular tissues such as choroid-RPE, uveal tract, iris ciliary bodies, can significantly affect the ocular bioavailability of the drug. Lipophilic beta-blockers such as betaxolol and metoprolol are known to accumulate in the pigment containing ocular structures [44]. In addition, mydriatic response of ephedrine diminishes with increase pigmentation in the iris [45]. Similarly, IOP lowering activity of timolol was shown to be dependent on the level of iris pigmentation of the subjects [46]. Therefore, New Zealand Red and Dutch-Belted rabbits (DB) are usually used in non clinical studies if the drug has the potential to bind to ocular melanin. Regulatory agencies in Europe call for the use of pigmented rabbits in non-clinical development of ophthalmic drugs [41].

Genotoxicity Studies: Genotoxicity studies are *in vitro* and *in vivo* tests designed to identity compounds that can cause direct or indirect damage to the genetic apparatus by various mechanisms. If compounds test positive they have the potential to be human carcinogens and/or mutagens [47]. Therefore, prior to human exposure, *in vitro* testing for gene mutation in bacteria and an *in vitro* testing for cytogenetic evaluation of chromosomal damage with mammalian cells or an *in vitro* mouse lymphoma tk assay are required. In addition to *in vitro* testing, an *in vivo* test for chromosomal damage using rodent hematopoietic cells is also required prior to initiation of phase 2 studies [47,48].

Carcinogenicity Studies: Carcinogenicity evaluations involve life-time exposure of the test animal to the drug. These studies are usually carried out in parallel with phase 3 studies. The purpose of these studies is to identify tumorigenic potential of drugs in animal and to evaluate the relevant risk in humans. These studies are required for drugs which will frequently be used to treat chronic or recurrent disorders. For ophthalmic drugs, these studies should be considered if there is a scientific cause for concern based on what is known about the drug candidate or if there is a significant systemic exposure of the drug [49].

Reproductive Toxicology Studies: Reproductive toxicology studies in animals evaluate the effect of the drug on fertility and early embryonic development to implantation, pre- and postnatal development, including maternal function and embryo-fetal development [50]. These studies should be carried out, as appropriate, in intended patient populations. In the United States, men may be enrolled in phase 1 and phase 2 clinical trials prior to male fertility studies. However, the effect of a drug candidate on male fertility needs to be studied prior to the initiation of phase 3 clinical trials. Women, not of child bearing potential, can be enrolled in clinical trials without reproductive toxicity studies provided effect of repeat dose toxicity on female reproductive organs has been studied. Women of child bearing potential may be enrolled in early clinical studies if appropriate measures are taken to minimize risks, including the use of pregnancy testing and abstinence during the study period. However, women of child bearing potential using birth control can only be enrolled in phase 3 trials after evaluation of female fertility and embryo-fetal development is complete. Data from all reproductive toxicity studies, genotoxicity studies and previous human exposure are needed for enrollment of pregnant women in clinical trials [38].

INVESTIGATIONAL NEW DRUG APPLICATION (IND) AND ITS REVIEW PROCESS

The use of a new or unapproved drug in clinical studies in the United States requires an IND. The Federal Food and Drug Cosmetic Act, (FD&C act Section 505) also prohibits the shipment of new drugs across state lines without an effective approved marketing application (*i.e.* an NDA or ANDA). An IND, or Notice of Claimed Investigational Exemption for a New Drug, is a regulatory submission to the U.S Food and Drug Administration (FDA) requesting permission to initiate a clinical study of a new or unapproved drug in the United States and to allow its interstate shipment [51,52]. A drug already approved by an NDA or ANDA may be considered to be a new drug and require IND filing. Therefore proper interpretation of the legal definitions of a new drug product as per the FD&C act is required [53]. An IND is also required for clinical studies in animals and should be submitted to the Center for Veterinary Medicine at FDA. Additionally, a large number of drugs used in ophthalmology were originally developed and approved for the systemic route of administration [37,54].

Therefore, it is imperative to understand when an IND is needed. For regulatory purposes, an IND is required if the drug is [37,55]:

- a new chemical entity

- a new derivative of an existing molecule *e.g.* Dipivefrin.

- not already approved for the therapeutic indication under investigation *e.g.* NSAID to inhibit miosis during cataract surgery.

- presented in a new dosage form and/or strength *e.g.* betaxolol and timolol for glaucoma.

- used in combination with another drug and the combination is not approved *e.g.* combination of tobramycin and dexamethasone.

- a component of new drug delivery system *e.g.* Retisert and Vitrasert

- delivered using a route other than that approved *e.g.* topical ocular dosage form of acetazolamide for IOP reduction.

An IND is not required for *in vitro* and/or preclinical studies, or, for a clinical trial of an approved drug product for an approved indication of use. In addition, clinical studies involving the use of placebos are exempted from IND regulations, as long as it would not otherwise require submission of an IND [56].

The regulations also exempt clinical studies of approved drugs from IND requirements if all of the following apply[56]:

1. The clinical study is not intended to be reported to FDA in support of new indications or to support other significant changes in labeling of the drug or advertisement of the prescription drug product;

2. The clinical study does not involve a route of administration, dose level , subject population or other factors that increase the risk associated with the use of the drug product;

3. The clinical study is conducted in conformity with the IRB review (21 CFR part 56) and informed consent (21 CFR part 50);

4.　The clinical study is conducted in conformity with the requirements involving the promotion and charging of the drug (21 CFR part 312.7)

FDA will not accept an IND application or review a clinical study that meets the above stated exemption provisions [56]. However, executing a clinical study without an effective IND would lead to a regulatory action by the FDA. Therefore, sponsors and investigators should consult with their regulatory affairs staff and their local IRB, respectively, to determine whether the study meets the exemption criteria and if an IND is required. The FDA may be consulted for clarification on the regulatory requirements, if needed [57].

Following receipt of the IND by the FDA, an IND number is assigned and the application is directed to an appropriate review division within FDA. In the case of ophthalmic drugs, the IND is directed to CDER (Center for Drug Evaluation and Research) for review [37]. The primary aim of the IND submission and the review process is "to ensure that subjects involved in the clinical studies will not face undue risk of harm" [58]. The FDA has 30 days to review the initial IND application. During this period the CDER review team critically reviews the preclinical animal pharmacology and toxicology data; chemistry, manufacturing and control (CMC) information; the clinical protocol and the qualifications of the proposed investigator(s) submitted in the IND application and decides if it is safe to proceed with the proposed clinical study [37,52].

Generally, a clinical study can be initiated 30 days after receipt of the application by the FDA or sooner if the FDA provides positive feedback on the application prior to the expiration of the 30 day review period. At this stage, the sponsor may ship the Investigational New Drug to the investigator [52]. However, the labeling of the Investigational New Drug should be in compliance with 21 CFR 312.6and the label should bear the following statement: "Caution: New Drug--Limited by Federal (or United States) law to investigational use" [59]. If significant issues related to safety of the subjects are observed by the reviewers, FDA can impose a "clinical hold". The hold may be a partial or a complete clinical hold. A clinical hold is an order from the FDA to suspend or delay a proposed clinical study or to suspend an ongoing study [60]. If the FDA decides to impose a clinical hold it will contact the sponsor of the IND and issue a clinical hold letter providing the reasons for the clinical hold. The clinical hold may be imposed on one or more phases of the clinical study covered by the IND. Some of the most common reasons for a clinical hold on a phase 1 study include [61]:

- Unreasonable and significant risk of illness or injury to the subjects;

- Investigators are not qualified to conduct the investigation described in the IND;

- Investigator brochure is erroneous;

- Insufficient information from an IND to assess risk;

A clinical hold may occur during phase 2 or 3 for any of the above reasons or if the study design is deficient in regard to meeting the stated objectives. In cases, where the subjects are not exposed to immediate and serious risk, if the FDA decides that there are grounds for issuing a clinical hold, the agency will discuss and resolve the matter before issuing a clinical hold order [61]. Following, receipt of the clinical hold the sponsor must submit a complete response, addressing the issues that led to the clinical hold. The FDA is required by the Food and Drug Modernization Act to respond in writing to the sponsor within 30 days of receipt of a complete response from the sponsor [60]. The FDA may lift the clinical hold, place a partial hold or continue with the hold until further clarification. Under no circumstances can the sponsor proceed with the clinical studies until the clinical hold is lifted by the FDA [52,60].

IND CONTENT AND FORMAT (21 CFR 312.23)

Table **1** outlines the IND content and format described under section 21 CFR 312.23 for submission to the FDA. The critical information that must be submitted in the IND application include the clinical development plan; chemistry, manufacturing and control information (CMC); pharmacology and toxicology information; and previous human experience with the investigational drug [62].

Table 1: IND content and format

1	Cover sheet (Form FDA-1571)
2	A Table of content
3	Introductory statement and general investigational plan
4	[Reserved]
5	Investigator's brochure
6	Protocol
7	Chemistry, manufacturing and control information
8	Pharmacology and toxicology information
9	Previous human experience with investigational drug
10	Additional information
11	Relevant information

Source: 21 CFR 312.23

Clinical Development

Protocols: The IND application may be submitted to the FDA for one or more phases of clinical investigations. A protocol for the conduct of each proposed clinical study needs to be submitted along with an overall summary of the clinical program. Phase 1 protocols need to provide an outline of the investigation - number of subjects to be included, a description of safety exclusion and a description of dosing plan or method to be used for determining dose. In addition, phase 1 protocols should also specify elements of the study that are critical to the safety of the subject. Phase 2 and Phase 3 protocols are required to be in much greater detail and should describe all aspects of the study. They should be designed in such a manner that if unexpected deviations occur, alternatives or contingencies are built into the plan [62].

Clinical protocols should contain the following, "with the special elements and details of the protocol reflecting the above distinctions depending of the phase of study" (21 CFR 312.23)[62]:

- Objective and purpose of the study

- Name and address of the investigator, the sub-investigator, the reviewing local IRB and qualifications of the investigator

- Criteria for patient selection or exclusion and estimate of number of subjects to be included in the clinical trial

- A description of the clinical study design, control group and method to be employed to minimize bias on part of the subjects, investigators and analysts

- Method for determining dose(s) and planned dosing regimen (dose, duration or exposure)

- Observations and measurements to be made to achieve the study objectives

- Description of clinical procedures, laboratory tests planned to monitor the effects of drug in the subject.

Clinical Study

In the United States formal written guidelines for clinical development of ophthalmic drugs are not available [63]. For new, previously untested agents introduced for the first time in human clinical development is generally divided into 3 phases. Although in general the phases are conducted sequentially, they may overlap [63].

Phase 1: During this phase the Investigational New Drug is tested in humans for the first time [64]. The primary goal of these studies is to determine ocular safety, tolerance, toxicity and comfort of the ophthalmic drug product [54,63]. Additionally, Phase 1 studies are designed to assess the ocular pharmacokinetics (absorption, distribution, excretion and metabolism), pharmacodynamics, pharmacology and early effectiveness of the drug [39,64,65]. These studies may also be used to determine structure-activity relationship and mechanism of action of the drug in humans [65]. Phase 1 studies are generally small (with less than hundred subjects (20-80)), closely monitored and form the basis for well-designed, scientifically sound, phase 2 studies [37,52,65]

Phase 1 studies start with a single low dose and the dose is then gradually increased in frequency, concentration and duration to establish the safety profile, comfort, side effects and toxicity of the ophthalmic product [54]. Generally, dose, dosing interval and duration with fewer side effects are chosen for further phases [66]. Following ocular administration, drug can enter into the systemic circulation and exert systemic side effects. Therefore, the rate and extent of systemic absorption, distribution and metabolism, is also determined for new ocular chemical entities during this phase [37]. If a drug approved for systemic or other routes of administration is being tested for ocular therapeutic potential, background information related to its ADME must be provided to the FDA. In general, Phase 1 studies are carried out in normal healthy human volunteers [67]. However, investigational drugs can be administered in a patient population if there is a significant risk associated with the administration of drug in normal volunteers or if the disease is "immediately life-threatening" and no further damage can be done by the drug. For example Lucentis®,intravitreal ranibizumab injection, phase 1 studies included patients with exudative age related macular degeneration because of safety issues associated with administration of intravitreal injection into healthy volunteers [66].

Phase 2: During this phase, the Investigational New Drug is tested in the intended patient population [39]. The primary objective of the phase 2 studies is to explore the therapeutic efficacy of the drug in the targeted patient population and to establish the dose(s) and regimen for Phase 3 studies [68]. Additionally, safety, efficacy, short-term side effects and risks associated with the drug in the patient population are further explored. Phase 2 may be divided into phase 2a and 2b [63,69]. Phase 2a studies are placebo controlled and are usually carried out in less than hundred patients [63]. This phase utilizes dose escalation regimen for early estimation of a dose-response relationship, efficacy and safety of the drug in intended patient population. Phase 2b studies can confirm the dose-response relationship by using parallel dose response design (can be deferred to phase 3). Confirmatory dose response studies may be conducted in phase 2 or left for phase 3 [68]. The dose used in phase 2 is usually, but not always, less than the highest dose in phase 1[68]. In the case of the development of Ocusert, this was accomplished by testing various doses and dosing regimen of pilocarpine for their ability to lower the intraocular pressure [37] Phase 2b studies are randomized, blinded and have a control group and one or more treatment groups [70]. These studies usually enroll several hundred patients. Another important objective of a phase 2 study is to evaluate potential clinically meaningful end points. In most of the ophthalmic clinical trials, improvement in the visual activity or function is an accepted clinically meaningful end point. In phase 2 studies, however, surrogate end points can be helpful in determining whether the therapy is efficacious and to justify larger phase 3 studies with clinically meaningful end points. Examples of surrogate end points in ophthalmics are reduction in the intraocular pressure (IOP) in glaucoma patients and leakage of fluorescein angiography and retinal thickness changes measured by optical coherence tomography in age-related macular degeneration [66,71]. In phase 3 studies clinically meaningful end points (*e.g.*vision) are considered as primary end points unless surrogate end points are thoroughly evaluated, validated and established [66].

Phase 3: The primary objective of phase 3 studies is to further confirm the efficacy and safety of the drug product [65,68]. For most of the drugs, FDA requires at least two phase 3 clinical trials to demonstrate the efficacy and safety of the drug [66,67,72]. These studies are carried out in multiple centers with the final drug product intended for commercialization. Phase 3 studies are well controlled, randomized and generally involve an active control (currently approved drug) for comparative assessment with the Investigational New Drug [69]. These studies involve several hundred to several thousands of patients and could last from several months to years, depending on the indication under consideration [65]. Data generated during this phase evaluates benefit-risk relationship of the drug and also provides the basis for appropriate labeling of the drug product [65].

Good Clinical Practice: Good clinical practice (GCP) is an ethical and scientific standard for conducting, designing, performing, monitoring, auditing, recording, analyzing and reporting of clinical trials. The goals of GCP are to protect the rights, safety and welfare of the human subjects involved in the clinical studies and to assure the quality and integrity of the data. Additionally, it provides guidelines and standards for conducting clinical research [73]. FDA regulations governing GCP are incorporated under Informed Consent of Human Subjects (21 CFR 50), the Institutional Review Board (IRB) (21 CFR 50) and the responsibilities of sponsors and investigators (21 CFR 312). GCP is dealt in extensive detail in ICH Harmonized Tripartite Guideline - Guideline for good clinical practice guidance document [74]. Each and every member involved in clinical trials is responsible for compliance with GCP. Some responsibilities of the sponsors, investigators and Institutional Review Board (IRB) in GCP compliance are presented here:

Responsibilities of the Sponsor

- Implement and maintain quality assurance and quality control systems to ensure that clinical trials are conducted and data generated, documented and reported in compliance with the protocol, GCP and applicable regulatory requirements

- Select well qualified, trained and experienced investigators to properly conduct the trial

- If the investigational drug posses a significant risk to the subject the sponsor should immediately discontinue those investigations and notify the FDA, IRB(s) and all investigators.

- Review and evaluate the safety and efficacy of the drug and prepare annual reports on the progress of the investigation in accordance with 21 CFR 312.33.

- Permit FDA officers or employees to have access, to copy and to verify records and reports concerning the clinical investigations.

Responsibilities of Investigators

- Conduct investigations according to the regulations, signed investigator statements (Form 1572) and investigational plan, to ensure the safety, rights and welfare of the subjects in the clinical trials

- Obtain informed consent of each subject to whom the drug is administered according to the provisions of 21 CFR Part 50

- Should not supply the investigational drug to any unauthorized person

- Maintain records of the disposition of the drug, including dates, quantity and use by subjects

- Maintain case histories that record all observations and data related to the investigations.

- Immediately report any adverse effect observed during the investigation to the sponsor

- Report changes in the research activity, unanticipated problems and risk to the human subjects to the IRB.

Responsibilities of IRB

IRB is an independent body, consisting of scientific and nonscientific members with diversity in experience, race, perspective, gender and ethnicity. Prior to initiation of the clinical trials an IRB, in addition to FDA, is also required to review and approve the clinical study protocol. FDA regulations that govern the IRB structure and function are described in provision 21 CFR 50, concerning IRB itselfand 21 CFR 56, concerning requirements of informed consent of human subjects. The responsibilities of the IRB are to protect the rights, safety and well-being of the human subjects involved in the clinical trials by approving, reviewingand providing continuing review of trials, of protocols and amendmentsand of the methods and material to be used in obtaining and documenting informed consent of the trial subject.

Chemistry, Manufacturing and Controls (CMC) (21 cfr 312.23 (a) (7)) [75]

Regulations require that an IND application submitted for each phase of the clinical investigation should contain sufficient CMC information to demonstrate proper identity, quality, potency and purity of the drug substance and drug product. The type and amount of information needed depends on the proposed phase of the investigation, duration of the study, nature and source of drug and dosage form of the product. Phase 1 CMC submission should provide sufficient information on the raw material, drug substance and drug product to evaluate the safety of the subject in the proposed study. If FDA identifies lack of data or potential concerns with respect to the safety of the subjects, a clinical hold based on the CMC section could be imposed. For later phase studies, which involve larger scale production of the drug substance and drug product, FDA expects CMC submissions to provide detailed characterization of the drug substance and drug product and greater control over the raw materials and manufacturing process. In addition, the focus of later phase CMC's should also be on safety issues [75]. A key aspect to assure the safety of subjects in clinical trials is adherence to current good manufacturing practices (cGMP). The GMP controls used to manufacture drug products for clinical trials should be consistent with the stage of developmentand they should be manufactured in suitable facilities, using appropriate production and control procedures to ensure the quality of the drug product. This section has be described in detail in guidelines for industry documents [76,77]

Drug Substance

- For phase 1 studies, a brief description of the drug substances and some evidence to support its chemical structure should be provided. For later-phase studies detailed description of physical, chemical and biological characteristics and chemical structures should be provided.

- Identification of all manufactures involved in the production of the drug substance should be provided.

- For a phase 1 study a general description of the manufacturing of the drug substance with a detailed flow diagram of the process with a list of chemicals and catalysts used should be provided. For later-phase studies a detailed description of the manufacturing process and controls should be provided. In addition, a process flow diagram with chemical structures and configurations, including stereo-chemical information, of the starting materials, intermediatesand significant side products should be identified.

- A description of the analytical methods and acceptable limits to assure the identity, strength, quality and purity of the drug substance should be provided. Validation data and established specifications are not required to be submitted for phase 1 studies. However, submission of the certificate of analysis is suggested. For later phase studies same type of information should be submitted. However, analytical methods and acceptable limits should be better defined and validation data should be provided if requested by the FDA.

- Data to support the shelf-life of the drug substance during the proposed clinical trials should be provided including a description of stability studies conducted and methods used to monitor stability. Detailed stability data and stability protocols are not required for phase 1 INDs. However, for later-phase studies stability protocols should be submitted including a list of all tests, stability indicating analytical procedures, sampling time points for each test and duration of the studies.

Drug Product

For IND applications a list of all drug substances and excipients used in the manufacturing of the drug product should be identified by their chemical name and their compendial status, if any, irrespective of the phase of clinical trials. For non-compendial components, the analytical procedures and acceptance criteria should be cited. For novel excipients, information submitted should be similar to that of the drug substance. A representative batch formula including the quantitative composition of the final drug product, on a per unit basis (*e.g.* milligram (mg)/milliliter (mL)) should be provided.

The name and address of the firm manufacturing the drug product should be provided.

A process flow-diagram representing a step-by-step description of the manufacturing procedure, packaging procedure and a description of the sterilization process, if applicable, should be provided for all phases of clinical testing.

Analytical tests used to characterize the drug product such as identity, assay, content uniformity, degradants, related impurities, viscosity, particle size, particle size distribution for suspensionsand biological assays for the drug product should be provided. Additionally, microbiological tests such as sterility and pyrogen or bacterial endotoxin tests for sterile products; antimicrobial preservative assays for multiple-dose sterile dosage forms should be provided. A description of the proposed container closure system and stability test methods and protocols must be provided including a list of all tests, stability indicating analytical procedures, sampling time points for each test and duration of stability studies for the drug products. The USP describes physiochemical and biological tests that are required to assess suitability of the use of plastics in ophthalmic containers [37].

Information on any placebo or marketed drug product used as a comparative product (name, strength, lot number and expiration date) that will be utilized in the proposed clinical trials should also be provided. Process flow diagrams and tabular summaries can be used to describe the composition, manufacture and control of the placebo.

Copies labeling that will be provided to the investigator should be submitted.

Pharmacology and Toxicology (21 CFR 312.23 (a) (8)) [78]

This section of the IND includes the non-clinical safety data generated by the sponsor during pre-clinical studies, to demonstrate reasonable safety of the new drug. The amount and kind of safety data needed depends on, the class of the new drug, intended human subjects, duration of the trial and proposed phase under investigation. Data from single and repeated dose toxicity studies, genotoxicity studies, reproductive toxicity studies are required for initiation of phase 1 studies [57,78]. As the development of drug advances, additional relevant safety data must be submitted to FDA in the form of an information amendment in accordance with 21 CFR 312.31.

The pharmacology and toxicology section of initial IND should contain the following:

- **Pharmacology:** A summary of the pharmacological effects, mechanism of action, ADME (absorption distribution, metabolism and excretion of drug) of the drug in animals. Absence of all of this information at the time of initial IND may not result in clinical hold.

- **Toxicology:** A combined summary of the toxicological evaluations of the drug substance in animals and *in vitro*, in the form of text and tables, should include:

- Date of study, design of the study and any deviations from the design in the conduct of the studies.

- Findings from the animal toxicology studies presented by tested organ systems.

- Name and qualification of the investigators who conducted the studies.

- A statement including geographic location of the experiments and availability of records for examination.

- A statement that the studies were carried out in accordance with Good Laboratory Practices (GLP) in accordance with 21 CFR 58. If the studies were not conducted in compliance with GLP the reason for noncompliance should be provided.

Previous Human Experience with the Investigational New Drug (21 CFR 312.23 (a) (9)) [79]

- If the Investigational New Drug is being administered in humans for the first time this section should be indicated as not applicable.

- However, in cases where the initial clinical trials are conducted in other countries or if the Investigational New Drug has been investigated or marketed previously in the U.S. or other countries, this section should provide information on the safety and effectiveness of the marketed drug products and experience from previous clinical trials that are relevant to the proposed investigation.

- A list of all countries where the drug product has been marketed and any countries in which the drug product has been withdrawn from the market due to safety issues must also be provided [79].

IND AMENDMENTS AND ADDITIONAL INFORMATION:

Protocol Amendments (21 CFR 312.30)[80]

The sponsor needs to submit protocol amendments to the FDA whenever (1) the sponsor wants to conduct a new clinical study under a new protocol, (2) changes are made to the existing clinical study protocol and (3) a new investigator is added to the existing protocol [80].

(i) New Protocol

If the sponsor wants to conduct a new study that is not covered by the protocol under the existing IND, a protocol amendment has to be submitted to the FDA. The sponsor may initiate the study once the IRB has approved the new protocol and if it has been submitted to the FDA for its review. However, if the FDA has safety concerns or if the protocol design does not meet the stated objectives a clinical hold on the study can be implemented.

(ii) Changes in Protocol

- Changes in phase 1 protocols that can significantly affect safety of the subjects in the study

- Changes in phase 2 and phase 3 studies that affect the safety of the subjects, the scope of the investigation, or the scientific quality of the study call for protocol amendment

Examples of changes include an increase in drug exposure (dose or duration), addition or deletion of a control group, or a change in the monitoring of safety. The sponsor may initiate the study once the IRB has approved the changes in the protocol as long as the changes have been submitted to the FDA for its review. However, a protocol amendment may be immediately implemented if the change is intended to eliminate an immediate hazard to subjects in accordance with 21 CFR 312.30 (b) (2) (ii), provided the FDA and the IRB are notified by a protocol amendment as soon as possible.

(iii) New Investigator

If a sponsor adds a new investigator to a previously approved protocol, a protocol amendment has to be submitted to the FDA within 30 days of the investigator being added to the study.

Information Amendments (21 CFR 312.31)[81]

Changes in essential information on the IND that are not covered under protocol amendments, IND safety reports, or annual reports should be reported in an Information Amendment. Information Amendments can include changes in essential information on the Investigational New Drug Product such as updates on toxicology, chemistry or other technical information; or a report indicating the termination of a clinical investigation [81].

IND Safety Reports (21 CFR 312.32)[82]

The sponsor is responsible for notifying the FDA, all participating investigators and the IRB about any "serious" and "unexpected adverse experience" associated with the use of the Investigational New Drug and any findings that suggests significant risk to human subjects, The notification should be done as soon as possible and no later than 15 calendar days after the sponsor receives the initial information. The written report must be made on form FDA 3500 A or in a narrative format and should be clearly labeled as "IND Safety Report". The sponsor is also responsible for notifying about any "unexpected fatal" or "life-threatening" adverse experience associated with the use of the Investigational New Drug to the FDA. The notification should be done no later than 7 calendar days after the sponsor receives the initial information. This should be done either by a telephone call or by facsimile transmission [82].

Annual Reports (21 CFR 312.33)[83]

The sponsor is responsible for submitting a brief progress report on all investigations included in the IND, to the FDA. This report must be submitted annually within 60 days after the IND becomes effective. The annual reports should include information such as:

- The title of the clinical study, total number of patients planned for inclusion in the study, total number of patient enrolled to date (by sex, race and age), total number of patients who completed the study, the number of subjects who dropped out for any reason and the results from the completed study if known.

- A summary of the IND safety report submitted during the past year, a list of subjects who died during the investigation with information on the cause of death, a list of patients who dropped out of study, a summary of any significant changes in the pharmacology, toxicology, or technical information and general investigation plan for the coming year [83].

THE NEW DRUG APPLICATION (NDA)

The sponsor collects data from the preclinical and clinical studies and if the data proves that the new ophthalmic drug product is safe and effective for the intended use in the intended population the sponsor submits a New Drug Application (NDA) to the FDA to obtain marketing approval for a drug in the United States. Section 505 (21 USC 355) of the Food, Drug and Cosmetic Act (FD&C Act) requires the FDA to obtain and review an NDA prior to marketing the product in the U.S in accordance with 21 CFR 314 [84]. Section 505 of the FD&C act describes two types of NDAs for new drugs [85].

- **505 (b) (1) NDA or Full NDA:** an application that consists of detailed reports of studies conducted by or for the applicant to support the safety and efficacy of a new drug product [85].

- **505 (b) (2) NDA:** an application in which at least part of the information required to support the safety and efficacy of a new drug product is based on studies that were not conducted on the new drug product by or for the applicant.

Section 505 (b) (2) was added to the FD&C act by the Drug price competition and patent restoration Act of 1984 (Hatch-Waxman Amendments) [85]. In this kind of application the applicant relies on the safety and effectiveness of a previously approved drug product in addition to or in lieu of preclinical or clinical studies on the New Investigational Drug. However due to the complexity of ophthalmic drug delivery systems, a sponsor should expect additional preclinical and clinical studies to be required to establish the safety and efficacy of a new ophthalmic drug product. Examples of when a 505 (b) (2) application has been used in the past or may be appropriate in the future include [85,86]:

- An application for a change of dosage form and dosage regimen but for similar indication. For example, Timoptic-XE (timolol gel-forming suspension) and Istalol (timolol maleate ophthalmic solution) relied on Timoptic (timolol maleate ophthalmic solution) [86].

- An application for change in dosage strength and route of administration.

- An application for change in the strength of the product

- An application for substitution of active ingredient in a combination product

The legal requirements of 505 (b) (1) and 505 (b) (2) NDAs are described in 21 CFR 314.50. Additional legal requirements of 505 (b) (2) NDAs are described in 21 CFR 314.54 and 21 CFR 314.50. These requirements include:

- The 505 (b) (2) NDA should identify any and all approved drug products on which the applicant is relying on to support the safety and efficacy of the new drug product by established name, proprietary name, dosage form, strength, route of administration, name of listed drug's sponsor and the approved drug product's application number in accordance with 21 CFR 314.54 (a) (1) (iii).

- If the 505 (b) (2) NDA applicant is seeking approval for new indications, a certification so stating is required in accordance with 21 CFR 314.54 (a)(1) (iv).

- The 505 (b) (2) NDA application requires a patent certification with respect to any relevant patents that claim the approved drug or that claim any other drugs on which investigations relied on by the applicant for approval of the application were conducted, (21 CFR 314. 54 (a) (1) (vi))

- 505 (b) (2) NDA application requires justification if the applicant believes the new drug product is entitled to marketing exclusivity in accordance with 21 CFR 324. 54 (a)(1)(vii).

New ophthalmic drug products approved under a 505 (b) (2) NDA application are eligible for market exclusivity. If the drug is a new ophthalmic drug 5 years exclusivity will be granted in accordance with 21 CFR 314.108 (b) (2). If the new drug product is an already approved drug, 3 years is granted, provided the application contains "new clinical investigations, other than Bioavailability/Bioequivalence studies . that are essential to the approval of the application or supplement and were conducted or sponsored by the applicant" in accordance with 21 CFR 314.50(j). In addition, a new ophthalmic drug product approved under a 505 (b) (2) NDA may also be eligible for orphan drug exclusivity in accordance with 21 CFR 314.20-316.36, or pediatric exclusivity in accordance with Section 505 A of the FD&C Act.

Contents of NDA

An NDA application should contain all investigational reports on the drug substance and the new drug product. Table **2** includes the regulations described in 21 CFR 314 (subpart B) for the submission of the NDA to the FDA. Some important regulations are summarized below

Content and Format of an NDA (21 CFR 314.50)

This section describes the requirements with respect to the content and format of the NDA. Briefly, it includes the application form, index, summary and technical sections. The application form (FDA 356 h) must be completed and signed by an official of the applicant or the applicant's attorney, agent or other authorized official. An index, by volume and page number, must be provided for all the elements of the application. The application summary consists of nine different sections. The summary should allow a reader to get a "good understanding of the data and information in the application, including an understanding of the quantitative aspects of the data" in accordance with 21 CFR 314.50 (c). The technical sections cover areas such as chemistry, manufacturing and controls (CMC), nonclinical pharmacology and toxicology, human pharmacokinetics and bioavailability, microbiology, clinical data and statistical analysis. The technical sections must contain data and information in sufficient detail for the agency to make an educated judgment towards approving or disapproving an application in accordance with 21 CFR 314. 50 (d) [87].

Table 2: New Drug Application 21 CFR 314 (subpart B)

314.50	Content and format of an application
314.52	Notice of certification of invalidity or noninfringement of a patent.
314.53	Submission of patent information.
314.54	Procedure for submission of an application requiring investigations for approval of a new indication for, or other change from, a listed drug.
314.55	Pediatric use information.
314.60	Amendments to an unapproved application, supplement, or resubmission.
314.65	Withdrawal by the applicant of an unapproved application.
314.70	Supplements and other changes to an approved application.
314.71	Procedures for submission of a supplement to an approved application.
314.72	Change in ownership of an application
314.80	Postmarketing reporting of adverse drug experiences.
314.81	Other postmarketing reports.
314.90	Waivers.
314.91	Obtaining a reduction in the discontinuance notification period

Source: 21 CFR 314 (subpart B)

Patent Certification (21 CFR 314. 52 and 21 CFR 314.50 (i))

If the applicant of a new drug product is aware of the possibility that the new drug product might infringe a patent owned by another party a Patent Certification must be included in the NDA application in accordance with 21 CFR 50 (i) (1) (i) (A) (4). The applicant must certify in the Patent Certification that they believe the patent(s) are invalid, unenforceable, or that their new drug product will not infringed the patent(s). In addition, the applicant is required to send notice of such certification to each patent assignee, NDA holder and specified interested parties [88].

Patent Information (21 CFR 314. 53)

The law requires that an applicant of an NDA include information on drug substance patents, drug product patents and method-of-use patents for the product for which the approval is sought and with respect to which a claim of patent infringement could reasonably be asserted. Such information, if the NDA is approved, is included in the "Orange Book" that is published on-line by FDA at http://www.accessdata.fda.gov/scripts/cder/ob/default.cfm. If an applicant believes that there are no relevant patents related to the drug product for which the NDA is approved, the applicant must so declare in FDA Forms 3542 or 3542a. This declaration must be signed by the patent owner, or the applicant's or patent owner's attorney, agent or other authorized official in accordance with 21 CFR 314. 53 [89].

Pediatric Use Information (21 CRF 314.55)

The pediatric use information provision requires that every NDA application filed after December 2002, for a new active ingredient, new indication, new dosage form, new dosage regimen or new route of administration, should include data on pediatric assessment for the claimed indication(s). This data helps the agency to evaluate the safety and effectiveness of the product in all relevant pediatric sub-populations. When the course of the disease or conditions are similar in both adult and pediatric population the agency may extrapolate the effectiveness of the drug in a pediatric population from the clinical studies conducted in adults. However, supplementary data on pharmacokinetics, dosing and safety data in a pediatric population may be required. If the clinical data can be extrapolated from one age group to another, studies in each pediatric age group will not be required [90,91].

An applicant may request from the FDA a deferral or a waiver of a pediatric assessment. If a deferral is granted, pediatric assessment data can be submitted after the submission of an NDA. According to 21 CFR 314.55, a waiver may be granted "if the applicant provides evidences that (1) the drug product does not provide a therapeutic advantage over existing pediatric treatments, (2) the product is not likely to be used in substantial number of pediatric population, (3) essential studies are not practical or impossible due to small or geographically dispersed patients, (4) drug product would be ineffective or unsafe in that age group" [91].

NDA Review Process

Before an NDA is formally submitted to the FDA the applicant can formally seek a "pre-NDA" meeting with the CDER reviewing staff. Some of the primary objectives of this meeting are to uncover any unresolved issues, to agree on format and content of the NDA or to determine the status of the ongoing studies to address pediatric safety and effectiveness in accordance with 21 CFR 312.47B(2). Additionally, early discussions on priority or standard review of the NDA and need for advisory committee meetings can be held during this meeting. Following receipt of the NDA, the FDA, within 60 days, decides either to file the application for its review or to send a refusal-to-file letter to the applicant. If the FDA decides to file the NDA, various sections of the application are forwarded to appropriate members of the review team. The team typically consists of pharmacologists, chemists, statisticians, microbiologists, clinicians and pharmacokineticists. In some cases the FDA can seek input from an outside the advisory committee. Once the safety, efficacy and CMC related issues are resolved by the applicant to FDA's satisfaction, the FDA will hold a preapproval inspection of the drug manufacturing, product development, preclinical studies and/or clinical sites, to evaluate compliance with GMPs and GCPs. FDA review and approval of proposed labeling for a new drug product is typically the last step in the approval process [92,93].

Once the review process is complete the FDA will either issue an approval letter or a complete response letter to the applicant in accordance with 21 CFR 314. 105 and 110. An approval letter indicates that FDA has determined the benefits of the drug product outweigh the risks and, under the conditions of use, the drug product will have the proposed effect indicated in the label. Receipt of a complete response letter indicates that the agency cannot accept the application in the present form. The complete response letter will describe the deficiencies identified by the FDA in the application and in some cases may also recommend the action that the applicant may take for gaining approval. After receiving a complete response letter the applicant can resubmit or withdraw the NDA, or can request a hearing from the FDA [94-96].

Prescription Drug User Fee Act (PDUFA) Fee

In order to file an NDA and begin the review process the applicant has to pay a prescription drug "user fee" under The Prescription Drug User Fee Act (PDUFA) enacted in 1992. For FY 2010, under the PUDFA, the applicant has to pay $1,405,500 for an application containing clinical data, $702,750 for application that does not contain clinical data and for an NDA supplement containing clinical data.

In addition the PUDFA can assess user fees such as establishment fees ($457,200) and product fees ($79,720) [97]. Discounted fees are available to small businesses.

POST-MARKETING STUDIES

Post-marketing studies, also known as Phase IV studies are conducted following the approval of the drug product and are usually designed to evaluate the safety, adverse reaction and efficacy of the product over time and to evaluate the drug product in other stages of disease, different forms of diseases and in other patient populations. These studies could also include trials of different doses or dosing schedules and comparison with a drug product already available in the market. Phase 4 studies may be required by the FDA as part of the NDA approval process or may be undertaken voluntarily by a company to support marketing efforts and to develop new label claims [54,72,98].

PROGRAMS DESIGNED TO EXPEDITE THE DEVELOPMENT AND FDA REVIEW PROCESS

Accelerated Approval (21 CFR 314 subpart H)

FDA regulations contained in 21 CFR 314 subpart H allow accelerated approval of a drug product indicated for the treatment of a serious or life-threatening illness or condition and that fills an unmet medical need based on surrogate end points rather than clinically meaningful end points [99]. For example, in the case of a drug product used to treat cancer instead of waiting to see whether the drug actually extends the survival of cancer patients (clinically meaningful end point), approval is provided based on evidence that the drug shrinks the tumor (surrogate end point), because tumor shrinkage is considered likely to predict the clinical benefit. 21 CFR 314.520 addresses drug products whose use is considered to be safe and effective only if distribution and use is restricted [100]. Accelerated approval is given on the condition that post-marketing clinical trials will be conducted by the sponsor to confirm the clinical benefit [99]. FDA may withdraw the product from the market if post marketing studies demonstrate that clinical benefit is not observed or if the sponsor did not conduct these studies or if post marketing restrictions are inadequate to assure safe use of the drug product [101].

Priority Review

Once an NDA is submitted to the FDA for review, under the PDUFA of 1992, the application is classified as standard review or priority review. Priority applications are reviewed within 6 months and standard applications are reviewed within 10 months from the filing date. Standard review is adopted if only minor improvements over the existing marketed product are observed. Priority review is adopted, for both serious and less serious diseases, if the product demonstrates increased effectiveness in treatment, prevention or diagnosis of diseases; eliminates or substantially reduces a treatment-limited drug reaction; enhanced patient willingness to take the medication according to the dosing regimen; and enhanced safety and effectiveness in children [102,103].

Fast Track of NDA Applications

This fast track approval mechanism was introduced in the FDA Modernization Act of 1997 (FDAMA). To qualify for a Fast track designation, the new drug product must be used for certain "serious" or "life-threatening" condition and should demonstrate the product has the potential to address an unmet medical need (Section 506, 21 U.S.C 356). The sponsor can request a "fast track" designation from FDA at any time before marketing approval. FDA will respond to the request within 60 days. If FDA grants fast track designation, frequent interactions with the FDA during the development of the product is encouraged. Sponsors whose new drug product is in the fast track program can also seek marketing approval under priority review, traditional and accelerated approval. In addition, a sponsor can submit portions of the NDA application to the FDA for review before the complete NDA is submitted [102].

EXPANDED ACCESS OF DRUG PRODUCTS

Orphan Drugs (21 CFR 316)

The Orphan Drug Act was passed in January 1983. This act provides financial and regulatory incentives for the development of treatments "for rare diseases and conditions". The original definition for rare disease and condition was refined and amended in 1984. "the term rare disease or condition means any disease or condition which (a) affects less than 200,000 persons in the U.S. or (b) affects more than

200,000 persons in the U.S. but for which there is no reasonable expectation that the cost of developing and making available in the U.S. a drug for such disease or condition will be recovered from sales in the U.S. of such drug" (Public law 98-551). The incentives for the development of orphan drugs include a 7 year marketing exclusivity to the first sponsor who obtains marketing approval, help with non-clinical and clinical investigations from the FDA, a tax credit covering 50% of the expenses incurred during clinical testing of the drug and federal funding through its grant program for clinical trials. To qualify for these benefits the sponsor must submit an application to the Office of Orphan Products Development (OOPD) requesting Orphan drug designation from the FDA [104,105]. The orphan drug product application process, approval process and regulations are described in 21 CFR 316.

Treatment Use of an Investigational New Drug (21 CFR 312.34)[106]

Treatment use of an Investigational New Drug is described in 21 CFR 312.34 [106]. These regulations allow the use of promising Investigational New Drugs in desperately ill patients who are not formally enrolled in the clinical trials. The investigational drug can be used for a treatment use if (1) the disease is serious or immediately life threatening, (2) there is no comparable treatments available for that specific disease stage, (3) the drug is currently in clinical trials under an IND or clinical trials have been completed and (4) the sponsor is actively seeking marketing approval for the Investigational New Drug FDA approval, IRB approval (21 CFR part 56) and informed consent (21 CFR part 50), are required before enrolling subjects.

Emergency Use of an Investigational New Drug (21 CFR 312.36)[107]

Emergency use of an Investigational New Drug is described in 21 CFR 312.36 [107], wherein the use of an Investigational New Drug may arise before an IND is submitted. In this case, FDA may authorize shipment of the Investigational New Drug prior to submission of an IND. However, the sponsor is required to submit the IND as soon as practicable after receiving.

ABBREVIATED NEW DRUG APPLICATION

Another regulatory route of approval for an ophthalmic drug product is *via* a 505(j) application commonly known as an abbreviated new drug application (ANDA). An ANDA contains the information required by FDA to show that the intended new drug product is identical in active ingredient, dosage form, strength, route of administration, labeling, quality, performance characteristics and intended use to a previously approved drug product, called the reference listed drug (RLD). In general an ANDA contains the same CMC information as contained in an NDA along with one or more pharmacokinetic studies demonstrating that the proposed drug product is bioequivalent to the RLD. The major difference between an NDA and an ANDA is that an ANDA does don't contain phase II/III clinical studies or safety studies. A drug product that is approved under an ANDA is referred to as a "generic drug". The ANDA process started under the Drug Price Competition and Patent Term Restoration Act of 1984, which is commonly known as the Hatch-Waxman Act.

CONCLUSION

In the last decade several non traditional approaches have been published that look promising. A major concern, however, is the novelty of these techniques, which throws up challenges in clinical trial design and the high costs. Moreover, in many cases these approaches do not take into account patient comfort, diminishing their marketing feasibility. Translation from animal models to humans is often times very challenging and may present totally different results in terms of performance of the ophthalmic formulations. The regulatory and safety guidelines need also be at the back of the minds of the inventors during the development of these strategies. Thus, although the field of drug delivery has advanced very rapidly in the last few years, a widely applicable successful delivery platform still remains elusive.

ACKNOWLEDGEMENT

Declared None.

CONFLICT OF INTEREST

The author(s) confirm that this chapter content has no conflict of interest.

REFERENCES

[1]   Mucke HA, Mucke P, Mucke E. International patenting in ophthalmology: An analysis of its structure and relevance for the development of drugs and diagnostics. Clin Ophthalmol 2009; 3: 103-109.
[2]   Roy S, Bowman M. Topical treatment for prevention of ocular Infections. US Patent 7056893, 2006.

[3]   Chong E, Burge C, Mizzen L. Formulations for treating eye disorders. US 20100010082 A1., 2010.

[4]   Mitra AK, Valagaleti P, Natesan S. Opthalmic compositions comprising calcineurin inhibitors or mTOR inhibitors. US 20090092665 A1. 2009.

[5]   Dai W, Funderburgh J, Schuman J, SundarRaj N. Inhibition of proliferation and fibrotic response of activated corneal stromal cells. US 20090239947 A1, 2009.

[6]   Lin HR, Sung KC. Ophthalmic drug delivery formulations and method for preparing the same. US Patent 6511660, 2003.

[7]   Xia E, Smerbeck RV. Reversible gelling system for ocular drug delivery. US Patent 6703039, 2004.

[8]   Bandyopadhyay P, Singh SK. Opthalmic formulation with gum system. US Patent 7128928, 2006.

[9]   Kunzler J, Schorzman D, Ammon D. Drug delivery systems based on catonic siloxanyl macromonomers. US 20090274745 A1, 2009.

[10]   Chauhan A, Gulsen D. Ophthalmic drug delivery system. US 20040241207 A1, 2004.

[11]   Byrne ME, Venkatesh S. Contact drug delivery system. US 20060177483 A1, 2006.

[12]   Abdulrazik M Enhancement of drug delivery to the central nervous system. US 20080131483 A1, 2007.

[13]   Higuchi JW, Tuitupou AL, Kochambilli RP, Li SK. Ocular delivery of triamcinolone acetonide phosphate and related compounds. US 20080009471 A1, 2008.

[14]   Yamada K, Kuwano M. Drug delivery system using subconjunctival depot. US 20060013859 A1, 2006.

[15]   Chang J, Hughes P. Oil-in-water method for making alpha-2 agonist polymeric drug delivery systems. US Patent 7589057, 2009.

[16]   Raiche AT, Salamone JC, Linhardt J. Method for the production of polymerized nanoparticles and microparticles by ternary agent concentration and temperature alteration induced immiscibility. US Patent 7495052, 2009.

[17]   Hofland H, Bongianni J, Wheeler T. Ophthalmic liposome compositions and uses thereof. US 20040224010 A1, 2004.

[18]   Karaoka K, Yasuhiro T, Harada A. Opthalmic drug delivery system using polymer micelle. US 20060110356 A1, 2006.

[19]   Del Amo EM, Urtti A. Current and future ophthalmic drug delivery systems. A shift to the posterior segment. Drug Discov Today 2008; 13(3-4): 135-143.

[20]   Robinson MR, Csaky KG, Yuan P, Sung C, Nussenblatt RB, Smith JA. Ocular therapeutic agent delivery devices and methods for making and using such devices. US Patent 6713081, 2004.

[21]   Asgharian B, Chowhan M. Devices and methods for opthalmic drug delivery. US 20080145406 A1, 2008.

[22]   Wong V Method for reducing neovascularization or edema. US 20080050420 A1, 2008.

[23]   Huang G, Nivaggioli T, Spada L, Sugimoto H, Blanda W, Chang J, Olejnik O. Methods for reducing neovascularization or edema. US 20080145407 A1, 2008.

[24]   Shiah JG, Bhagat R, Blanda WM, Nivaggioli T, Peng L, Chou D, Weber DA. Ocular implant made by a double extrusion process. US 20080107712 A1, 2008.

[25]   Burkstrand MJ, Erickson SR, Chudzik SJ, Reed PJ. Biodegradable ocular implants and methods for treating ocular conditions. US 20080089923 A1, 2008.

[26]   Hughes PM Hypotensive lipid-containing biodegradable intraocular implants and related methods. US 20080131481 A1, 2008.

[27]   Kohn J, Khan I, Iovine C. Compositions and methods for treating ophthalmic diseases. US 20090238858 A1, 2009.

[28]   Meng E, Humayun M, Lo R, Li PY, Saati S. Implantable drug delivery devicesand apparatus and methods for refilling the devices. US 20090192493 A1, 2009.

[29]   Santini JT, Cima MJ, Langer RS, Ausiello D, Sheppard NF, Herman SJ. Flexible microchip devices for ophthalmic and other applications. US Patent 6796982, 2005.

[30]   Pardridge WM Non-invasive gene targeting to ocular cells. US Patent 7090864, 2006.

[31]   Lyons RT, Ma H. Methods and compositions for intraocular delivery of therapeutic siRNA. US 20090226531 A1, 2009.

[32]   FDA. Code of Federal Regulations Title 21 Section 211.167. (Cited on: 23 March 2010).Available from: http://www.accessdata.fda.gov/scripts/cdrh/cfdocs/cfcfr/CFR Search.cfm

[33]   FDA. Code of Federal Regulations Title 21 Section 200.50. (Cited on: 23 March 2010).Available from: http://www.accessdata.fda.gov/scripts/cdrh/cfdocs/cfcfr/CFR Search.cfm

[34]   FDA. Guidance for Industry, Sterile drug products produced by aseptic processing - Current good manufacturing practice, September 2004. (Cited on: 23 March 2010).Available from: http://www.fda.gov/downloads/Drugs/GuidanceComplianceRegulatoryInformation/Guidances /ucm070342.pdf

[35]   Federal Register 56 (198); 51354, October 11, 1991.

[36]   Lang CJ, Roehrs ER, Rodeheaver PD, Missel JP, Jain R, Chowhan AM. Design and Evaluation of Ophthalmic Pharmaceutical Products. In Banker SG, Rhodes TC, editors. Modern Pharmaceutics, Fourth ed.: Marcel Dekker, Inc. p 415-479.

[37]   Roehrs ER, Krueger SD. 2003. Regulatory Considerations. In Mitra AK, editor Ophthalmic Drug Delivery Systems, Second ed.: Marcel Dekker, Inc. p 663-693.

[38]   ICH Harmonized Tripartite Guideline. Maintenance of the ICH guideline on non-clinical safety studies for the conduct of human clinical trials for pharmaceuticals M3(R1), November 9, 2000. (Available from: http://www.pmda.go.jp/ich/m/m3r1_00_12_27e.pdf

[39]   Gryziewicz JL, Whitcup SM. 2006. Regulatory Issues in Drug Delivery to the Eye. In Jaffe JG, Ashton P, Pearson AP, editors. Intraocular Drug Delivery, ed.: Taylor and Francis Group. p 59-70.

[40]   FDA. Code of Federal Regulations Title 21 Section 58. (Cited on: 23 March 2010).Available from: http://www.accessdata.fda.gov/scripts/cdrh/cfdocs/cfcfr/CFRSearch.cfm?CFRPart=58

[41]   Short BG. Safety evaluation of ocular drug delivery formulations: techniques and practical considerations. Toxicol Pathol 2008; 36(1): 49-62.

[42]   Note for guidance on non-clinical local tolerance testing of medicinal products, March 1, 2001 CPMP/SWP/2145/00. (Cited.Available from: http://www.ema.europa.eu/pdfs /human/swp/ 214500en.pdf

[43]   Kaila T, Salminen L, Huupponen R. Systemic absorption of topically applied ocular timolol. J Ocul Pharmacol 1985; 1(1): 79-83.

[44]   Pitkanen L, Ranta VP, Moilanen H, Urtti A. Binding of betaxolol, metoprolol and oligonucleotides to synthetic and bovine ocular melaninand prediction of drug binding to melanin in human choroid-retinal pigment epithelium. Pharm Res 2007; 24(11): 2063-2070.

[45]   Patil PM, Jacobowitz D. Unequal accumulation of adrenergic drugs by pigmented and nonpigmented iris. Am J Ophthalmol 1974; 78(3): 470-477.

[46]   Katz IM, Berger ET. Effects of iris pigmentation on response of ocular pressure to timolol. Surv Ophthalmol 1979; 23(6): 395-398.

[47]   FDA. Guidance for Industry, S2B Genotoxicity: A standard battery for genotoxicity testing of pharmaceuticals, 1997. (Cited on: 23 March 2010).Available from: http://www.fda.gov/ downloads/Drugs/GuidanceComplianceRegulatoryInformation/Guidances/ucm074929.pdf

[48]   ICH Draft Consensus Guideline. Guidance on genotoxicity testing and data interpretation for pharmaceuticals intendend for human use S2 (R1), March 6, 2008. (Cited.Available from: http://www.ich.org/LOB/media/MEDIA4474.pdf

[49]   ICH Harmonised Tripartite Guideline. Guideline on the need for carcinogenicity studies of pharmaceuticals (S1A), November 29,1995. (Available from: http://www.ich.org /LOB/media /MEDIA489.pdf

[50]   ICH Harmonized Tripartite Guideline. Detection of toxicity to reproduction for medicinal products and toxicity to male fertility S5(R2), November 2005. (Cited.Available from: http://www.ich.org/LOB/media/MEDIA498.pdf

[51]   FDA. Code of Federal Regulations Title 21 Section 312.3. (Cited on: 23 March 2010).Available from: http://www.accessdata.fda.gov/scripts/cdrh/cfdocs/cfcfr/CFRSearch. cfm?fr=312.3

[52]   Holbein ME. Understanding FDA regulatory requirements for investigational new drug applications for sponsor-investigators. J Investig Med 2009; 57(6): 688-694.

[53]   FDA. Federal Food, Drug and Cosmetic act Chapter II Section 201 (g) (1). (Cited on: 23 March 2010).Available from: http://www.fda.gov/RegulatoryInformation/Legislation/ FederalFoodDrugandCosmeticActFDCAct/FDCActChaptersIandIIShortTitleandDefinitions/uc m086297.htm

[54]   Novack GD. The development of new drugs for ophthalmology. Am J Ophthalmol 1992; 114(3): 357-364.

[55]   Ali Y, Lehmussaari K. Industrial perspective in ocular drug delivery. Adv Drug Deliv Rev 2006; 58(11): 1258-1268.

[56]   FDA. Code of Federal Regulations Title 21 Section 312.2. (Cited on: 23 March 2010).Available from: http://www.accessdata.fda.gov/scripts/cdrh/cfdocs/cfcfr/CFRSearch. cfm?fr=312.2

[57]   Hamrell RM. 2008. What is IND? In Pisano JD, Mantus SD, editors. FDA Regulatory Affairs A guide for prescription drugs, medical devicesand biologics, Second ed.: Informa Health Care USA, Inc. p 33-69.

[58]   FDA. Guidance for Industry, Investigatorsand Reviewers, Exploratory IND Studies. (Cited on: 23 March 2010).Available from: http://www.fda.gov/downloads/Drugs/Guidance ComplianceRegulatoryInformation/Guidances/ucm078933.pdf

[59]   FDA. Code of Federal Regulations Title 21 Section 312.6. (Cited on: 23 March 2010).Available from: http://www.accessdata.fda.gov/scripts/cdrh/cfdocs/cfcfr/CFRSearch. cfm?fr=312.6

[60]   FDA. Manual of Policies and Procedures (MAPP) 6030.1- IND Process and Review Procedures (Including Clinical Holds). (Cited on: 23 March 2010).Available from: http://www.fda.gov/downloads/AboutFDA/ReportsManualsForms/StaffPoliciesandProcedures /ucm082022.pdf

[61]   FDA. Code of Federal Regulations Title 21 Section 312.42. (Cited on: 23 March 2010).Available from: http://www.accessdata.fda.gov/scripts/cdrh/cfdocs/cfcfr/CFRSearch. cfm?fr=312.42

[62] FDA. Code of Federal Regulations Title 21 Section 312.23. (Cited on: 23 March 2010).Available from: http://www.accessdata.fda.gov/scripts/cdrh/cfdocs/cfcfr/CFR Search.cfm?fr=312.23

[63] Novack GD. Ophthalmic drug development: procedural considerations. J Glaucoma 1998; 7(3): 202-209.

[64] Howland RH. How are drugs approved? Part 3. The stages of drug development. J Psychosoc Nurs Ment Health Serv 2008; 46(3): 17-20.

[65] FDA. Code of Federal Regulations Title 21 Section 312.21 [(Cited on: 23 March 2010).Available from: http://www.accessdata.fda.gov/scripts/cdrh/cfdocs/cfcfr/CFR Search.cfm?fr=312.21

[66] Lloyd R, Harris J, Wadhwa S, Chambers W. Food and Drug Administration approval process for ophthalmic drugs in the US. Curr Opin Ophthalmol 2008; 19(3): 190-194.

[67] Robuck PR, Wurzelmann JI. Understanding the drug development process. Inflamm Bowel Dis 2005; 11 Suppl 1: S13-16.

[68] ICH Harmonised Tripartite Guideline, General Considerations for Clinical Trials, E8, July 17, 1997. Available from: http://www.ich.org/LOB/media/MEDIA484.pdf

[69] DiFeo TJ. Safety and efficacy: the role of chemistry, manufacturingand controls in pharmaceutical drug development. Drug Dev Ind Pharm 2004; 30(3): 247-257.

[70] Moore SW. An overview of drug development in the United States and current challenges. South Med J 2003; 96(12): 1244-1255; quiz 1256.

[71] Coleman AL. Applying evidence-based medicine in ophthalmic practice. Am J Ophthalmol 2002; 134(4): 599-601.

[72] Lipsky MS, Sharp LK. From idea to market: the drug approval process. J Am Board Fam Pract 2001; 14(5): 362-367.

[73] FDA. Guidance for Industry, E6 Good Clinical Practice: Consolidated Guidance. (Cited on: 23 March 2010). Available from: http://www.fda.gov/downloads/regulatoryinformation/ guidances/UCM129515.pdf

[74] ICH Harmonized Tripartite Guideline - Guideline for Good Clinical Practice, E6(R1), June 10, 1996. Available from: http://www.ich.org/LOB/media/MEDIA482.pdf

[75] FDA. Code of Federal Regulations Title 21 Section 312.23 (a) (7). (Cited on: 23 March 2010).Available from: http://www.accessdata.fda.gov/scripts/cdrh/cfdocs/cfcfr/CFRS earch.cfm?fr=312.23

[76] FDA. Guidance for Industry, Content and Format of Investigational New Drug Applications (INDs) for phase 1 Studies of Drugs, Including Well-Characterized, Therapeutics, Biotechnology-derived Products, November 1995. (Cited on: 23 March 2010).Available from: http://www.fda.gov/downloads/Drugs/GuidanceCompliance RegulatoryInformation/Guidances/ucm071597.pdf

[77] FDA. Guidance for Industry, INDs for Phase 2 and Phase 3 Studies: Chemistry, Manufacturing and Controls Information, May 2003. (Cited on: 23 March 2010).Available from: http://www.fda.gov/downloads/Drugs/GuidanceComplianceRegulatoryInformation /Guidances /ucm070567.pdf

[78] FDA. Code of Federal Regulations Title 21 Section 312.23 (a) (8). (Cited on: 23 March 2010).Available from: http://www.accessdata.fda.gov/scripts/cdrh/cfdocs/cfcfr/CFRSearch. cfm?fr=312.23

[79] FDA. FDA, Code of Federal Regulations Title 21 Section 312.23 (a) (9). (Cited on: 23 March 2010).Available from: http://www.accessdata.fda.gov/scripts/cdrh/cfdocs/cfcfr /CFRSearch. cfm?fr=312.23

[80]   FDA. Code of Federal Regulations Title 21 Section 312.30 (Cited on: 23 March 2010).Available from: http://www.accessdata.fda.gov/scripts/cdrh/cfdocs/cfcfr/CFRSearch.cfm

[81]   FDA. Code of Federal Regulations Title 21 Section 312.31. (Cited on: 23 March 2010).Available from: http://www.accessdata.fda.gov/scripts/cdrh/cfdocs/cfcfr/CFRSearch.cfm

[82]   FDA. Code of Federal Regulations Title 21 Section 312.32. (Cited on: 23 March 2010).Available from: http://www.accessdata.fda.gov/scripts/cdrh/cfdocs/cfcfr/CFRSearch.cfm

[83]   FDA. Code of Federal Regulations Title 21 Section 312.33 (Cited on: 23 March 2010).Available from: http://www.accessdata.fda.gov/scripts/cdrh/cfdocs/cfcfr/CFRSearch.cfm

[84]   FDA. Code of Federal Regulations Title 21 Section 314. (Cited on: 23 March 2010).Available from: http://www.accessdata.fda.gov/scripts/cdrh/cfdocs/cfcfr/CFRSearch.cfm

[85]   FDA. Guidance for Industry (Draft), Applications covered by section 505 (b) (2). (Cited on: 23 March 2010).Available from: http://www.fda.gov/downloads/Drugs/Guidance Compliance RegulatoryInformation/Guidances/ucm079345.pdf

[86]   Novack GD. Ophthalmic drug delivery: development and regulatory considerations. Clin Pharmacol Ther 2009; 85(5): 539-543.

[87]   FDA. Code of Federal Regulations Title 21 Section 314.50. (Cited on: 23 March 2010).Available from: http://www.accessdata.fda.gov/scripts/cdrh/cfdocs/cfcfr/CFRSearch.cfm

[88]   FDA. FDA, Code of Federal Regulations Title 21 Section 314.52 and 314.50 (i) (Cited on: 23 March 2010).Available from: http://www.accessdata.fda.gov/scripts/cdrh/cfdocs/cfcfr/CFRSearch.cfm

[89]   FDA. Code of Federal Regulations Title 21 Section 314.53. (Cited on: 23 March 2010).Available from: http://www.accessdata.fda.gov/scripts/cdrh/cfdocs/cfcfr/CFRSearch.cfm?fr=314.53

[90]   FDA. Guidance for Industry, Recommendations for complying with the pediatric rule (21 CFR 314.55 (a) and 601.27 (a)), November 2000. (Cited on: 23 March 2010).Available from: http://www.fda.gov/downloads/Drugs/GuidanceComplianceRegulatoryInformation/Guidances/ucm072034.pdf

[91]   FDA. Code of Federal Regulations Title 21 Section 314.55. (Cited on: 23 March 2010).Available from: http://www.accessdata.fda.gov/scripts/cdrh/cfdocs/cfcfr/CFRSearch.cfm

[92]   Department of Health and Human service, Office of Inspector General. FDA's Review process for new drug applications, March 2003. ed.

[93]   Monahan C, Babiraz CJ. 2008. The New Drug Application. In Pisano JD, Mantus SD, editors. FDA Regulatory Affairs A guide for prescription drugs, medical devicesand biologics, ed.: Informa Health Care USA, Inc. [. p 69-109.

[94]   Federal Register, Vol 73, No 133, July 2008/ rules and regulations. (Available from: http://edocket.access.gpo.gov/2008/pdf/E8-15754.pdf

[95]   FDA. Code of Federal Regulations Title 21 Section 314.105. (Cited on: 23 March 2010).Available from: http://www.accessdata.fda.gov/scripts/cdrh/cfdocs/cfcfr/CFRSearch.cfm

[96]   FDA, Code of Federal Regulations Title 21 Section 314.110, viewed 23 March 2010. (Cited.Available from: < http://www.accessdata.fda.gov/scripts/cdrh/cfdocs/cfcfr/CFR Search.cfm>

[97]   FDA. Prescription Drug User Fee Rates for Fiscal Year 2010, Federal Register Doc.E9-18457, (Vol 74, Number 147). (Cited on: 23 March 2010).Available from: http://edocket.access.gpo.gov/2009/E9-18457.htm

[98]   Gerhard N. 2009. Dictionary of Pharmaceutical Medicine. ed.: Springer.

[99]   FDA. Code of Federal Regulations Title 21 Section 314.510. (Cited on: 23 March 2010).Available   from: http://www.accessdata.fda.gov/scripts/cdrh/cfdocs/cfcfr/CFR Search.cfm

[100]   FDA. Code of Federal Regulations Title 21 Section 314.520. (Cited on: 23 March 2010).Available from: http://www.accessdata.fda.gov/scripts/cdrh/cfdocs/cfcfr/CFRSearch.cfm

[101]   FDA. Code of Federal Regulations Title 21 Section 314.530. (Cited on: 23 March 2010).Available from: http://www.accessdata.fda.gov/scripts/cdrh/cfdocs/cfcfr/CFRSearch.cfm

[102]   FDA. Fast Track, Accelerated Approval and Priority Review: Accelrating availability of new drugs for patients with serious diseases. (Cited on: 23 March (2010).Available from: http://www.fda.gov/ForConsumers/ByAudience/ForPatientAdvocates/SpeedingAccesstoImpor tantNewTherapies/ucm128291.htm#priorityreview

[103]   FDA. Center for Drug Evaluation and Review. Manual of Policies and Procedures, MAPP 6020. 3, Review Classification Policy: Priority (P) and Standard (S). Available from: http://www.fda.gov/AboutFDA/CentersOffices/CDER/ManualofPoliciesProcedures/default.ht m

[104]   Villarreal AM. CRS Report for Congress, Orphan Drug Act: Background and Proposed Legislation in the 107th Congress. (Cited on: 23 March 2010).Available from: https://www.policyarchive.org/bitstream/handle/10207/3490/RS20971_20010725.pdf

[105]   FDA. Code of Federal Regulations Title 21 Section 316. (Cited on: 23 March 2010).Available from: http://www.accessdata.fda.gov/scripts/cdrh/cfdocs/cfcfr/CFRSearch.cfm?CFRPart=316

[106]   FDA. Code of Federal Regulations Title 21 Section 312.34. (Cited on: 23 March 2010).Available from: http://www.accessdata.fda.gov/scripts/cdrh/cfdocs/cfcfr/CFRSearch.cfm

[107]   FDA. Code of Federal Regulations Title 21 Section 312.36. (Cited on: 23 March 2010).Available from: http://www.accessdata.fda.gov/scripts/cdrh/cfdocs/cfcfr/CFRSearch.cfm

Send Orders of Reprints at reprints@benthamscience.net

CHAPTER 10

Application of Nanotechnology in Ocular Drug Delivery

Xiaoyan Yang, Ashaben Patel, Aswani Dutt Vadlapudi and Ashim K. Mitra[*]

Division of Pharmaceutical Sciences, School of Pharmacy, University of Missouri-Kansas City, 2464 Charlotte Street, Kansas City, MO 64108-2718, USA

Abstract: Drug delivery to treat ocular diseases is one of the most challenging fields, due to complex anatomy of eye and its physiological barriers like precorneal loss and the presence of biological barriers, especially in the posterior segment of the eye. Although topical eye drop administration is usually preferred to treat disorders of the eye, the biological protecting factors lead to low ocular absorption and poor bioavailability (1–10%). An efficient ocular drug delivery system, which can provide maximum precorneal residence time, overcome ocular barriers and sustain delivery of drugs following topical administration is desirable. Nanotechnology is an emerging field in drug delivery and considerable research is taking place towards the development of nanotechnology-based ocular drug delivery systems. Because of their ability to avoid various biological barriers and providing targeted and sustained drug delivery to various ocular tissues, nanotechnology-based formulations paved the approaches for efficient ophthalmic drug delivery for both the anterior and posterior segments of eye. This review discusses a variety of nanocarriers, such as nanoparticles, nanosuspension, liposomes, niosomes, discomes, micelles, dendrimers and microemulsion developed for the ocular delivery of many drugs. Some of them have shown promising results for improving ocular bioavailability. This review also attempts to extend the information on recently issued and filed patents on nanotechnology-based ocular drug delivery systems in the last few years.

Keywords: Nanotechnology, ocular, drug delivery, nanocarriers, nanoparticles, nanosuspensions, liposomes, niosomes, discomes, micelles, dendrimers, microemulsion, patents.

INTRODUCTION

Developing a delivery system that can deliver active agents to the target site in therapeutic amounts with minimal or no side effect is a goal for pharmaceutical scientists. Previously, numerous approaches to drug delivery and formulation

---
*****Address correspondence to Ashim K. Mitra:** University of Missouri Curators' Professor of Pharmacy, Chairman, Division of Pharmaceutical Sciences, Vice-Provost for Interdisciplinary Research, University of Missouri - Kansas City, School of Pharmacy, 2464 Charlotte Street, Kansas City, MO 64108, USA; Tel: 816-235-1615; Fax: 816-235-5779; E-mail: mitraa@umkc.edu

development utilizing nanotechnology have been investigated. Nanotechnology (also referred to as nanotech) is the engineering of functional systems by design, characterization, productionand application of structures, devicesand systems by controlled manipulation of size and shape at an atomic and molecular scale [1]. In recent years, nanotechnology has been applied to a diverse set of problems associated with delivery of various small and macromolecules with poor solubility, poor stability, enzymatic degradation and poor permeability through biological membranes. Moreover, targeted and controlled drug delivery properties have led to improved efficacy and reduced side effects. The chronic nature of many ocular diseases coupled with complex anatomy of eye renders drug delivery to ocular tissues one of the most challenging tasks. Various anatomical and physiological barriers like precorneal loss and presence of biological barriers limit attainment of therapeutic drug concentrations at target site (Fig. **1**). Nanotechnology-based delivery systems are gaining momentum in the field of ocular drug delivery primarily due to advantages in overcoming ocular barriers and enabling localized controlled drug delivery. At present, many nanotechnology-based ocular drug delivery systems such as nanoparticles, niosomes, liposomes, dendrimers and micelles are preferred mode of delivery (Fig. **2**).

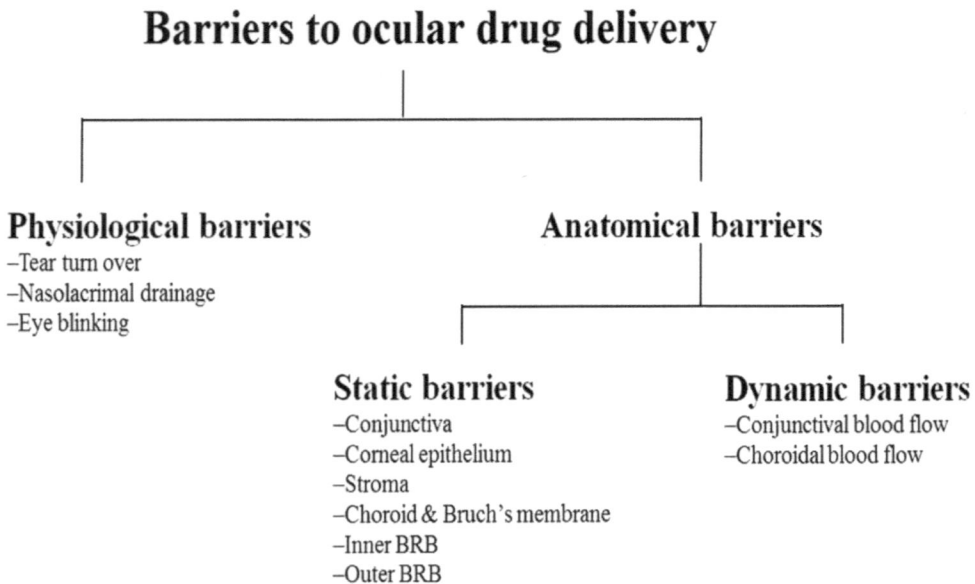

Barriers to ocular drug delivery

Physiological barriers
–Tear turn over
–Nasolacrimal drainage
–Eye blinking

Anatomical barriers

Static barriers
–Conjunctiva
–Corneal epithelium
–Stroma
–Choroid & Bruch's membrane
–Inner BRB
–Outer BRB

Dynamic barriers
–Conjunctival blood flow
–Choroidal blood flow

Figure 1: Barriers to ocular drug delivery.

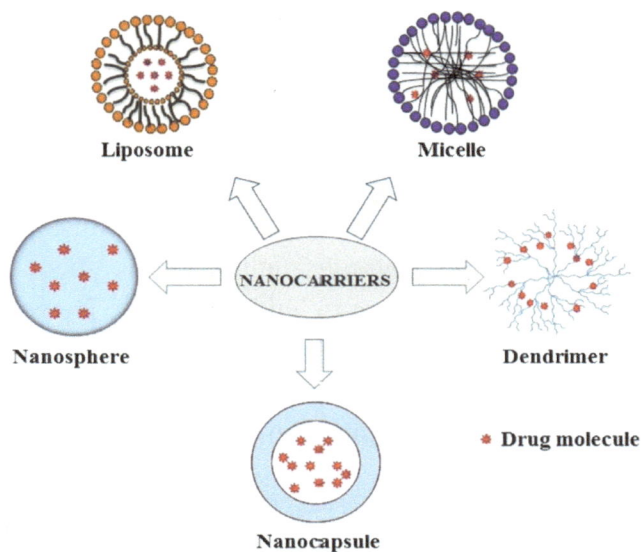

Figure 2: Nanocarriers for ocular drug delivery.

SIGNIFICANCE OF NANOTECHNOLOGY IN OCULAR DRUG DELIVERY

Ocular diseases can best be treated by conventional ophthalmic dosage forms, such as aqueous solutions, ointments and suspensions than systemic administration. The advantages include rapid onset of action especially from solution or drop formulation of lower dose, no or minimal systemic toxicity, ease of administrationand high patient compliance. Although topical administration is usually preferred to treat disorders of anterior segment, the biological protecting layers lead to low ocular absorption and poor bioavailability (1–10%). Numerous approaches have been examined to improve ocular bioavailability of topically applied drugs, such as viscosity enhancers, penetration enhancers, prodrugsand drug delivery devices like collagen shields and ocular inserts. Among these approaches, viscosity enhancers and prodrug derivatization suffer from disadvantages of precorneal loss of liquid formulation. In the case of penetration enhancers, care should be taken in the selection of the agent due to high sensitivity of ocular tissues. Ocular devices, such as collagen shields and inserts may lead to tissue irritation, surgical complications and poor patient compliance as these materials must remain in the site of application for hours to days [2].

Treatment of diseases affecting the posterior segments, *i.e.* retina, choroid, vitreous humorand optic nerve, involves greater challenges. Achieving therapeutic drug concentrations in the posterior segment eye by topical drug administration is a daunting task, because of corneal and conjunctival epithelia barriers and the lacrimal drainage. Furthermore, blood-retinal barriers (BRB) prevent therapeutics from entering posterior segment following systemic administration. As a result, only options remaining are invasive approaches, such as intravitreal, subconjunctival, sub-Tenon's and, suprascleral injections. However, due to rapid elimination from ocular tissues, frequent injections may be necessary. Repeated injections may lead to discomfort, as well as complications, such as cataracts, vitreous hemorrhage, retinal detachmentand endophthalmitis.

Hence, an efficient ocular drug delivery system, which can provide maximum precorneal residence time, overcome ocular barriers and sustain drug delivery following topical administration, is desirable [3]. A variety of nanocarriers, including liposomes and nanoparticles, can be formulated into eye drops for delivery of both hydrophilic and lipophilic molecules. Nanocarriers can be specifically taken up by the cornea by endocytosis. Thus the cornea can act as a reservoir and release the active slowly to the surrounding tissues [4, 5]. To overcome impermeable corneal barriers, a nanotechnology-based approach is plausible. Additionally, encapsulation provides protection of drugs and prodrugs from enzymatic degradation. It can also prolong exposure due to controlled release [6]. Targeted drug delivery by surface modification of nanocarriers with various targeting moieties has also been investigated [7].

Nanotechnology-based drug delivery systems may be applied for the treatment of chronic ocular diseases, in which frequent drug administration is necessary, for example, chronic cytomegalovirus (CMV) retinitis, age related macular degeneration (AMD) and diabetic macular edema (DME). Although an intravitreal implant releases agents for up to six months, it is restricted due to the need of surgery during insertion and removal and several side effects such as astigmatism and vitreous hemorrhage [8-10]. Intravitreal injection of polylactide (PLA) nanoparticles (NPs) can eventually localize to RPE cells and provide sustained drug release for four months [11]. Therefore, NP can be a potential carrier for targeted and controlled localized drug delivery to the posterior segment following intravitreous injection. Once delivered to the ocular vitreous space, nanoparticles may not induce inflammatory responses in the retinal tissue or alter the structures of surrounding ocular tissues [12].

Thus, nanotechnology-based formulations are being developed for efficient ocular drug delivery for both the anterior and posterior segments. Nanotechnology based systems with an appropriate particle size (narrow size range usually <10 μm) can be designed to ensure low irritation, adequate bioavailabilityand ocular tissue compatibility. In this chapter, different nanocarriers for ocular drug delivery based on published literature including patents are discussed.

NANOCARRIERS IN OCULAR DRUG DELIVERY

In a last few decades, many approaches have been utilized for the treatment of ocular diseases. Nanotechnology based ophthalmic formulations are one of the approaches which is currently being heavily pursued for both anterior, as well as posterior segment indications. Several nanocarriers, such as nanoparticles, nanosuspension, liposomes, niosomes, discomes, nano micelles, dendrimers and microemulsion, have been developed for ocular delivery. Some of them have shown promising results for improving ocular bioavailability.

Nanoparticles

Nanoparticles are colloidal drug carrier systems comprised of macromolecules that vary in size from 10 nm to 1000 nm. The particles can be classified as nanospheres or nanocapsules, depending upon whether the active molecules are uniformly dispersed into the polymeric material or coated within the polymeric shell (Fig. **2**) [7, 13]. Nanoparticles for ophthalmic drugs have been formulated with various biodegradable, non-biodegradable and naturally occurring polymers, such as polylactides (PLAs), polycyanoacrylate, poly (D, L-lactides), chitosan, gelatin, sodium alginateand albumin. Table **1** shows recent developments in ocular delivery systems based on nanoparticles. Following topical administration, nanoparticles primarily reside in the precorneal area for longer time periods and are taken up by the corneal cells. The particles form a depot intracellularly and release the cargo in a sustained manner. Sustained drug release and prolonged therapeutic effects can be achieved with nanoparticle formulations [14]. Calvo *et* *al.* observed that after topical administration, cyclosporine loaded poly-ε-caprolactone nanocapsules were taken up by corneal epithelial cells and a five-fold higher drug level was achieved compared to the drug-loaded oily solution [15]. Ocular pharmacokinetics of pilocarpine-loaded polybutylcyanoacrylate nanoparticles for the treatment of glaucoma were investigated in rabbit eyes. The AUC of pilocarpine in the aqueous humor was elevated by 23% with the nanoparticle suspension compared to reference aqueous solution. Moreover, a significantly prolonged reduction in intraocular pressure was observed [16]. Recently, Boddu *et al.* from our laboratory have developed PLGA nanoparticles of dexamethasone (DEX), hydrocortisone acetate (HA)and prednisolone acetate (PA), suspended in thermosensitive gels for the treatment of macular edema (ME) [17]. Higher entrapment was noted with o/w emulsion solvent evaporation compared to the dialysis method. Irrespective of the preparation method, nanoparticles exhibited a biphasic release pattern with an initial burst phase followed by a sustained release phase. After suspending nanoparticles in thermosensitive PLGA-PEG-PLGA gel, a zero-order drug release for approximately 25 days was observed. Moreover, a sustained release of DEX from nanoparticles suspended in thermosensitive gel was observed in e*x vivo* permeability studies with rabbit sclera.

Nanoparticles are primarily endocytosed by the corneal cells generating higher ocular bioavailability. However, a part of the formulation is washed away by nasolacrimal drainage because of nano size. The residence time of nanoparticles in cul-de-sac can be improved by coating nanoparticles with PEG, chitosan (CS) and hyaluronic acid, or by fabricating with mucoadhesive polymer. PEG coated acyclovir-PLA nanospheres significantly improved ocular bioavailability after topical administration in rabbits. AUC values for aqueous humor were 1.8- and 12.6-fold greater for PEG-coated PLA nanospheres compared to uncoated particles and free drug suspension, respectively. Improved ocular bioavailability of acyclovir provided by PEG-coated PLA nanospheres may be due to mucoadhesion [18].

For improvement in cyclosporine A delivery, Angela *et al.* prepared cyclosporine A (CyA) loaded chitosan nanoparticles. *In vivo* studies on rabbit eye showed that animals treated with CyA-loaded chitosan nanoparticles had significantly higher corneal and conjunctival drug levels (2–6-fold increase) than those treated with a suspension of CyA in a chitosan aqueous solution [19].

Albumin nanoparticles may be fairly effective for drug delivery to the posterior segment of the eye. Moreover, a high content of charged amino acids render them suitable for absorption both for positively charged ganciclovir and negatively charged oligonucleotides. Arnedo *et al.* developed albumin nanoparticles for intravitreal delivery of anti-sense oligonucleotide (phosphodiester) for the treatment of CMV. Albumin nanoparticles promoted nuclear accumulation of phosphodiester and oligonucleotides into MRC-5 fibroblasts. Moreover, nanoparticle formulation significantly raised antiviral activity of free PO in MRC-5 fibroblasts infected with human cytomegalovirus [20]. To avoid organic solvents and polymer toxicity, solid lipid nanoparticles have also been attempted in ocular drug delivery. Due to extremely small dimension, solid lipid nanoparticles (SLN) are presumably entrapped and retained in the mucin layer covering the corneal epithelium. Recently, phospholipon 90 G surface-modified solid SLN of timolol have been examined for permeation through bioengineered human cornea [21]. Surface-modified SLN exhibited high entrapment efficiency compared to unmodified SLN. No burst release was observed with surface modified SLN, which is usually observed with unmodified SLN. In a permeation study across regenerated human cornea, high and sustained permeation of timolol was observed in surface modified relative to unmodified SLN.

Even though nanoparticles are a promising tool for enhancing ocular bioavailability, various developmental issues, such as formulation stability, large scale production of sterile formulationand rate control of drug release still need to be considered.

Table 1: Recent Developments in Nanoparticle Based Ocular Drug Delivery

Drug	Polymer	Features	References
Tobramycin	Hexadecyl Phosphate	Tobramycin-loaded SLN produced higher in C_{max} (1.5-fold), t_{max} (eight-fold) and AUC (four-fold) compared to eye drops.	[22]
Carboplatin	Chitosan, Sodium alginate	Carboplatin loaded in NP demonstrated elevated and sustained antiproliferative activity with IC_{50} of 0.56 µg/ml and 0.004 µg/ml for free carboplatin and carboplatin loaded nanoparticles respectively in a retinoblastoma cell line (Y79).	[23]

Table 1: contd...

Flurbiprofen	PLGA	Flurbiprofen-loaded nanospheres enhanced drug penetration about two times more than commercial eye drops containing poly (vinyl alcohol) and about four times more than flurbiprofen at pH 7.4 phosphate buffer in an *ex vivo* rabbit corneal permeation study.	[24]
Sparfloxacin	PLGA	Sparfloxacin-loaded nanoparticles were retained for a longer duration on the corneal surface as opposed to an aqueous solution, which was drained rapidly from the corneal surface. An extended drug release was observed.	[25]
Pilocarpine	Chitosan/Carbopol	Of all the polymers, chitosan/carbopol nanoparticles displayed longest lasting antimitotic effects in rabbit eyes.	[26]
Dexamethasone (DEX)	PLGA	Intravitreal injection of DEX-NPs provided sustained drug release with improved ocular bioavailability over 50 days in rabbits and a relatively steady vitreous drug level for up to 30 days.	[27]
Cyclosporine A (CyA)	Poly-ε-caprolactone (PCL)	High CyA level was achieved in rabbit corneas for a nanosphere formulation, with 5.9–15.5 ng/mg tissue level with poly-epsilon-caprolactone (PCL)/benzalkonium chloride (BKC) and 11.4–23.0 ng/mg tissue for HA coated PCL/BKC nanospheres within the first 24 hrs.	[28]
Brimonidine Tartrate (BT)	Sodium alginate	Topical instillation of BT-loaded nanoparticles in albino rabbits demonstrated continuous drug release over eight hrs.	[29]
Amphotericin-B	Eudragit RL 100	Nanoparticle formulation showed good antifungal activity against *Fusarium solani* as examined by the disk diffusion methodand no ocular irritation was observed.	[30]
Ganciclovir (GCV)	Albumin	GCV loaded albumin nanoparticles inhibited viral replication with nearly two-fold higher efficacy than aquous ganciclovir, in human corneal fibroblasts (CHN).	[31]
Diclofenac (DS)	PLGA	Diclofenac-loaded biopolymeric (poly (lactide-*co*-glycolide) and poly (lactide-*co*-glycolide-leucine)) nanosuspension exhibited drug release with no ocular irritation for 24 hrs.	[32]
Pilocarpin	Chitosan–PAA	Both *in vivo* and *in vitro* studies suggested that nanosuspension was more effective in sustaining drug release relative to commercial eye drops.	[33]

Table 1: contd...

Cloricromene	Eudragit	Nanosuspension improved both shelf life and ocular bioavailability of cloricromene.	[34]
Methylprednisolone acetate (MPA)	Copolymer of poly(ethylacrylate, methyl-methacrylate and chlorotrimethyl-ammonioethyl methacrylate)	MPA-loaded nanosuspension showed a significant inhibition of endotoxin- induced ocular inflammation in rabbit relative to a microsuspension of MPA.	[35]
Ibuprofen	Eudragit RS 100	A higher drug level was achieved in aqueous humor after application of a nanosuspension compared to eye drops.	[36]

Nanosuspensions

Nanosuspensions represent a colloidal dispersion of nano sized drug particles stabilized by surfactants. Such formulations provide advantages for easy eye drop preparation, enhanced solubility, lower dosage and improved physical stability. These formulations can be designed successfully for compounds, which are insoluble in either water or oil [37]. Nano-sized particles offer many other advantages, such as a higher surface area for dissolution, a faster dissolution rate, improved bioadhesion, and rapid corneal penetrationand reduced ocular irritation. Kassem *et al.* compared ocular bioavailability of various glucocorticoids (prednisolone, dexamethasone and hydrocortisone) formulated as nanosuspensions, solutions and microcrystalline suspensions. This study reported that a higher extent of drug absorption and more intense drug effect from nanosuspensions (Tables **2** and **3**) [38].

Table 2: Pharmacodynamic Parameters for Prednisolone Solution and as well as Micro- and Nanosuspensions

Prednisolone preparations	% IOP_{max}	T_{max} (h)	AUC_{0-11h} (% increase in IOP.h)	HVD (h)	HVDR (h)	MRT (h)
(A) Dexamethasone solution	11.49 ± 0.83 ***	$1.80 \pm 0.08^\dagger$	34.60 ± 2.64***	3.11 ± 0.31*	3.11 ± 0.31***	2.88 ± 0.08*
(B) Dexamethasone nanosuspension of mean particle diameter 930 nm	25.70 ± 1.24	1.85 ± 0.07	103.18 ± 7.21	3.87 ± 0.28	5.82 ± 0.27	3.71 ± 0.07
(C) Dexamethasone microsuspension of mean particle diameter 2.46 μm	18.38 ± 0.43***	$2.00 \pm 0.13^\dagger$	66.44 ± 2.84***	$3.20 \pm 0.19^\dagger$	4.85 ± 0.29*	$3.50 \pm 0.08^\dagger$

Table 2: contd...

(D) Dexamethasone microsuspension of mean particle diameter 4.89 µm	13.30 ± 1.03***	1.90 ± 0.06†	44.95 ± 2.92***	3.60 ± 0.16†	4.17 ± 0.18***	3.06 ± 0.09***

* *p*= 0.05 significant.
*** *p*= 0.001very highly significant.
† Insignificant.

Table 3: Pharmacodynamic Parameters for Dexamethasone Solution and as well as Micro- and Nanosuspensions

Dexamethasone preparations	% IOP$_{max}$	T_{max} (h)	AUC$_{0-11h}$ (% increase in IOP.h)	HVD (h)	HVDR (h)	MRT (h)
(A) Dexamethasone solution	13.87 ± 1.05 ***	1.55 ± 0.09†	66.02 ± 5.85***	4.82 ± 0.33*	4.82 ± 0.33***	4.33 ± 0.11*
(B) Dexamethasone nanosuspension of mean particle diameter 930 nm	24.97 ± 1.27	1.75 ± 0.08	148.05 ± 7.69	6.10 ± 0.29	8.39 ± 0.17	4.95 ± 0.30
(C) Dexamethasone microsuspension of mean particle diameter 2.46 µm	19.95 ± 0.43***	1.90 ± 0.06†	101.49 ± 7.43***	5.00 ± 0.49*	6.56 ± 0.47***	4.78 ± 0.15†
(D) Dexamethasone microsuspension of mean particle diameter 4.89 µm	17.35 ± 0.81***	1.80 ± 0.08†	88.92 ± 8.59***	4.69 ± 0.42*	6.05 ± 0.50***	4.83 ± 0.14†

* *p*= 0.05 significant.
*** *p*= 0.001very highly significant.
† Insignificant.

Hence nanosuspensions represent an efficient ophthalmic drug delivery system with the advantages of lower dosage requirement, less frequent instillation, prolonged releaseand negligible ocular irritation. However, actual performance depends on intrinsic solubility and dissolution rate of drug in lacrimal fluid, which can fluctuate, due to constant in and outflow. As a consequence, a nanosuspension may fail to provide consistent performance. However, nanosuspension represents an ideal approach for ocular delivery of poorly soluble drugs owing to the inherent ability of the dosage form to increase saturation solubility. Moreover, to achieve sustained drug release, nanosuspension can be incorporated into a hydrogel, a mucoadhesive base, or ocular inserts.

Liposomes

Liposomes are small lipid vesicles (0.08 μm to 10 μm) containing an aqueous core enclosed by phospholipid bilayers (Fig. **2**). Depending upon size and number of bilayers, liposomes are referred to as small unilamellar vesicles (SUV, 10–100 nm), large unilamellar vesicles (LUV, 100–3000 nm), oligolamellar vesicles (OLV, 100–1000 nm), or multilamellar vesicles (MLV, >1 μm) (Fig. **3**). Because of their amphiphilic properties, such vesicles can entrap both hydrophilic and hydrophobic drugs.

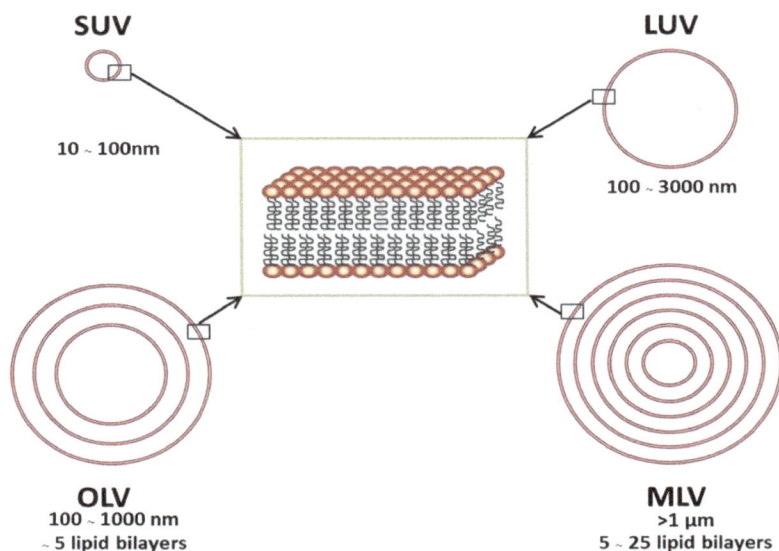

Figure 3: Schematic representation of the commonly applied classification scheme for liposomes in ocular drug delivery.

Dehydrated-rehydrated vesicles (DRV) have been prepared to explore small unilamellar vesicles. A thin lipid film is first formed on the inner side of flask by evaporating organic solvents under vacuum in a rotary evaporator. This film is then dissolved in drug solution and sonicated to obtain small unilamellar vesicles [39]. The suspension is freeze-dried overnight. Li *et al.* has prepared chitosan-coated liposome by injection method. Briefly, an aliquot of ethanol containing lipid components and the active agent is injected slowly through a 21-gauge needle into a calcium acetate solution with stirring at 60°C under a nitrogen flow. After evaporating the ethanol, the suspension is homogenized and dialyzed with

0.9% NaCl to create a calcium acetate gradient across the lipid bilayer [40]. This suspension is then freeze-dried overnight. Reversed-phase evaporation technique is applied to prepare large unilamellar liposomes [41]. The mixture of lipid film was redissolved in ether and then drug solution in acetone together with phosphate-buffered saline (PBS, pH 7.4). The mixture is sonicated and the organic solvent is evaporated. The formed liposomes are equilibrated at room temperature and PBS is added to the liposomal suspension and filtered five times through 4.5 μm and then ten times through 2.2 μm microporous filter for purification. The final formulation is kept overnight at 4°C. The process of preparing oligolamellar vesicles is very similar to unilamellar under the reverse-phase evaporation technique [42]. The only difference is that the process of evaporation under rotary evaporator is applied after the sonication to remove organic solvent. Formed liposomes are equilibrated at room temperature and stored in PBS overnight at 4°C. For preparation of multilamellar veisicles (MLV), different liposome preparation procedures are adopted. Most common method for MLV is reversed-phase evaporation technique [39, 42-44]. A mixture of lipid film in diethyl ether and drug solution is emulsified by sonication. Any residual organic solvent present in the emulsion is removed by rotary evaporation. The resulting viscous gel is resuspended in PBS (pH 7.4). Large MVL is prepared by a thin-layer evaporation technique (TLE) under an atmosphere of nitrogen by hydrating (vortex mixing) lipid films with drug solution [39, 45, 46]. Frozen and thawed multilamellar vesicles are obtained by freezing the MLVs in liquid nitrogen and thawing samples in a warmed water bath. Under lipid film hydration (LFH) technique, liposomes are prepared by dispersing the lipid film in drug (pH 7.4) solution by mechanical stirring [41, 42, 47-50]. The liposomal suspension is left to mature overnight at 4°C to ensure full lipid hydration. Finally, the liposomal suspension is passed through microporous filters for purification.

The application of liposomes in ophthalmology was first explored by Smolin, *et al.* in 1981 [51]. Topical drop of liposomal iodoxouridine was prepared for the treatment of herpes simplex keratitis. In ocular drug delivery, liposomes offer numerous advantages including prolonged drug retention, improved drug absorption and protection of active molecules from metabolic enzymes at the tear/corneal epithelium interface. Table **4** summarizes some recent developments

Table 4: Recent Developments in Liposomal Ocular Drug Delivery

No.	Drug	Type of Liposomes	Formulation Charge	Method of Preparation	Result	Reference
1.	Acyclovir	Oligolamellar Multilamellar	Positive Negative Neutral	Dehydrated-rehydrated vehicles preparation (DRV) Reverse-phase evaporation Thin-layer evaporation technique (TLE)	Uptake of positively charged liposomes by the cornea was highest, with lesser uptake in the case of negatively charged liposomes and least with neutral liposomes.	[39]
2.	Diclofenac sodium (DS)	Chitosan-coated liposomes	Positive Negative	Injection method	*In vitro* drug release was significantly prolonged by the liposome encapsulation (61% at 24 hrs) and further by low molecular weight chitosan (LCH) coating (55% after 24 hrs).	[40]
3.	Ofloxacin	Thermosensitive liposomal hydrogel(multilamellar and unilamellar)	Neutral Positive Negative	Lipid film hydration technique, reverse-phase evaporation	Liposomal *in situ* thermosensitive hydrogel produced seven-fold higher transcorneal permeation.	[41]
4.	Acetazolamide	Multilamellar, Unilamellar	Positive, Negative, Neutral	Lipid film hydration, reverse-phase evaporation	Multilamellar liposomes produced a more significant lowering in IOPand showed a more sustained therapeutic activity than REV liposomes.	[42]
5.	Chloramphenicol (CAP)	Multilamellar	Neutral	Reverse-phase evaporation	Encapsulated CAP liposomes generated highest antibacterial and antibiotic activity compared to absorbed CAP liposomes and partitioned CAP liposomes.	[43]
6.	Demeclocycline	Multilamellar	Positive Negative Neutral	Reverse-phase evaporation	A higher drug concentration was achieved (69-95%). The drug concentrations in the cornea, aqueous humorand conjunctiva	[44]

Table 4: contd….

					were 4.76, 2.18and 23.32 µg/g of tissue respectively.	
7.	Ciprofloxacin	Hydrogel multilamellar			Thin-film hydration method	Hydrogel ensured liposomes to provide steady and prolonged *in vitro* release with 50% in 4600 min in presence of 0.1% dipalmitoyl phosphatidylcholine (DPPC)/ phorbol myristate acetate (PMA) and 5507 min for 15% Poly(vinyl alcohol) (PVA).	[45]
8.	Vasoactive intestinal peptide	Pegylated liposomes			Thin-film hydration, then lyophilization–rehydration method	Liposomal formulation showed 15 times higher drug concentration in ocular fluids than solution after 24 hrs.	[46]
	Povidone-iodine	Multilamellar	Negative	Lipid film hydration	Liposomal povidone-iodine formulations demonstrated lower cytotoxicity and better tolerability compared with the aqueous solution.	[47]
9.	16-Mer oligonucleotides	Multilamellar		Lipid film hydration	With intravitreal injection of liposomes, the residual concentration of the oligonucleotide within the ocular tissues was significantly elevated relative to a simple solution. Also, sustained levels were observed in the vitreous and retina-choroid with lower distribution to nontarget tissues, *i.e.* lens sclera.	[48]
10.	Bevacizumab (Avastin)			Lipid film hydration with dehydration-rehydration method	Mean free drug concentrations in ocular tissue from liposomes were two (48 *vs.* 28 µg/ml) and five (16 *vs.* 3.3 µg/ml) times higher at days 28 and 42 respectively compared with drug solution.	[49]

Table 4: contd….

11.	Fluorescence probe (Coumarin-6)	Submicron-sized liposomes(ssLips) and multilamellar		Lipid film hydration	Following topical administration of submicron-sized liposomes (ssLips), drug was delivered to the posterior segment including the retina.	[50]
12.	Glycoprotein B and DTK peptides	Multilamellar	Positive	Lipid film hydration	Liposomes can quantitatively encapsulate gB1s and around 30% the DTK peptides.	[59]
13.	Diclofenac sodium		Positive	Reverse-phase evaporation	Ocular bioavailability of liposomes in the aqueous humor was 211% relative to the eye drops.	[60]
14.	Ganciclovir (GCV)		Negative	Reverse-phase evaporation	*In vitro* studies demonstrated 3.9-fold higher transcorneal permeability with liposomal formulation. Moreover, ocular tissue levels (sclera, cornea, iris, lensand vitreous humor) of GCV were two to ten times higher with liposomes compared with solution dosing.	[61]

in ocular liposomal drug delivery. Properties of liposomes vary substantially with lipid composition, size, surface chargeand methods of preparation. Several studies indicated that multilamellar liposomes demonstrate higher encapsulation efficiency and prolonged release than unilamellar liposomes after topical administration. The lipid composition of liposomes can lowering tear-driven dilution in the conjunctival sac and thereby enhances drug sustained release [45]. Liposomes can also enhance drug absorption by improving contact time with corneal and conjunctival surfaces. Positively charged liposomes possess a higher binding affinity to negatively charged corneal surface compared to negatively charged or neutral liposomes. Negatively charged liposomes exhibit lowest loading efficiency and most rapid drug release, while positively charged liposomes shows the highest entrapment efficiency and slowest drug release rate. Therefore, positively charged liposomes demonstrate better therapeutic effectiveness and a more prolonged effect than neutral and negatively charged ones [42, 52]. However, a few studies have demonstrated that positively charged liposomes containing positive charged cargo, such as cationic lipid stearylamine may cause ocular irritation [53]. Therefore, chitosan, a cationic polymer obtained from natural sources with favorable biocompatibility and mucoadhesiveness, has been introduced into the liposome formulation. Chitosomes are mucoadhesive biocompatible chitosan-coated liposomes. Coating enhances ocular drug permeation with increased and prolonged drug effect [54, 55]. These chitosan-coated liposomes demonstrate an improved physicochemical stability, rapid transcorneal penetration with prolonged retention, relative to non-coated liposomes [40]. Exact location of drug molecules in the liposomal formulation plays an important role in the encapsulation efficiency, drug release and therapeutic effectiveness [43].

The polymer hydrogel in liposomal formulation ensured steady, as well as prolonged transcorneal permeation [56]. The gelation time could be further decreased by the addition of liposomes into the hydrogel. The prepared liposomal hydrogel enhanced transcorneal permeation several-fold compared to the aqueous solution [41]. Site-specific and sustained release immunoliposomes containing antiviral drugs, like ganciclovir and 5-iododeoxyuridine, can improve therapy of ocular herpes simplex virus infection [54, 57]. The magnitude of fluorescence emission of coumarin-6 encapsulated liposomes indicated that vesicle rigidity and particle size were related to delivery of drugs to the posterior segment by eye drop administration [58].

Niosomes

Niosomes are formed by self-assembly of non-ionic amphipathic molecules in aqueous media and have a bilayered structure physically similar to liposomes (Fig. **4**). These vesicles have been used to encapsulate both hydrophilic and lipophilic drugs, either in an aqueous layer or in a lipid membrane [62]. To prepare niosomes vehicles, a particular class of amphiphiles such as nonionic surfactants with cholesterol are required to prevent less leakage. Additionally, stabilizers are also added to prevent vesicle aggregation by repulsive, steric, or electrostatic effect. Niosomes for topical ocular drug delivery provide numerous advantages over liposomes, such as greater stability and ease of storage, low toxicity, structural flexibility, fluidity, size, biodegradability, biocompatibility and non-immunogenicity [63]. Unlike liposomes, niosomes are a promising and suitable delivery system, not only for lipophilic compounds, but also for hydrophilic drug molecules. Niosomes enhance the ocular bioavailability of hydrophilic drugs preferentially by modifying the permeability characteristics of conjunctival and scleral membranes [64-66].

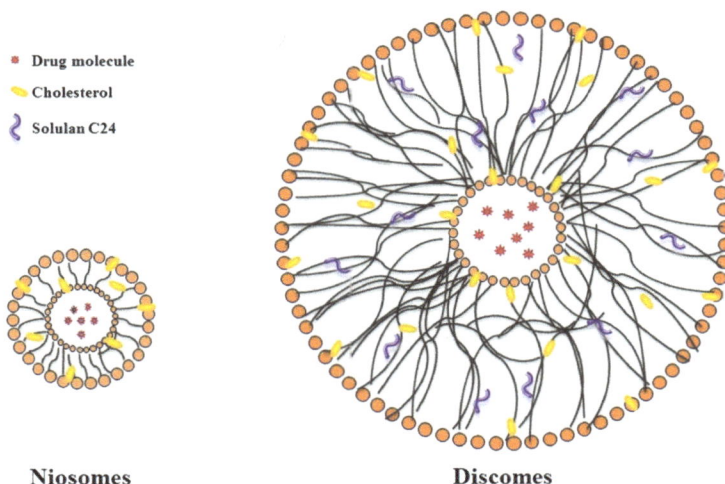

Figure 4: Structures of niosomes and discomes

Timolol maleate, a water-soluble drug was encapsulated in niosomes by Vyas *et al.* [67]. Ocular bioavailability of timolol maleate was improved 2.48 times compared to a timolol maleate solution. In another study, chitosan or carbopol coated niosomal formulations containing timolol maleate were prepared by reversed-phase evaporation (REV) [68]. In an *in vitro* study, release of timolol maleate from niosomes was extended significantly. In pharmacodynamic studies in albino rabbits, a niosome formulation containing 0.25% timolol maleate showed similar effects as that obtained by 0.5% marketed gel formulation. Hence, niosomal formulations can be exploited for reduction in cardiovascular side effects associated with ocular timolol maleate therapy. Recently, niosomal formulation containing water-soluble gentamicin sulfate was prepared in the presence of cholesterol and a negatively charge inducer dicetyl phosphate (DCP) by a thin film hydration technique [69]. Ninety two percent entrapment efficiency was achieved when an optimized molar ratio of Tween 60, cholesterol and DCP

1:1:0.1 was incorporated. *In vitro* drug release from niosomes was much more sustained relative to drug solution.

In another study, carbopol-coated niosomes containing acetazolamide were prepared to achieve enhanced bioadhesive effect [70]. Pharmacodynamic studies indicated an ideal sustained effect for 6 hrs after instillation in rabbit model. In addition, duration of therapeutically effective concentration was also significantly prolonged.

A five-fold increase in entrapment efficiency for naltrexone hydrochloride was achieved with 2%–5% mol/mol additives [71]. The volume diameters and shapes of niosomes were significantly dependent on the additive used. The shape of most niosomes is typically spherical, whereas niosomes with additive C24 are usually oval giant niosomes (discomes). This type of niosomes controls naltrexone hydrochloride release rate and extended drug release. Such niosomes can also enhance drug permeation as shown by *ex vivo* transcorneal permeation studies. These niosomal formulations do not cause ocular irritation in rabbit model [69, 71].

Discomes

Discomes represent a modified form of niosomes, which have large disc shaped structures (12-60 µm). These vesicles are derived from niosomes by the addition of a non-ionic surfactant, such as Solulan C24, which partitions into lipid bilayers leading to formation of larger flattened disc-like structures (Fig. **4**) [67, 71-72]. Larger size of discomes prevents drainage into systemic pooland disc shape provides a better fit in ocular cul-de-sac [72-73]. Discomes can be selected as a carrier for controlled ocular administration of water-soluble drugs [67]. Such formulation can yield higher entrapment efficiency (25%) of the water-soluble compound timolol maleate relative to niosomes (14%). Moreover, ocular bioavailability was found to be approximately 3.07-fold higher with discomes in comparison to timolol maleate solution. Moreover, discomes prolonged duration of action from 1.5 hrs to 5 hrs [67].

Micelles

Micelles are self-assembling amphiphiles and orient to form supramolecular core-shell structures in the aqueous milieu. Hydrophobic interactions in these carriers force assembly of amphiphiles in aqueous environment when concentrations exceed critical micelle concentration, resulting in the formation of micelles within the size range of less than 200 nm (Fig. **2**) [74-76]. These nanosized micellar drug delivery systems are composed of amphiphilic polymers containing a low molecular-weight hydrophobic core-forming block. A minimum monomer concentration, in equilibrium with micelles, reduces toxicity in addition to providing sufficient thermodynamic stability. High thermodynamic stability offers slow drug release and high penetration enhancing activity thereby improving drug permeability across ocular tissues [74]. Polymeric micelles composed of a copolymer of *N*-isopropylacrylamide (NIPAAM), vinyl pyrrolidone (VP)and acrylic acid (AA) having cross-links with *N*, *N'*-methylene *bis*-acrylamide (MBA), were prepared as a host carrier, in which up to 30% w/w ketorolac was entrapped. This formulation is stable for eight to ten days at room temperature. A two-fold increase in ocular bioavailability with no corneal damage was observed in excised rabbit corneal permeation studies, compared to an aqueous suspension containing the same amount of drug [77]. Recent studies showed utilization of three copolymers of polyhydroxyethylaspartamide (PHEA), with side chains of polyethylene glycol (PEG) and/or hexadecylamine (C16) (PHEA-PEG, PHEA-PEG-C16 and PHEA-C16 respectively). *In vivo* bioavailability studies with PHEA-PEG-C16 micelles loaded with dexamethasone provided greater drug bioavailability in rabbits, when compared to an aqueous suspension [78]. J Liaw et.al achieved stable and efficient transfer of plasmid DNA with lacZ gene *in vivo* using PEO-PPO-PEO non-ionic copolymeric micelles.

More recently, our research group in collaboration with Lux Biosciences, Inc., developed a novel, clear micellar formulation of voclosporin, a calcineurin inhibitor for keratoconjunctivitis sicca. Voclosporin, an analog of cyclosporine, is four times more potent and patient compliant than Restasis®, currently Food and Drug Administration (FDA) approved in U.S. for the treatment of dry eye syndrome. Voclosporin poses a major challenge in terms of formulation of a clear aqueous eye drop, since the drug is very hydrophobic. We developed a clear, mixed nano micellar solution of voclosporin, comprised of amphiphilic polymers, *i.e.* Vit E TPGS and Octoxynol-40, mixed at optimum ratios. These compositions exhibited superior tolerability in rabbit models, with mean irritation scores much lower than Restasis® (Fig. **5**).

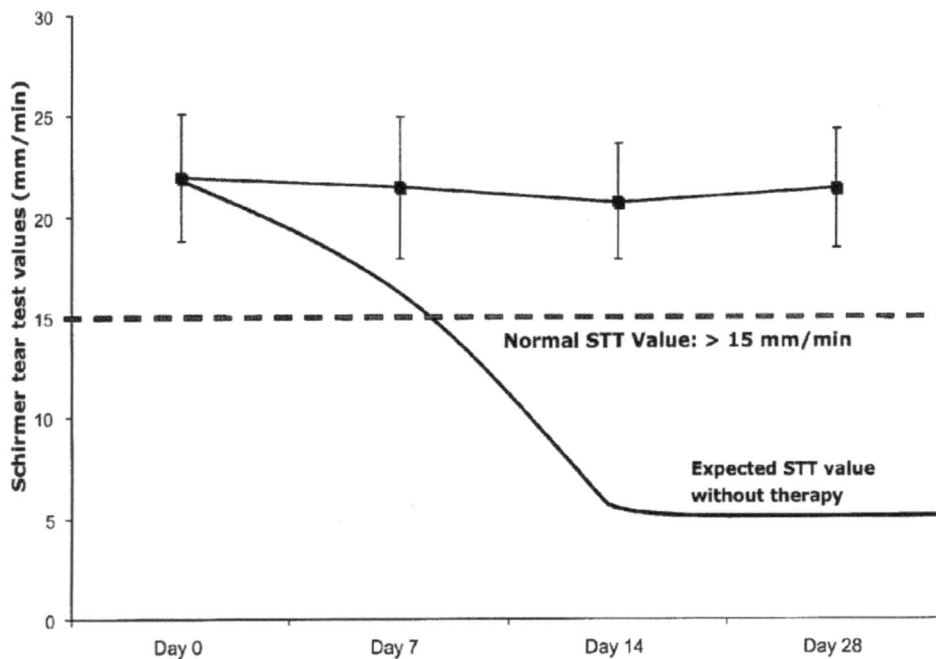

Figure 5: The graphical representation of mean Shirmer Tear Test (STT) values of canine KCS patients through 30 days of treatment using 0.2% voclosporin mixed micellar formulation.

Moreover, high drug levels were achieved in rabbit ocular tissues for up to and beyond 24 hrs, especially in the posterior segment (retina/choroid and optic nerve), in addition to the tissues in the anterior eye (cornea, conjunctiva, sclera). This formulation showed feasibility of treating posterior eye diseases (*e.g.* retinal diseases involving the optic nerve, such as glaucoma) with topical administration [79]. This novel mixed micellar formulation shown opens new possibilities for delivering drugs to the back of the eye topical administration (Fig. **6**).

Dendrimers

Dendrimers represent a unique class of synthetic macromolecules that comprise a series of branches around an inner core (Fig. **2**). These molecules have countless cavities within their branches, which can carry therapeutic agents. Dendrimers selected for drug delivery are usually 10 to 100 nm in diameter with multiple surface-functional groups (typically amines, carboxylic acid and hydroxyl

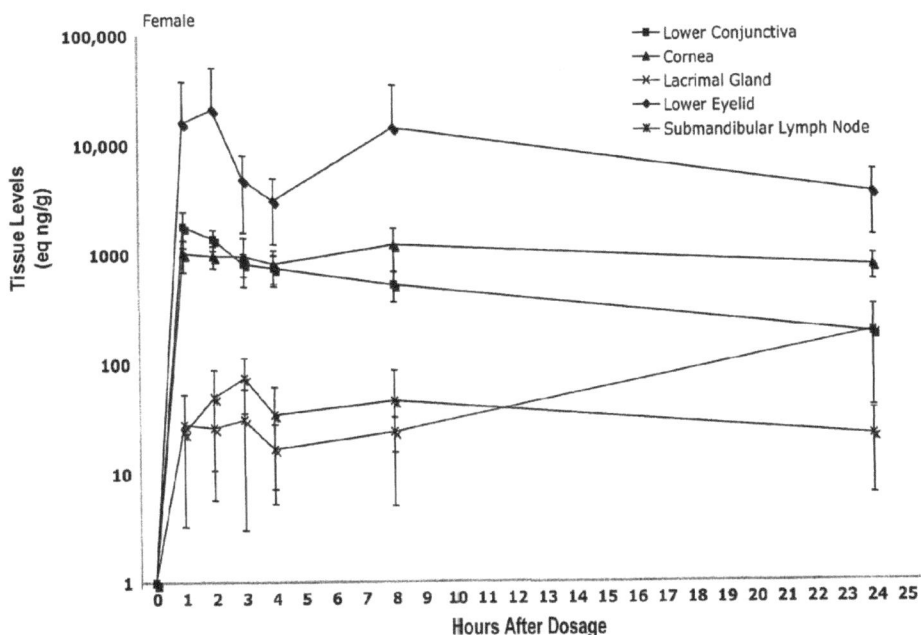

Figure 6: The therapeutically achieved ocular tissue levels of voclosporin after a single topical administration of mixed micellar formulation to female New Zealand white rabbits.

groups). These functional groups are responsible for high reactivity of dendrimers and provide the ability to conjugate multiple surface groups for biological recognition [80]. It is also possible to control the molecular size, shape, dimension, density, polarity, flexibilityand solubility of dendrimers by selecting different building blocks and surface-functional groups during synthesis [7, 81]. To overcome various side effects and poor ocular residence time associated with different types of polymeric formulations such as bioadhesive polymers and colloidal formulations, poly (amidoamine) dendrimers (PAMAM) were introduced. Vandamme *et al.* evaluated a series of poly (amidoamine) (PAMAM) (G0, G1, G2, G4 and G6) dendrimers for controlled ocular drug delivery in rabbits. These PAMAM dendrimers have the capability to entrap and solubilize both hydrophilic and lipophilic drugs. The residence time is evaluated with fluorescein as a model drug. Mean ocular residence times of aqueous solutions containing 0.25% of G1 2.5, 2.0% of G2 (OH) and 2.0% of G4 (OH) dendrimers are comparable to that of the 0.2% w/v carbopol solution. With the same *in vivo* model, prolonged mitotic or mydriatic effects of dendrimer solutions containing pilocarpine nitrate or tropicamide, have been noted. Improved ocular bioavailability with eye drops contains aqueous G1.5 and G4 (OH) dendrimers with carboxylate and hydroxyl surface groups, respectively [82]. Shaunak *et al.* synthesized PAMAM (G3.5) - glucosamine (DG) and PAMAM (G3.5) - glucosamine 6-sulfate (DGS) with immuno-modulatory and anti-angiogenic properties, respectively. In rabbit models of wound healing following glaucoma filtration surgery, subjects treated with DG and DGS showed minimal scar tissue formation, compared to placebo-treated animals [83]. Wimmer *et al.* synthesized lipid–lysine dendrimers for improving the delivery of anti-VEGF ODN-1 into the nuclei of retinal cells. Oligonucleotide ODN1- dendrimer complexes were highly efficient in transfecting human cells (d-407) and a significant reduction in the hVEGF-levels was observed after 24 hrs, compared to a control. *In vivo* efficacy of these complexes was evaluated in a laser-induced, choroidal neovascularization (CNV) rat model. *In vivo* results showed a significant reduction in the severity of CNV. After intravitreal injection, these complexes remained active up to two months and maintained anti-CNV activity [84-85]. Moreover, no significant tissue damage or toxicity was observed in rat eyes. A series of phosphorus-containing dendrimers, with a quaternary ammonium salt as core and carboxylic acid terminal groups [(from generation 0 (3 carboxylic acid terminal groups) to generation 2 (12 carboxylic acid terminal groups)] were also synthesized for the delivery of carteolol [86]. These dendrimers were designed in such a manner that the carboxylic group can interact with the amino group of carteolol to render cationic speciesand the quaternary ammonium group could replace benzalkonium chloride. No significant difference was observed in the aqueous humor level of carteolol, either after administration of carteolol alone, or after the administration of carteolol entrapped within the generation G0 dendrimer in rabbit eye. In case of second generation G2, due to their low solubility, the quantity of carteolol instilled was lower, but the quantity of carteolol penetrated inside the eyes was 2.5 times higher compared with carteolol alone. Even though solubility is a problem, on the basis of pharmacodynamics, these types of dendrimers can be a good vehicle for ocular drug delivery [86].

Microemulsions

For the past few decades, microemulsions have been investigated for topical ocular drug delivery. It is a thermodynamically stable dispersion of water and oil, with the aid of a surfactant and co-surfactant. Microemulsions provide several advantages over conventional ocular drug delivery systems, such as stability, a high capacity of dissolving drugs and high ocular bioavailability. Moreover, the ease of formulating into eye drops, the ability to accommodate both hydrophilic and lipophilic drugs and the easy production and sterilization make microemulsions more attractive than other ocular drug delivery systems [7, 87-88]. Moreover, the presence of surfactants provides microemulsions the ability to act as penetration enhancers, thus increasing corneal permeability and facilitating the passage of drugs through the corneal membrane. Hence, these dosage forms have the potential to improve ocular bioavailability after topical application. A few microemulsion-based formulations have already been approved for ocular drug delivery, and are available on the market. Restasis® was the first anionic lipid emulsion containing cyclosporine A 0.05% (Allergan®, Irvine, CA, USA), approved for the treatment of chronic dry eye disease by FDA in December 2002 [5]. Refresh Enduraw®, a non-medicated anionic emulsion, is used in the United States for eye lubricating purposes for moderate-to-severe dry eye syndrome [89]. Pilar Calvo *et al.* observed a 300% increase in ocular bioavailability after instillation of a submicron emulsion relative to a commercial solution. This study reported a four-fold increase in indomethacin concentration in the cornea and aqueous humor at one hr post instillation with a submicron emulsion compared to a commercial solution [4]. Higher timolol bioavailability from microemulsion was observed, compared to an aqueous drop. After instillation of microemulsion, the area under the curve for timolol in aqueous humor was 3.5 times higher compared to an aqueous solution instillation [90].

Further, with a positively-charged microemulsion, it is possible to improve corneal residence time, as the cornea is negatively charged. It also prolongs drug release from a topical application, as nanodroplets can act as a drug reservoir. The oil droplets can also adhere to the cornea and are not quickly washed away by lacrimal drainage. It reduces the frequency of administration and renders these formulations more attractive for ocular drug delivery [88]. Azithromycin lipid emulsion improved drug residence time in the conjunctiva and reduced precorneal loss [91]. Naveh *et al.* found a prolonged, progressive decrease in IOP in normotensive rabbits for up to 29 hrs, from a single application of 1.7% pilocarpine emulsion [92]. Two daily administrations of pilocarpine microemulsion were equivalent to four daily administrations of conventional eye drops [93].

Moreover, low surface tension of microemulsion can enhance its spreadability and thus, improves contact between drug molecules and cornea. Microemulsions also produce lower irritation to ocular tissues. Ocular irritation test on rabbit eyes with dexamathasone microemulsion showed no significant alteration in ocular structure of the cornea, conjunctiva, iris and ciliary body [94]. Further, no ocular irritation has been observed with microemulsions containing adaprolol maleate in humans [95]. High ocular bioavailability and low toxicity with less frequent administrations render microemulsions an attractive alternative to conventional ocular drug delivery systems.

RECENT PATENTS ON NANOTECHNOLOGY BASED OCULAR DRUG DELIVERY

Nanotechnology is an emerging field in drug delivery. Considerable research is currently in progress regarding the development of nanotechnology-based ocular drug delivery systems. Because of their ability to cross biological barriers, provide targeted and sustained drug delivery to various ocular tissues, nanotechnology-based formulations are gaining popularity in the field of ocular drug delivery. Interest in nanotechnology-based ocular drug delivery systems reflects an increasing number of US patents issued and/or filed in the last few years. Table **5** provides the list of some recently issued and filed patents on nanotechnology-based ocular drug delivery systems.

Table 5: Recent Patents on Nanotechnology-based Ocular Drug Delivery

No	Title	Type of Nano Formulation	Issue/ Application Date	Publication No	Reference
1.	Ophthalmic Drug Delivery System	Nanoparticles in contact lens	Dec. 29, 2009	US20040096477	[96]
2.	Methods and Composition for Intraocular Delivery of Therapeutic SiRNA	Nanoparticles	Sep. 10, 2009	US20090226531	[97]

Table 5: contd…

No	Title	Type of Nano Formulation	Issue/ Application Date	Publication No	Reference
3.	Use of Compacted Nucleic Acid Nanoparticles in Non-viral Treatments of Ocular Diseases	Nanoparticles	Jan. 8, 2009	US20090011040	[98]
4.	Pharmaceutical Compositions Suitable for the Treatment of	Solid lipid nanoparticles	Feb. 2, 2006	US20060024374	[99]

	Ophthalmic Diseases				
5.	Integrin Inhibitors for the Treatment of Eye Diseases	Nanoparticles	Dec. 21, 2006	US20060287225	[100]
6.	Ophthalmic Formulation of a Selective cyclooxygenase-2 inhibitory drug	Nanoparticles	Mar. 21, 2002	US20020035264	[101]
7.	Use of a Cationic Colloidal Preparation for the Diagnosis and Treatment of Ocular Diseases	Liposome	Feb. 11, 2010	US20100034749	[102]
8.	Formulations Containing Alkylphosphocholines Using Novel Negative Charge Carriers	Liposomes	Apr. 17, 2008	US20080090781	[103]
9.	Non-invasive Gene Targeting to Ocular Cells	Liposomes	Aug. 15, 2006	US20020054902	[104]
10.	Ophthalmic Liposome Compositions and Uses Thereof	Liposomes	Nov. 11, 2004	US20040224010	[105]
11.	Ophthalmic Emulsions Containing Prostaglandins	Microemulsion	May 8, 2008	US20080107738	[106]
12.	Dispersions of Microemulsions in Hydrogels for Drug Delivery	Microemulsion	Mar. 27, 2008	US20080075757	[107]
13.	Ophthalmic Oil-in-Water Type Emulsion with Stable Positive Zeta Potential	Microemulsion	Oct. 25, 2007	US20070248645	[108]
14.	Use of Emulsions for Intra and Periocular Injections	Microemulsion	Jan. 5, 2006	US20060002963	[109]

FUTURE PERSPECTIVES

Drug delivery to treat ocular diseases is a very challenging task for scientists working in the field of ophthalmology. The nature of diseases and the presence of ocular barriers, especially to the posterior segment, pose difficulties. Therefore, newer strategies are required for delivering drugs to the eye. This led to the development of nanotechnology, which is continuous to play a critical role in recent science and technology developments. Nanotechnology and its applications pave the way for developing newer ophthalmic drug delivery systems. The vital application of nano drug delivery systems is to develop clinically useful formulations for treating ocular infections. Emerging nanotechnology based approaches can aid in the development of new classes of bioactive macromolecules that need precise intracellular delivery. Nanodevices can be designed for complex eye surgeries, including glaucoma and retinal vascular surgeries. Moreover, nanocomposites can also be used to develop new lens material for cataract treatment. Colloidal nanocarriers can significantly improve drug delivery by different methods, including injectable, oral, implantable, preocular, intravitreal and transscleral administrations. Nanotechnology-based formulations can resolve solubility issuesand improve drug bioavailability. Multidisciplinary approaches have recently been applied to improve bioavailability, such as *in situ* gelling systems, microneedles, iontophoresis and magnetic resonance imaging. Also, generally acquired blindness and eye disorders can also be effectively treated by developing robust DNA nanoparticulate therapy. Nanotechnology can assist in the production of scaffolds for tissue bioengineering, such as neural stem cells. It can also improve gene delivery for treating a wide array of ocular pathologies. However, technologies involving the controlled and sustained drug release will likely continue to have the greatest clinical impact for a foreseeable future in the field of ophthalmology. A clear, understanding of anatomical and physiological constraints of the eye, ocular barriers and its compartmental pharmacokinetics would greatly hasten the development of nanotechnology based ocular drug delivery systems.

ACKNOWLEDGEMENTS

This work has been supported by NIH grants RO1 EY 09171 and RO1 EY 10659.

CONFLICT OF INTEREST

The author(s) confirm that this chapter content has no conflict of interest.

REFERENCES

[1]   Bawa R. Patents and nanomedicine. Nanomed 2007; 2(3): 351-74.
[2]   Kaur IP, Kanwar M. Ocular preparations: the formulation approach. Drug Dev Ind Pharm 2002; 28(5): 473-93.
[3]   Bourlais CL, Acar L, Zia H, Sado PA, Needham T, Leverge R. Ophthalmic drug delivery systems--recent advances. Prog Retin Eye Res 1998; 17(1): 33-58.
[4]   Calvo P, Alonso MJ, Vila-Jato JL, Robinson JR. Improved ocular bioavailability of indomethacin by novel ocular drug carriers. J Pharm Pharmacol 1996; 48(11): 1147-52.
[5]   Lallemand F, Felt-Baeyens O, Besseghir K, Behar-Cohen F, Gurny R. Cyclosporine A delivery to the eye: a pharmaceutical challenge. Eur J Pharm Biopharm 2003; 56(3): 307-18.

[6]   Kayser O, Lemke A, Hernandez-Trejo N. The impact of nanobiotechnology on the development of new drug delivery systems. Curr Pharm Biotechnol 2005; 6(1): 3-5.

[7]   Sahoo SK, Dilnawaz FS, Krishnakumar F. Nanotechnology in ocular drug delivery. Drug Discov Today 2008; 13(3-4): 144-51.

[8]   Morley MG, Duker JS, Reichel E. Ganciclovir intraocular implant. Ophthalmology 1996; 103(10): 1517.

[9]   Dunn JP, Van NM, Foster G, *et al.* Complications of ganciclovir implant surgery in patients with cytomegalovirus retinitis: the Ganciclovir Cidofovir Cytomegalovirus Retinitis Trial. Retina 2004; 24(1): 41-50.

[10]   Guembel HO, Krieglsteiner S, Rosenkranz C, Hattenbach LO, Koch FH, Ohrloff C. Complications after implantation of intraocular devices in patients with cytomegalovirus retinitis. Graefes Arch Clin Exp Ophthalmol 1999; 237(10): 824-9.

[11]   Bourges JL, Gautier SE, Delie F, *et al.* Ocular drug delivery targeting the retina and retinal pigment epithelium using polylactide nanoparticles. Invest Ophthalmol Vis Sci 2003; 44(8): 3562-9.

[12]   Irache JM, Merodio M, Arnedo A, Camapanero MA, Mirshahi M, Espuelas S. Albumin nanoparticles for the intravitreal delivery of anticytomegaloviral drugs. Mini Rev Med Chem 2005; 5(3): 293-305.

[13]   Sahoo SK, Labhasetwar V. Nanotech approaches to drug delivery and imaging. Drug Discov Today 2003; 8(24): 1112-20.

[14]   Nagarwal RC, Kant S, Singh PN, Maiti P, Pandit JK. Polymeric nanoparticulate system: a potential approach for ocular drug delivery. J Control Release 2009; 136(1): 2-13.

[15]   Calvo P, Sanchez A, Martinez J, *et al.* Polyester nanocapsules as new topical ocular delivery systems for cyclosporin A. Pharm Res 1996; 13(2): 311-5.

[16]   Zimmer A, Mutschler E, Lambrecht G, Mayer D, Kreuter J. Pharmacokinetic and pharmacodynamic aspects of an ophthalmic pilocarpine nanoparticle-delivery-system. Pharm Res 1994; 11(10): 1435-42.

[17]   Boddu SH, Jwala J, Vaishya R, *et al.* Novel nanoparticulate gel formulations of steroids for the treatment of macular edema. J Ocul Pharmacol Ther 2010; 26(1): 37-48.

[18]   Giannavola C, Bucolo C, Maltese A, *et al.* Influence of preparation conditions on acyclovir-loaded poly-d,l-lactic acid nanospheres and effect of PEG coating on ocular drug bioavailability. Pharm Res 2003; 20(4): 584-90.

[19]   De Campos AM, Sanchez A, Alonso MJ. Chitosan nanoparticles: a new vehicle for the improvement of the delivery of drugs to the ocular surface. Application to cyclosporin A. Int J Pharm 2001; 224(1-2): 159-68.

[20]   Arnedo A, Irache JM, Merodio M, Espuelas Millán MS. Albumin nanoparticles improved the stability, nuclear accumulation and anticytomegaloviral activity of a phosphodiester oligonucleotide. J Control Release 2004; 94(1): 217-27.

[21]   Attama AA, Reichl S, Müller-Goymann CC. Sustained release and permeation of timolol from surface-modified solid lipid nanoparticles through bioengineered human cornea. Curr Eye Res 2009; 34(8): 698-705.

[22]   Cavalli R, Gasco MR, Chetoni P, Burgalassi S, Saettone MF. Solid lipid nanoparticles (SLN) as ocular delivery system for tobramycin. Int J Pharm 2002; 238(1-2): 241-5.

[23]   Parveen S, Mitra M, Krishnakumar S, Sahoo SK. Enhanced antiproliferative activity of carboplatin-loaded chitosan-alginate nanoparticles in a retinoblastoma cell line. Acta Biomater 2010; 6(8): 3120-31.

[24]   Vega E, Gamisans F, García ML, Chauvet A, Lacoulonche F, Egea MA. PLGA nanospheres for the ocular delivery of flurbiprofen: drug release and interactions. J Pharm Sci 2008; 97(12): 5306-17.

[25]   Gupta H, Aqil M, Khar RK, Ali A, Bhatnagar A, Mittal G. Sparfloxacin-loaded PLGA nanoparticles for sustained ocular drug delivery. Nanomedicine 2010; 6(2): 324-33.

[26]   Kao HJ, Lin HR, Lo YL, Yu SP. Characterization of pilocarpine-loaded chitosan/Carbopol nanoparticles. J Pharm Pharmacol 2006; 58(2): 179-86.

[27]   Zhang L, Li Y, Zhang C, Wang Y, Song C. Pharmacokinetics and tolerance study of intravitreal injection of dexamethasone-loaded nanoparticles in rabbits. Int J Nanomedicine 2009; 4: 175-83.

[28]   Yenice I, Mocan MC, Palaska E, et al. Hyaluronic acid coated poly-epsilon-caprolactone nanospheres deliver high concentrations of cyclosporine A into the cornea. Exp Eye Res 2008; 87(3): 162-7.

[29]   Singh KH, Shinde UA. Development and Evaluation of Novel Polymeric Nanoparticles of Brimonidine Tartrate. Curr Drug Deliv 2010.

[30]   Das S, Suresh PK, Desmukh R. Design of Eudragit RL 100 nanoparticles by nanoprecipitation method for ocular drug delivery. Nanomedicine 2010; 6(2): 318-23.

[31]   Merodio M, Espuelas MS, Mirshahi M, Arnedo A, Irache JM. Efficacy of ganciclovir-loaded nanoparticles in human cytomegalovirus (HCMV)-infected cells. J Drug Target 2002; 10(3): 231-8.

[32]   Agnihotri SM, Vavia PR. Diclofenac-loaded biopolymeric nanosuspensions for ophthalmic application. Nanomedicine 2009; 5(1): 90-5.

[33]   Lin HR, Yu SP, Kuo CJ, Kao HJ, Lo YL, Lin YJ. Pilocarpine-loaded chitosan-PAA nanosuspension for ophthalmic delivery. J Biomater Sci Polym Ed 2007; 18(2): 205-21.

[34]   Pignatello R, Ricupero N, Bucolo C, Maugeri F, Maltese A, Puglisi G. Preparation and characterization of eudragit retard nanosuspensions for the ocular delivery of cloricromene. AAPS PharmSciTech 2006; 7(1): E27.

[35]   Adibkia K, Omidi Y, Siahi MR, et al. Inhibition of endotoxin-induced uveitis by methylprednisolone acetate nanosuspension in rabbits. J Ocul Pharmacol Ther 2007; 23(5): 421-32.

[36]   Pignatello R, Bucolo C, Ferrara P, Maltese A, Puleo A, Puglisi G. Eudragit RS100 nanosuspensions for the ophthalmic controlled delivery of ibuprofen. Eur J Pharm Sci 2002; 16(1-2): 53-61.

[37]   Rabinow BE. Nanosuspensions in drug delivery. Nat Rev Drug Discov 2004; 3(9): 785-96.

[38]   Kassem MA, Abdel Rahman AA, Ghorab MM, Ahmed MB, Khalil RM. Nanosuspension as an ophthalmic delivery system for certain glucocorticoid drugs. Int J Pharm 2007; 340(1-2): 126-33.

[39]   Fresta M, Panico AM, Bucolo C, Giannavola C, Puglisi G. Characterization and in vivo ocular absorption of liposome-encapsulated acyclovir. J Pharm Pharmacol 1999; 51(5): 565-76.

[40]   Li N, Zhuang C, Wang M, Sun X, Nie S, Pan W. Liposome coated with low molecular weight chitosan and its potential use in ocular drug delivery. Int J Pharm 2009; 379(1): 131-8.

[41]   Hosny KM. Preparation and evaluation of thermosensitive liposomal hydrogel for enhanced transcorneal permeation of ofloxacin. AAPS PharmSciTech 2009; 10(4): 1336-42.

[42]   Hathout RM, Mansour S, Mortada ND, Guinedi AS. Liposomes as an ocular delivery system for acetazolamide: in vitro and in vivo studies. AAPS PharmSciTech 2007; 8(1): 1.

[43] Mahmoud SS, Gehman JD, Azzopardi K, Robins-Browne RM, Separovic F. Liposomal phospholipid preparations of chloramphenicol for ophthalmic applications. J Pharm Sci 2008; 97(7): 2691-701.

[44] Afouna MI, Khattab IS, Reddy IK. Preparation and characterization of demeclocycline liposomal formulations and assessment of their intraocular pressure-lowering effects. Cutan Ocul Toxicol 2005; 24(2): 111-24.

[45] Budai L, Hajdú M, Budai M, et al. Gels and liposomes in optimized ocular drug delivery: studies on ciprofloxacin formulations. Int J Pharm 2007; 343(1-2): 34-40.

[46] Lajavardi L, Bochot A, Camelo S, et al. Downregulation of endotoxin-induced uveitis by intravitreal injection of vasoactive intestinal Peptide encapsulated in liposomes. Invest Ophthalmol Vis Sci 2007; 48(7): 3230-8.

[47] Wutzler P, Sauerbrei A, Klöcking R, et al. Virucidal and chlamydicidal activities of eye drops with povidone-iodine liposome complex. Ophthalmic Res 2000; 32(2-3): 118-25.

[48] Bochot A, Fattal E, Boutet V, et al. Intravitreal delivery of oligonucleotides by sterically stabilized liposomes. Invest Ophthalmol Vis Sci 2002; 43(1): 253-9.

[49] Abrishami M, Zarei-Ghanavati S, Soroush D, Rouhbakhsh M, Jaafari MR, Malaekeh-Nikouei B. Preparation, characterizationand in vivo evaluation of nanoliposomes-encapsulated bevacizumab (avastin) for intravitreal administration. Retina 2009; 29(5): 699-703.

[50] Inokuchi Y, Hironaka K, Fujisawa T, et al. Physicochemical Properties Affecting Retinal drug/coumarin-6 Delivery from Nanocarrier Systems via Eyedrop Administration. Invest Ophthalmol Vis Sci 2010; 51(6): 3162-70.

[51] Smolin G, Okumoto M, Feiler S, Condon D. Idoxuridine-liposome therapy for herpes simplex keratitis. Am J Ophthalmol 1981; 91(2): 220-5.

[52] Shafaa MW, Sabra NM, Fouad RA. The extended ocular hypotensive effect of positive liposomal cholesterol bound timolol maleate in glaucomatous rabbits. Biopharm Drug Dispos 2011; 32(9): 507-17.

[53] Taniguchi K, Yamamoto Y, Itakura K, Miichi H, Hayashi S. Assessment of ocular irritability of liposome preparations. J Pharmacobiodyn 1988; 11(9): 607-11.

[54] Mehanna MM, Elmaradny HA, Samaha MW. Mucoadhesive liposomes as ocular delivery system: physical, microbiologicaland in vivo assessment. Drug Dev Ind Pharm 2010; 36(1): 108-18.

[55] Li N, Zhuang CY, Wang M, Sui CG, Pan WS. Low molecular weight chitosan-coated liposomes for ocular drug delivery: in vitro and in vivo studies. Drug Deliv 2012; 19(1): 28-35.

[56] Hosny KM. Optimization of gatifloxacin liposomal hydrogel for enhanced transcorneal permeation. J Liposome Res 2010; 20(1): 31-7.

[57] Norley SG, Huang L, Rouse BT. Targeting of drug loaded immunoliposomes to herpes simplex virus infected corneal cells: an effective means of inhibiting virus replication in vitro. J Immunol 1986; 136(2): 681-5.

[58] Hironaka K, Inokuchi Y, Tozuka Y, Shimazawa M, Hara H, Takeuchi H. Design and evaluation of a liposomal delivery system targeting the posterior segment of the eye. J Control Release 2009; 136(3): 247-53.

[59] Cortesi R, Argnani R, Esposito E, et al Cationic liposomes as potential carriers for ocular administration of peptides with anti-herpetic activity. Int J Pharm 2006; 317(1): 90-100.

[60] Sun KX, Wang AP, Huang LJ, Liang RC, Liu K. Preparation of diclofenac sodium liposomes and its ocular pharmacokinetics. Yao Xue Xue Bao 2006; 41(11): 1094-8.

[61] Shen Y, Tu J. Preparation and ocular pharmacokinetics of ganciclovir liposomes. AAPS J 2007; 9(3): E371-7.

[62] Muzzalupo R, Tavano L, Trombino S, Cassano R, Picci N, La Mesa C. Niosomes from alpha,omega-trioxyethylene-bis(sodium 2-dodecyloxy-propylenesulfonate): preparation and characterization. Colloids Surf B Biointerfaces 2008; 64(2): 200-7.

[63] Perini G, Saettone MF, Carafa M, Santucci E, Alhaique F. Niosomes as carriers for ophthalmic drugs: *in vitro/in vivo* evaluation. Boll Chim Farm 1996; 135(2): 145-6.

[64] Keller N, Moore D, Carper D, Longwell A. Increased corneal permeability induced by the dual effects of transient tear film acidification and exposure to benzalkonium chloride. Exp Eye Res 1980; 30(2): 203-10.

[65] Burstein NL. Preservative alteration of corneal permeability in humans and rabbits. Invest Ophthalmol Vis Sci 1984; 25(12): 1453-7.

[66] Kaur IP, Smitha R. Penetration enhancers and ocular bioadhesives: two new avenues for ophthalmic drug delivery. Drug Dev Ind Pharm 2002; 28(4): 353-69.

[67] Vyas SP, Mysore N, Jaitely V, Venkatesan N. Discoidal niosome based controlled ocular delivery of timolol maleate. Pharmazie 1998; 53(7): 466-9.

[68] Aggarwal D, Kaur IP. Improved pharmacodynamics of timolol maleate from a mucoadhesive niosomal ophthalmic drug delivery system. Int J Pharm 2005; 290(1-2): 155-9.

[69] Abdelbary G, El-Gendy N. Niosome-encapsulated gentamicin for ophthalmic controlled delivery. AAPS PharmSciTech 2008; 9(3): 740-7.

[70] Aggarwal D, Pal D, Mitra AK, Kaur IP. Study of the extent of ocular absorption of acetazolamide from a developed niosomal formulation, by microdialysis sampling of aqueous humor. Int J Pharm 2007; 338(1-2): 21-6.

[71] Abdelkader H, Ismail S, Kamal A, Alany RG. Design and evaluation of controlled-release niosomes and discomes for naltrexone hydrochloride ocular delivery. J Pharm Sci 2011; 100(5): 1833-46.

[72] Kaur IP, Garg A, Singla AK, Aggarwal D. Vesicular systems in ocular drug delivery: an overview. Int J Pharm 2004; 269(1): 1-14.

[73] Aggarwal D, Garg A, Kaur IP. Development of a topical niosomal preparation of acetazolamide: preparation and evaluation. J Pharm Pharmacol 2004; 56(12): 1509-17.

[74] Torchilin VP. Structure and design of polymeric surfactant-based drug delivery systems. J Control Release 2001; 73(2-3): 137-72.

[75] Matsumura Y. Poly (amino acid) micelle nanocarriers in preclinical and clinical studies. Adv Drug Deliv Rev 2008; 60(8): 899-914.

[76] Talelli M, Rijcken CJ, Van Nostrum CF, Storm G, Hennink WE. Micelles based on HPMA copolymers. Adv Drug Deliv Rev 2010; 62(2): 231-9.

[77] Gupta AK, Madan S, Majumdar DK, Maitra A. Ketorolac entrapped in polymeric micelles: preparation, characterisation and ocular anti-inflammatory studies. Int J Pharm 2000; 209(1-2): 1-14.

[78] Civiale C, Licciardi M, Cavallaro G, Giammona G, Mazzone MG. Polyhydroxyethylaspartamide-based micelles for ocular drug delivery. Int J Pharm 2009; 378(1-2): 177-86.

[79] Mitra AK, Velagaleti PR, Natesan S. Ophthalmic Compositions Comprising Calcineurin Inhibitors or MTOR Inhibitors. US Patent Application 20110300195.

[80] Cheng Y, Xu Z, Ma M, Xu T. Dendrimers as drug carriers: applications in different routes of drug administration. J Pharm Sci 2008; 97(1): 123-43.

[81]   Tomalia DA, Naylor AM, Goddard WA. Starburst Dendrimers: Molecular-Level Control of Size, Shape, Surface Chemistry, Topologyand Flexibility from Atoms to Macroscopic Matter. Angew Chem Int Ed Engl 1990; 29(2): 138-175.

[82]   Vandamme TF, Brobeck L. Poly(amicoamine) dendrimers as ophthalmic vehicles for ocular delivery of pilocarpine nitrate and tropicamide. J Control Release 2005; 102(1): 23-38.

[83]   Shaunak S, Thomas S, Gianasi E, *et al*. Polyvalent dendrimer glucosamine conjugates prevent scar tissue formation. Nat Biotechnol 2004; 22(8): 977-84.

[84]   Parekh HS, Marano RJ, Rakoczy EP, Blanchfield J, Toth I. Synthesis of a library of polycationic lipid core dendrimers and their evaluation in the delivery of an oligonucleotide with hVEGF inhibition. Bioorg Med Chem 2006; 14(14): 4775-80.

[85]   Marano RJ, Wimmer N, Kearns PS, *et al*. Inhibition of *in vitro* VEGF expression and choroidal neovascularization by synthetic dendrimer peptide mediated delivery of a sense oligonucleotide. Exp Eye Res 2004; 79(4): 525-35.

[86]   Spataro G, Malecaze F, Turrin CO, *et al*. Designing dendrimers for ocular drug delivery. Eur J Med Chem 2010; 45(1): 326-34.

[87]   Lawrence MJ, Rees GD. Microemulsion-based media as novel drug delivery systems. Adv Drug Deliv Rev 2000; 45(1): 89-121.

[88]   Vandamme TF. Microemulsions as ocular drug delivery systems: recent developments and future challenges. Prog Retin Eye Res 2002; 21(1): 15-34.

[89]   Sasaki H, Yamamura K, Nishida K, Nakamura J, Ichikawa M. Delivery of drugs to the eye by topical application. Prog Retin Eye Res 1996; 15(2): 583-620.

[90]   Gasco MR, Gallarate M, Trotta M, Bauchiero L, Gremmo E, Chiappero O. Microemulsions as topical delivery vehicles: ocular administration of timolol. J Pharm Biomed Anal 1989; 7(4): 433-9.

[91]   Liu Y, Lin X, Tang X. Lipid emulsions as a potential delivery system for ocular use of azithromycin. Drug Dev Ind Pharm 2009; 35(7): 887-96.

[92]   Naveh N, Muchtar S, Benita S. Pilocarpine incorporated into a submicron emulsion vehicle causes an unexpectedly prolonged ocular hypotensive effect in rabbits. J Ocul Pharmacol 1994; 10(3): 509-20.

[93]   Garty N, Lusky M. Pilocarpine in submicron emulsion formulation for treatment of ocular hypertension: A phase II clinical trial. Invest Ophth Vis Sci 1994; 35(4): 2175-9.

[94]   Fialho SL, Da Silva-Cunha A. New vehicle based on a microemulsion for topical ocular administration of dexamethasone. Clin Experiment Ophthalmol 2004; 32(6): 626-32.

[95]   Melamed S, Kurtz S, Greenbaum A, Haves JF, Neumann R, Garty N. Adaprolol maleate in submicron emulsion, a novel soft /8-blocking agent, is safe and effective in human studies. Invest Ophthalmol Vis Sci 1994; 35(4): 1387.

[96]   Chauhan A, Gulsen D. Ophthalmic drug delivery system. US Patent Application 20040096477.

[97]   Lyons R, Ma H. Methods and composition for intraocular delivery of therapeutic SIRNA. US Patent Application 20090226531.

[98]   Naash M, Cooper M. Use of compacted nucleic acid nanoparticles in non-viral treatments of ocular diseases. US Patent Application 20090011040.

[99]   Gasco MR, Saettone MF, Zara GP. Pharmaceutical compositions suitable for the treatment of ophthalmic diseases. US Patent Application 20060024374.

[100] Bender H, Haunschild J, Lang U, Wiesner M, Friedlander M. Integrin inhibitors for the treatment of eye diseases. US Patent Application 20060287225.

[101] Kararli TT, Bandyopadhyay R, Singh SK, Hawley LC. Ophthalmic formulation of a selective cyclooxygenase-2 inhibitory drug. US Patent Application 20020035264.

[102] Schulze B, Michaelis U, Hansen L, *et al*. Use of a cationic collodal preparation for the diagnosis and treatment of ocular diseases. US Patent Application 20100034749.

[103] Eibl HJ, Wieland-Berghausen SC, Steffan J. Formulations containing alkylphosphocholines using novel negative charge carriers. US Patent Application 20080090781.

[104] Pardridge WM. Non-invasive gene targeting to ocular cells. US Patent Application 20020054902.

[105] Hofland H, Bongianni J, Wheeler T. Ophthalmic liposome compositions and uses thereof. US Patent Application 20040224010.

[106] Philips B, Bague S, Lambert G, Rabinovich-Guilatt L. Ophthalmic emulsions containing prostaglandins. US Patent Application 20080107738.

[107] Chauhan A, Onbilger DG, Li C, Kapoor Y. Dispersions of microemulsions in hydrogels for drug delivery. US Patent Application 20080075757.

[108] Bague S, Philips B, Rabinovich-Guilatt L, Lambert G. Ophthalmic oil-in-water type emulsion with stable positive zeta potential. US Patent Application 20070248645.

[109] Rabinovich-Guilatt L, Kozak YD, Lambert G, Benita S. Use of emulsions for intra and periocular injections. US Patent Application 20060002963.

INDEX

A

Acyclovir (ACV) 153-154

Age related macular degeneration 114, 121, 128

Albumin nanoparticles 259

Alginates 96, 107, 108

Anatomical barriers 21-22

Anterior segment 42, 44, 49, 51, 53, 56, 58-59

Anterior segment microdialysis 166,169

Aqueous humor 8-9, 162, 164-171, 173, 180-181, 185-187, 192-193

B

Benzalkonium chloride 28, 46

Betaxolol 182

Bevacizumab 184-186

Biocompatibility 99,100,124, 134

Biodegradable matrix implant 117

Biodegradable polymers 96- 98, 103, 107, 109

Biotin-ganciclovir 82

Blood retinal barrier (BRB) 20, 31, 78

Blood-aqueous barrier 20, 31

Bruch's membrane- choroid 72-73

C

Carbopol-coated niosomes 270

Chemistry manufacturing and control 223- 225, 230, 239

Chitosan 96, 106-107

Chitosan-coated liposomes 268

Choroidal blood flow 77-78

Clinical Study 226

Collagen 96, 103, 104, 105

Conjunctiva 5-6, 75

Conjunctival blood flow 76

www.ingramcontent.com/pod-product-compliance
Lightning Source LLC
Chambersburg PA
CBHW050813220326
41598CB00006B/193